Radiology 101

The Basics and Fundamentals of Imaging

Second Edition

Radiology 101

The Basics and Fundamentals of Imaging

Second Edition

EDITOR

William E. Erkonen, M.D.

Associate Professor Emeritus
Department of Radiology
Carver College of Medicine
University of Iowa Hospitals and Clinics
Iowa City, Iowa

ASSOCIATE EDITOR

Wilbur L. Smith, M.D.

Professor and Chairman
Department of Radiology
Wayne State University/Detroit Medical Center
Detroit, Michigan

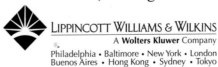

LIPPINCOTT WILLIAMS & WILKINS
A **Wolters Kluwer** Company

Philadelphia • Baltimore • New York • London
Buenos Aires • Hong Kong • Sydney • Tokyo

Acquisitions Editor: Lisa McAllister
Developmental Editor: Matthew Kory
Project Manager: Alicia Jackson
Senior Manufacturing Manager: Benjamin Rivera
Marketing Manager: Angela Panetta
Designer: Bess Kiethas
Production Service: TechBooks
Printer: Maple Press

Library of Congress Cataloging-in-Publication Data

Radiology 101 : the basics and fundamentals of imaging / editor, William E. Erkonen; associate
   editor, Wilbur L. Smith. — 2nd ed.
       p. ; cm.
   Includes bibliographical references and index.
   ISBN 0-7817-5198-5 (pbk. : alk. paper)
   1. Radiography, Medical.   2. Diagnosis, Radioscopic.
3. Diagnostic imaging.   I. Erkonen, William E. II. Smith, Wilbur L.
   [DNLM: 1. Diagnostic Imaging.   2. Radiology.   WN 180 R1295 2005]
RC78.R242   2005
616.07′54—dc22
                                                                    2004023820

Care has been taken to confirm the accuracy of the information presented and to describe generally accepted practices. However, the authors, editors, and publisher are not responsible for errors or omissions or for any consequences from application of the information in this book and make no warranty, expressed or implied, with respect to the currency, completeness, or accuracy of the contents of the publication. Application of the information in particular situation remains the professional responsibility of the practitioner.

The authors, editors, and publisher have exerted every effort to ensure that drug selection and dosage set forth in this text are in accordance with current recommendations and practice at the time of publication. However, in view of ongoing research, changes in government regulations, and the constant flow of information relating to drug therapy and drug reactions, the reader is urged to check the package insert for each drug for any change in indications and dosage and for added warnings and precautions. This is particularly important when the recommended agent is a new or infrequently employed drug.

Some drugs and medical devices presented in the publication have Food and Drug Administration (FDA) clearance for limited use in restricted research settings. It is the responsibility of the health care provider to ascertain the FDA status of each drug or device planned for use in their clinical practice.

10 9 8 7 6 5 4 3 2 1

To the students and practitioners in all the medical sciences who seek basic information about the subject of radiology.

CONTENTS

CONTRIBUTING AUTHORS

John W. Boardman, M.D.
Associate, Department of Radiology, Carver College of
Medicine, University of Iowa Hospitals and Clinics,
200 Hawkins Road, Iowa City, Iowa

Carol A. Boles, M.D.
Professor, Department of Radiology, Wake Forest
University School of Medicine, Winston-Salem,
North Carolina

David L. Bushnell, Jr., M.D.
Chief of Diagnostic Imaging, Veterans Administration
Hospital, Iowa City, Iowa; Associate Professor, Carver
College of Medicine, University of Iowa Hospitals
and Clinics, 200 Hawkins Road,
Iowa City, Iowa

William E. Erkonen, M.D.
Associate Professor Emeritus, Department of Radiology,
Carver College of Medicine, University of Iowa Hospitals
and Clinics, 200 Hawkins Road, Iowa City, Iowa

Laurie L. Fajardo, M.D.
Professor and Head, Department of Radiology, Carver
College of Medicine, University of Iowa Hospitals
and Clinics, 200 Hawkins Road,
Iowa City, Iowa

Thomas A. Farrell, M.B.
Attending Radiologist, Department of Radiology,
Evanston Hospital, 2650 Ridge Avenue, Evanston, Illinois

Edmund A. Franken, Jr., M.D.
Professor, Department of Radiology, Carver College of
Medicine, University of Iowa Hospitals and Clinics,
200 Hawkins Road, Iowa City, Iowa

Monte L. Harvill, M.D.
Assistant Professor, Department of Radiology, and Chief
of Interventional Radiology, Wayne State University,
Detroit Medical Center, 4201 St. Antoine Boulevard,
Detroit, Michigan; Chief of Department of Radiology,
Harper University Hospital, 3990 John R Street,
Detroit, Michigan

Yutaka Sato, M.D.
Professor, Director of Pediatric Radiology, Department of
Radiology, Carver College of Medicine, University of Iowa
Hospitals and Clinics, 200 Hawkins Road,
Iowa City, Iowa

Wilbur L. Smith, M.D.
Professor and Chairman, Department of Radiology,
Wayne State University, Detroit Medical Center, Detroit
Receiving Hospital (3L8), 4201 St. Antoine Boulevard,
Detroit, Michigan

PREFACE

The specialty of radiology has been around for over 100 years and has played a critical role in patient diagnosis and care. However, during the last thirty years the role of radiology in patient diagnosis and care has soared on the wings of extraordinary technologic advances.

The purpose of this book is to give the reader a feel for radiologic anatomy and the radiologic manifestations of some common disease processes. After reading this book, the reader will be better prepared for consultation with the radiologist, and this usually leads to an appropriate diagnostic workup. As the reader develops an understanding of what radiology has to offer, improved patient diagnosis and care are likely to follow. In addition, the reader will be able to approach an image without feeling intimidated. You might say, "it will prepare you for the wards and boards." The book is not intended to transform the reader into a radiologist look-alike. Rather, it is designed to be a primer or general field guide to the basics of radiology.

Anatomy is the language of radiology. A solid foundation in old-fashioned normal radiologic anatomy is essential for understanding the various manifestations of diseases on radiologic images. This book places heavy emphasis on images, stressing normal anatomy and commonly encountered radiologic pathology. We present clearly labeled images of normal anatomy from a variety of angles, not only on radiographs but also on other commonly used imaging modalities such as computed tomography, magnetic resonance imaging, and ultrasonography.

Section One presents basic understandable discussions of how major imaging modalities function. Understanding how radiologic images are produced by the various imaging modalities is extremely helpful in understanding what their images portray. The strengths and weaknesses of the various modalities are described in clinical tips within the text (e.g., What are the basic differences between T-1 and T-2 images and what are the clinical indications for each?)

Section Two systematically examines the imaging of anatomic areas and major organ systems and contains extensive presentations of normal anatomy, normal anatomic variants, and commonly encountered pathology. Each chapter begins with an outline to make topics easier to locate, and the chapter concludes with a summary list of key points to remember. In general, the writing tends to be informal and dispenses common-sense tips and pointers freely (e.g., how to systematically examine or approach a chest radiograph and how to correctly position an image on the viewbox). We have attempted to make each chapter user-friendly by adding practical tips on how to radiographically approach common clinical problems such as abdominal trauma. This work should be an excellent resource for any beginner in any medical-allied field.

We call the reader's attention to Chapter Four, which combines pediatric chest and abdomen, as they are the most frequently ordered pediatric images. All other pediatric images and text are located in their appropriate chapters.

New to this second edition are many updates to keep pace with this rapidly changing specialty. These changes will be found especially in the chapters involving nuclear imaging, the abdomen, mammography, and interventional radiology.

ACKNOWLEDGEMENTS

A deep debt of gratitude is owed to the entire Radiology faculty and resident staff at the University of Iowa for providing images and advice for this book. Special thanks to Doctors Monzer Abu-Yousef, Thomas Barloon, Eric Brandser, Bruce Brown, Robert C. Brown, Daniel Crosby, Rommel Dhadha, William Daniel, Gerald Decker, J. G. Fletcher, Jeffrey Galvin, Charles Jacoby, Elvira Lang, Charles Lu, Mark Madsen, Hoang Nyguyen, Retta Pelsang, Scott Pretorius, Patrick Rheingans, Parvez Shirazi, William Sickels, William Stanford, Allan Stolpen, Shiliang Sun, Brad Thompson, and Donald C. Young. We are also indebted to the technologists of the Radiology Department, especially Stephanie Ellingson, Mary Burr, Scot Heery, Deborah Troyer, and Heidi Berns. Librarian Nicole Jenkins was extremely helpful with references.

A special thank you is owed to Doctor William E. Ehling, who reviewed the book from the standpoint of an experienced family physician, and to Doctors Brian Mullan and James Choi, who reviewed the book from the standpoint of Directors of Medical Student Teaching. Their advice is truly appreciated and helped to reshape this work.

A very special thanks to George El-Khoury, Ronald Bergman, and Kathy Martensen, RTR, for their persistent encouragement, suggestions, and general advice.

The skillful illustrations of Shirley Taylor and the late Frank J. Sindelar are greatly appreciated. Brian Clarke provided the original drawings for Figures 9-1, 9-2, 9-18, 9-21, and 9-23.

SECTION I

Basic Principles

Radiography, Computed Tomography, Magnetic Resonance Imaging, and Ultrasonography: Principles and Indications

William E. Erkonen

Very few of us take the time to study, let alone enjoy, the physics of the technology that we use in our everyday lives. Almost everybody drives an automobile, for instance, but only a few of us have working knowledge about what goes on under our car hoods. The medical technology that produces imaging studies is often met with a similar reception: we all want to drive the car, so to speak, but we don't necessarily want to understand the principles underlying the computed tomograms or magnetic resonance images that we study. Yet a basic understanding of imaging modalities is extremely important because you will most likely be reviewing images with a radiologist during radiologic consultations throughout your professional life, and the results of these consultations will at times profoundly affect your clinical decision making. Add to this the fact that the interpretation of imaging studies is to a considerable degree dependent on understanding how the images are produced. Here is where our analogy breaks down: One doesn't necessarily have to be a mechanic to be a skilled driver, but reaching a basic understanding of how imag-

ing studies are produced is a necessary first step to viewing the studies themselves. This chapter is designed to demonstrate the elementary physics of radiologic diagnostic imaging.

RADIOGRAPHY

Radiographs are the most common imaging consultations requested by clinicians. So let's set off on the right foot by referring to radiologic images as *radiographs*, *images*, or *films*, but not *x-rays*. After all, x-rays are electromagnetic waves produced in an x-ray tube. It is acceptable for a layperson to refer to a radiograph as an x-ray, but the knowledgeable clinician and health care worker should avoid the term. Your usage of appropriate terminology demonstrates *savoir-faire* (the ability to say and do the right thing) to your colleagues and patients.

Whenever possible, radiographs are accomplished in the radiology department. The number of views obtained

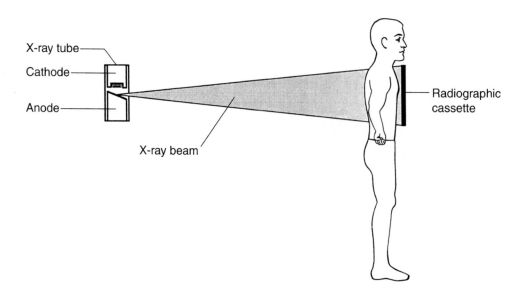

FIGURE 1-1. A posteroanterior chest radiograph. The patient's chest is pressed against the cassette with hands on the hips. The x-ray beam emanating from the x-ray tube passes through the patient's chest in a posterior-to-anterior or back-to-front direction. The x-rays that pass completely through the patient eventually strike the radiographic film and screens inside the radiographic cassette.

during a standard or routine study depends on the anatomic site being imaged. The common radiographic views obtained are referred to as posteroanterior (PA), anteroposterior (AP), oblique, and lateral views.

The chest will be used to illustrate these basic radiographic terms, but this terminology applies to almost all anatomic sites. PA indicates that the central x-ray beam travels from posterior to anterior or back to front as it traverses the chest or any other anatomic site (Fig. 1-1). Lateral indicates that the x-ray beam travels through the patient from side to side (Fig. 1-2). When the patient is unable to cooperate for these routine views, a single AP upright or supine view is obtained. AP means that the x-ray beam passes through the chest or other anatomic site from anterior to posterior or front to back (Fig. 1-3). PA and AP radiographs have similar appearances. When the patient cannot tolerate a transfer to the radiology facility, a portable study is obtained, which means that a portable x-ray machine is brought to the patient wherever he or she is located. AP is the standard portable technique with the patient sitting or supine (Fig. 1-4).

Radiographs have traditionally been described in terms of shades of black, white, and gray. What causes a structure to appear black, white, or gray on a radiograph? Actually,

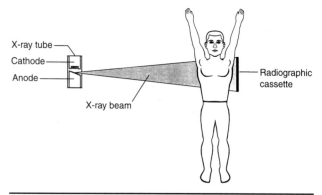

FIGURE 1-2. A lateral chest radiograph. The x-ray beam passes through the patient's chest from side to side. The x-rays that pass completely through the patient eventually strike the radiographic film and screens. Note that the patient's arms are positioned as not to project over the chest.

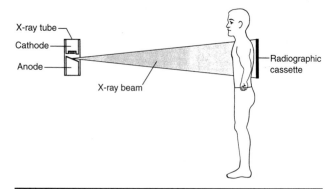

FIGURE 1-3. An anteroposterior chest radiograph. The x-ray beam passes through the patient's chest in an anterior-to-posterior or front-to-back direction. Note that the hands are on the hips.

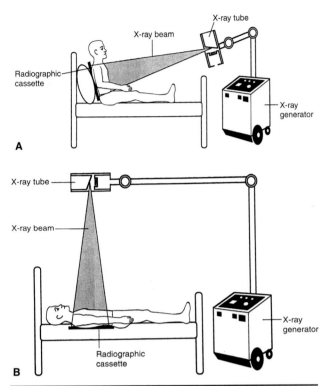

FIGURE 1-4. An anteroposterior portable chest radiograph with the patient either sitting (**A**) or supine (**B**). The x-ray beam passes through the patient's chest in an anterior-to-posterior direction. The x-ray machine has wheels, and that allows it to be used wherever needed throughout the hospital.

it is the density of the object being imaged that determines how much of the x-ray beam will be absorbed or attenuated (Fig. 1-5). In other words, as the density of an object increases, fewer x-rays pass through it. It is the variable density of structures that results in the four basic radiographic classifications: air (black), fat (black), water (gray), and metallic or bone (white; Table 1-1). For example, the lungs primarily consist of low-density air, which absorbs very little of the x-ray beam. Thus, air allows a large amount of the x-ray beam to strike or expose the radiographic film. As a result, air in the lungs will appear black on a radiograph. Similarly, fat has a low density, but its

▶ **TABLE 1-1 Basic Radiograph Film Densities or Appearances**

Object	Film Density
Air	Black
Fat	Black
Bone	White
Metal	White
Calcium	White
Organs, muscles, soft tissues	Shades of gray

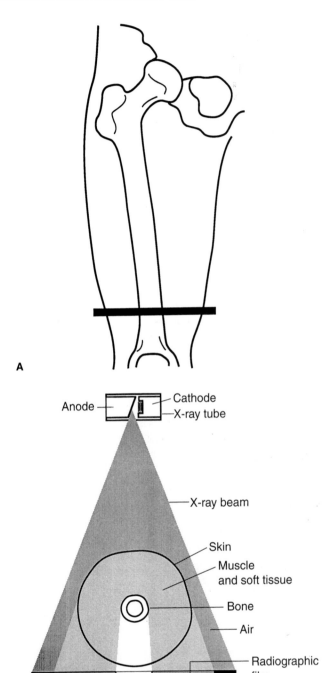

FIGURE 1-5. A: The level in the distal thigh through which the x-ray beam is passing in B. **B:** Cross section of the distal thigh at the level indicated in A. Notice that when the x-ray beam passes through air, the result is a black area on the radiograph. When the x-ray beam strikes bone, the result is a white area on the radiograph. If the x-ray beam passes through soft tissues, the result is a gray appearance on the film.

density is slightly greater than air. Fat will appear black on a radiograph but slightly less black than air. High-density objects such as bones, teeth, calcium deposits in tumors, metallic foreign bodies, right and left lead film markers, and intravascularly injected contrast media absorb all or nearly all of the x-ray beam. As a result, the radiographic film receives little or no x-ray exposure, and these dense structures appear white. Muscles, organs (heart, liver, spleen), and other soft tissues appear as shades of gray, and the shades of gray range somewhere between white and black depending on the structure's density. These shades of gray are referred to as *water density*.

Radiographic screens are positioned on either side of the radiographic film inside the light-tight cassette or film holder (Fig. 1-6A). The chemical structure of the screens

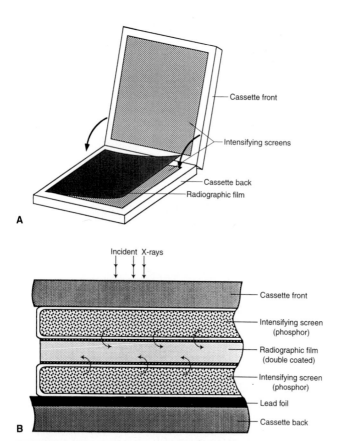

FIGURE 1-6. A: An open radiographic cassette containing one sheet of radiographic film and two intensifying screens. A radiographic screen is positioned on each side of the film, and the screens emit a light flash (fluoresce) when struck by an x-ray. Also, some x-rays directly strike the radiographic film. This combination of light flashes from the screens and x-rays directly striking the film causes the radiographic film to be exposed. This is similar to photographic film. **B:** Cross-sectional illustration of a radiographic cassette. Note the lead foil in the back of the cassette that is designed to stop any x-rays that have penetrated the full thickness of the cassette. The *curved arrows* represent light flashes that are created when x-rays strike the screens.

causes them to emit light flashes or to fluoresce when struck by x-rays (Fig. 1-6B). Actually, it is the fluoresced light from the screens on both sides of the film that accounts for the major exposure of the radiographic film. The direct incident x-rays striking the radiographic film account for a small proportion of the film exposure. The use of screens decreases the amount of radiation required to produce a radiograph, and this in turn decreases the patient's exposure to radiation. *It is important to remember that both radiographic and photographic film respond in a similar manner to light and x-rays.*

Computed Radiography

In conventional radiography, the radiographic image is recorded on film that goes through chemical processing for development. Computed radiography (CR) is the process of producing a *digital* radiographic image. A special phosphor plate (instead of film) is exposed to the x-ray beam. The image information is obtained by scanning the phosphor plate with a laser beam that causes light to be released from the phosphor plate. The intensity of the emitted light depends on the local radiation exposure. This emitted light is intensified by a photomultiplier tube and subsequently is converted into an electron stream. The electron stream is digitized, and the digital data are converted into an image by computer. The resulting image can be viewed on a monitor or transferred to radiographic film. The beauty of this system is that the digital image can be transferred via networks to multiple sites in or out of the hospital, and the digital images are easily stored in a computer or server. For example, a digital chest radiograph obtained in an intensive care unit (ICU) can be transmitted to the radiology department for consultation and interpretation in a matter of minutes. Then the radiologist can send this image via a network back to the ICU or to the referring physician's office. Of course, this digital information would be stored in a computer (server) for future recall. As this technology improves, it will become more and more important to the routine practice of medicine.

Contrast Media

Because soft tissues (muscles, blood vessels, organs) appear approximately the same on a radiograph, we often need a way to distinguish between these structures and their surroundings. Thus, high-density contrast agents are injected intravascularly to enhance organs and other soft tissues. It is this enhancement (which increases their density or makes them whiter) that enables the viewer to detect subtle differences between normal and abnormal soft tissues and between an organ and the surrounding tissues on a radiograph. Contrast media usage varies from a simple injection into a fistulous tract to an invasive procedure such as an angiogram, and this will be discussed in greater detail in Chapter 11.

Another type of contrast media is used for the gastrointestinal (GI) tract. To accomplish a GI contrast examination, barium sulfate suspension is introduced into the GI tract either by oral ingestion (upper GI series), or through an intestinal tube (small bowel series), or as an enema (barium enema). When air is introduced into the GI tract along with the barium, the result is called a double-contrast study. Barium studies are safer, better tolerated by patients, and relatively inexpensive compared to the more invasive GI endoscopic studies. Barium studies can be effective in diagnosing a wide variety of GI pathology as they are quite sensitive and specific.

When the integrity of the GI tract is in question, there exists a potential for catastrophic extravasation of the barium into the mediastinum or peritoneum. In these situations, barium studies are contraindicated and a water-soluble iodinated compound should be used. As a general rule, images produced with water-soluble contrast agents are less informative than barium studies because the water-soluble agents are less dense than barium and result in poorer contrast.

Oral ingested tablets containing iodinated compounds can be used to visualize the gallbladder (oral cholecystogram). These compounds are removed from the blood by the hepatic cells, then excreted into the biliary tree and concentrated in the gallbladder. This study provides information about gallbladder function and the presence or absence of filling defects such as calculi and tumors.

Often it is necessary to visualize the urinary tract *(excretory urogram)* when searching for a wide variety of pathologic conditions and when seeking anatomic and physiologic information. This study uses intravenously injected ionic high and low osmolar iodinated compounds that are excreted by the kidneys. These same compounds are used in angiography, arthrography, and computed tomography (CT).

Angiography is merely the injection of contrast media directly into a vein or artery via a needle and/or catheter (see Chapter 11). *Arthrography* is the injection of contrast media and/or air into a joint. Air may be used alone or in combination with these compounds to improve contrast. Arthrography has been used to image multiple joints such as rotator cuff injuries of the shoulder and to assess meniscus injuries in the knee. Since the advent of CT and magnetic resonance imaging (MRI), the arthrogram has become less important.

Myelography is the placement of contrast media in the spinal subarachnoid space, usually via a lumbar puncture. This procedure is useful for diagnosing diseases in and around the spinal canal and cord. Because of the advent of the less invasive CT and MRI modalities, the use of myelogram studies has been decreasing. Gadolinium will be discussed in the MRI section.

COMPUTED TOMOGRAPHY

Computed tomography involves sectional anatomy imaging, or anatomy in the sagittal, coronal, and axial (cross-sectional, transverse) planes. These terms, which can be confusing, are clearly illustrated in Fig. 1-7. Sectional anatomy has always been important to the physician and health care worker, but the newer imaging modalities of computed tomography (CT), magnetic resonance imaging (MRI), and ultrasonography (US) demand an in-depth understanding of anatomy displayed in this manner.

Computed tomography (CT or CAT scan) technology was developed in the 1970s, and the rock group The Beatles gave a big boost to CT development when they invested a significant amount of money in a business called Electric Musical Instruments Limited (EMI). It was EMI engineers who subsequently developed CT technology. Initially, EMI scanners were used exclusively for brain imaging, but this technology was rapidly extended to the abdomen, thorax, spine, and extremities.

CT imaging is best understood if the anatomic site to be examined is thought of as a loaf of sliced bread; an image of each slice of bread is created without imaging the other slices (Fig. 1-8). This is in contradistinction to a radiograph, which captures the whole loaf of bread as in a photograph.

The external appearance of a typical CT unit or machine is illustrated in Fig. 1-9. CT images are produced by a combination of x-rays, computers, and detectors. A computer-controlled couch transfers the patient in short increments

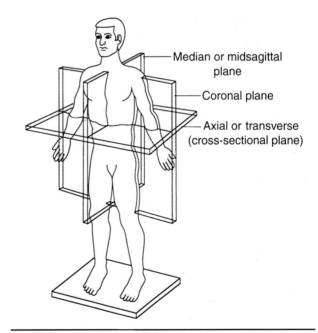

FIGURE 1-7. Sagittal, coronal, and axial anatomic planes.

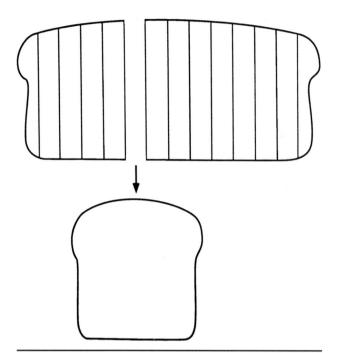

FIGURE 1-8. Illustration of how CT technology creates an image of a single slice of bread from a loaf of sliced bread without imaging the other slices.

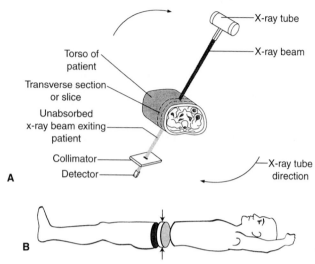

FIGURE 1-10. A: Illustration of how the x-ray tube circles the patient's abdomen to produce an image (slice) as shown in B. **B:** Demonstration of how a CT scan creates a thin-slice axial image of the abdomen (*arrows*) without imaging the remainder of the abdomen.

through the opening in the scanner housing. In the standard CT unit, the x-ray tube located in the housing (gantry) rotates around the patient, and each anatomic slice to be imaged is exposed to a pencil-thin x-ray beam (Fig. 1-10). Each image or slice requires only a few seconds; therefore breath holding is usually not an issue. The thickness of

these axial images or slices can be varied from 1 to 10 mm depending on the indications for the study. For example, in the abdomen and lungs we commonly use a 10-mm slice thickness because the structures are large. A slice thickness of only a few millimeters is used to image small structures like those found in the middle and inner ear. An average CT study takes approximately 10 to 20 minutes depending on the circumstances.

As in a radiograph, the amount of the x-ray beam that passes through each slice or section of the patient will be inversely proportional to the density of the traversed tissues. The x-rays that pass completely through the patient eventually strike detectors (not film), and the detectors subsequently convert these incident x-rays to an electron stream. This electron stream is digitized or converted to numbers referred to as CT units or Hounsfield units (HU); then computer software converts these numbers to corresponding shades of black, white, and gray. A dense structure, such as bone, will absorb most of the x-ray beam and allow only a small amount of x-rays to strike the detectors. The result is a white density on the film. On the other hand, air will absorb little of the x-ray beam, allowing a large number of x-rays to strike the detectors. The result is a black density on the image. Soft tissue structures appear gray on the image.

This CT digital information can be displayed on a video monitor, stored on magnetic tape, transmitted across computer networks, or printed on radiographic film via a format camera.

Because CT technology uses x-rays, the image densities of the anatomic structures being examined are the same

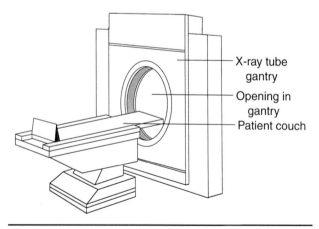

FIGURE 1-9. A standard CT scanner or machine. The patient couch or cradle is fed through the opening in the x-ray tube gantry or housing, and the anatomic part to be imaged is centered in this opening. The x-ray tube is located inside the gantry and moves around the patient to create an image.

▶ **TABLE 1-2 Some Common Indications
for CT Imaging**

Trauma
Intracranial hemorrhage (suspected or known)
Abdominal injury, especially to organs
Fracture detection and evaluation
Spine alignment
Detection of foreign bodies (especially in joints)
Diagnosis of primary and secondary neoplasms (liver, renal, brain,
    lung, and bone)
Tumor staging

on both CTs and radiographs. In other words, air appears black on both a CT image and a radiograph and bone appears white on both modalities. One major difference between a radiograph and a CT image is that a radiograph displays the entire anatomic structure, whereas a CT image allows us to visualize the same structure in slices. Another major difference is that in radiography the x-rays that pass through an object are recorded on film, whereas in CT the x-rays are recorded by devices called detectors and converted to digital data.

CT imaging is accomplished with and/or without intravenously injected contrast media. The intravenous contrast media enhance or increase the density of blood vessels, vascular soft tissues, organs, and tumors as in a radiograph. This enhancement assists in distinguishing between normal tissue and a pathologic process. Contrast media are not needed when searching for intracerebral hemorrhage or a suspected fracture or for evaluating a fracture fragment within a joint. However, contrast is used when evaluating the liver, kidney, and brain for primary and secondary neoplasms. A few of the common indications for CT imaging are listed in Table 1-2. Whenever possible, oral GI contrast agents are administered prior to an abdominal CT to delineate the contrast-filled GI tract from other abdominal structures.

High-resolution Computed Tomography

High-resolution computed tomography (HRCT) refers to CT studies that result in thin slices that are approximately 1.0 to 2.0 mm thick. This technology has become very useful in the diagnosis of parenchymal lung diseases.

Helical or Spiral Computed Tomography

Helical or spiral CT imaging is a relatively recent development. This technology is similar to standard CT but with a few new twists. In helical or spiral CT, the patient continuously moves through the gantry while the x-ray tube continuously encircles the patient (Fig. 1-11). This combination of the patient and x-ray tube continuously moving results in a spiral configuration. This technology can produce 1 slice per second, and the slice can vary in thickness from 1 to 10 mm. The resolution and contrast of these images are better than on standard CT images, resulting in improved images in areas such as the thorax and abdomen.

Multislice Computer Tomography

Conventional CT scanners have a single row of detectors; thus only one tomographic slice is generated for each rotation of the x-ray tube around the patient. In multislice CT there are multiple contiguous rows of detectors that yield multiple tomographic slices or images with each rotation of the x-ray tube. There can be as many as sixteen detector rows in one CT machine, resulting in reduced acquisition time. Some advantages and disadvantages of multidetector CT are listed in Table 1-3.

Computed Tomographic Angiography

This term refers to noninvasive angiography using either a multislice or a helical CT scanner. The procedure produces 3-mm slices during the rapid injection of contrast media.

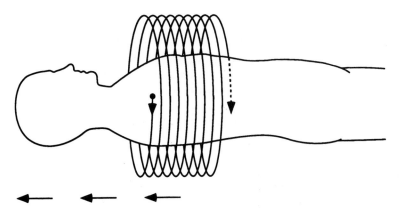

FIGURE 1-11. A helical or spiral CT scanner. The x-ray tube continuously circles the patient while the patient couch moves continuously through the opening in the x-ray tube gantry. The combination of continuous patient and x-ray tube movement results in a spiral configuration; hence the name "helical." In a standard CT or nonhelical scanner, the patient couch moves in short increments toward the gantry opening and stops intermittently to allow the x-ray tube to move around the patient. Thus, the x-ray tube moves around the patient only when the couch is stationary.

▶ **TABLE 1-3 Advantages and Disadvantages of Multislice CT**

Advantages
Static and cine or movie images
Noninvasive
Rapid filming results in decreased motion artifact
Good spatial resolution

Disadvantages
Expensive
Limited availability

This information can be used to create three-dimensional reconstructed images.

MAGNETIC RESONANCE IMAGING

Magnetic resonance imaging (MRI or MR) is another method for displaying anatomy in the axial, sagittal, and coronal planes. The slice thicknesses of the images vary between 1 and 10 mm. MRI is especially good for coronal and sagittal imaging, whereas axial imaging is the forte of CT. One of the main strengths of MRI is its ability to detect small changes (contrast) within soft tissues, and MRI soft tissue contrast is better than that found on CT images and radiographs.

CT and MR imaging modalities are digital-based technologies that require computers to convert digital information to shades of black, white, and gray. The major difference in the two technologies is that in MRI the patient is exposed to external magnetic fields and radio frequency waves, whereas the patient is exposed to x-rays during a CT study. The magnetic fields used in MRI are believed to be harmless. MR scanning can be a problem for people who are prone to develop claustrophobia because they are surrounded by a tunnel-like structure for approximately 30 to 45 minutes. Some of the advantages and disadvantages of MRI are summarized in Table 1-4. There are a few

▶ **TABLE 1-4 Advantages and Disadvantages of MRI**

Advantages
Static and cine or movie images
Multiple plane images
Good contrast
No known health hazards
Good for soft tissue injuries of the knee, ankle, and shoulder joints

Disadvantages
More expensive than CT
Long scan times may result in claustrophobia and motion artifacts
Limited availability

▶ **TABLE 1-5 Contraindications for MRI Studies**

Pregnancy unless an emergency
Cerebral aneurysms clipped by ferromagnetic clips
Cardiac pacemakers
Inner ear implants
Metallic foreign bodies in and around the eyes

contraindications for an MRI study, and these are listed in Table 1-5.

The external appearance of an MRI scanner or machine is similar to a CT scanner with the exception that the opening in the MR gantry is more tunnel-like (Fig. 1-12). As in CT, the patient is comfortably positioned supine, prone, or decubitus on a couch. The couch moves only when examining the extremities. The patient hears and feels a jackhammer-like thumping while the study is in progress.

The underlying physics of MRI is complicated, and strange-sounding terms proliferate. Let's keep it simple: *MRI is essentially the imaging of protons.* The most commonly imaged proton is hydrogen, as it is abundant in the human body and is easily manipulated by a magnetic field. However, other nuclei can be imaged. Because the hydrogen proton has a positive charge and is constantly spinning at a fixed frequency, called the *spin frequency,* a small magnetic field with a north and south pole surrounds the proton. Remember that a moving charged particle creates a surrounding magnetic field. Thus, these hydrogen protons act like magnets and align themselves within an external magnetic field much like nails in a magnetic field or the needle of a compass.

In the MR scanner, or magnet, short bursts of radio-frequency waves are broadcast into the patient from radio transmitters. The broadcast radio wave frequency is the same as the spin frequency of the proton being imaged (hydrogen in this case). The hydrogen protons absorb the broadcast radio wave energy and become energized, or

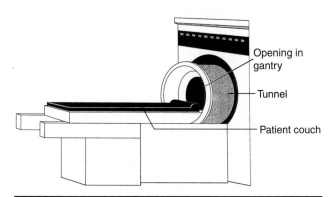

FIGURE 1-12. Illustration of an MRI scanner. Notice that its external appearance is similar to that of a CT scanner. The main difference, of course, is that there is a magnetic field, rather than an x-ray tube around the gantry opening.

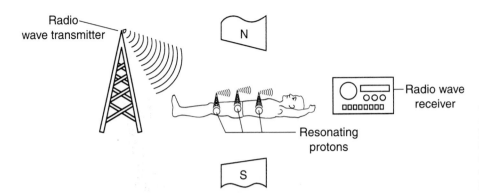

FIGURE 1-13. The general principles of MRI physics. The frequencies of the radio wave transmitter, the radio wave receiver, and the spin frequency of hydrogen atom protons are the same.

resonate. Hence the term *magnetic resonance*. Once the radio-frequency wave broadcast is discontinued, the protons revert or decay back to their normal or steady state that existed prior to the radio wave broadcast. As the hydrogen protons decay back to their normal state or relax, they continue to resonate and broadcast radio waves that can be detected by a radio wave receiver set to the same frequency as the broadcast radio waves and the hydrogen proton spin frequency (Fig. 1-13). The intensity of the radio wave signal detected by the receiver coil indicates the numbers and locations of the resonating hydrogen protons. For example, there are many hydrogen atoms and protons present in fat, and the received radio wave signal will be intense or very bright. However, there is much less hydrogen in bone cortex, and the received radio wave signal is of low intensity or black. The overall result is a three-dimensional proton density plot or map of the anatomic slice being examined. This analog (wave) data received by the receiver coil is subsequently converted to numbers (digitized), and the numbers are converted to shades of black, white, and gray by computers.

Now comes the complicated part. The received radio wave signal intensity from the patient is determined not only by the number of hydrogen atoms but by the T1 and T2 relaxation times. If the radio receivers listen early during the decay following the discontinuance of the radio wave broadcast, it is called a T1-weighted sequence. In a T1 image, the fat is white and the gray soft tissue detail is excellent. If the radio receivers listen late during the decay, it is called a T2-weighted sequence wherein the water in soft tissues is now a lighter gray and fat appears gray. The simplest way to think of T1 and T2 is as two different technical ways to look at the same structure. This is analogous to the PA and lateral radiographs being two different ways to view a bone or the chest. We tend to use T1 imaging when seeking anatomic information. T2 imaging is helpful when searching for pathology, because most pathology tends to contain considerable amounts of water or hydrogen and T2 causes water to light up like a light bulb. In general, T1 images have good resolution and T2 images have better contrast than T1 images.

Although human anatomy is always the same no matter what the imaging modality, the appearances of anatomic structures are very different on MR and CT images. Sometimes it is difficult for the beginner to differentiate between a CT and an MR image. The secret is to *look to the fat.* If the subcutaneous fat is black, it is a CT image as fat appears black on studies that use x-rays. If the subcutaneous fat is white (high-intensity signal), then it has to be an MR. Next, *look to the bones.* Bones should have a gray medullary canal and a white cortex on radiographs and CT images. The medullary canal contains bone marrow, and the gray is due to the large amount of fat in bone marrow. On a T1 MR image, nearly all of the bone appears homogeneously white as the bone marrow is fat that emits a high-intensity signal and appears white. Also, on MR the cortex of the bone will appear black (dark or low-intensity signal), whereas on CT images the cortex is white. Soft tissues and organs appear as shades of gray on CT and MR. Air appears black on CT and has a low-intensity signal (black or dark) on MR. Table 1-6 compares the appearances of various structures on MR and CT images.

Standard iodinated contrast agents are of no use in MRI. Instead, we use magnetically active substances (paramagnetic) such as gadolinium to enhance imaging certain disease processes. Gadolinium does not produce an MR signal, but it shortens the T1 relaxation time in tissues where it has localized. Gadolinium creates improved contrast between tissues, especially on T1 images, and it is useful for imaging tumors, infections, and acute stroke. Gadolinium is safer than the iodinated contrast media.

Magnetic Resonance Angiography (MRA)

MRA is a special noninterventional study that can image vessels without using needles, catheters, or iodinated contrast media. As a general rule, flowing blood appears black on most MR images, but by using a special imaging technique (gradient-echo pulse sequence) the arterial and venous blood appears as a high-intensity signal, or bright (Fig. 1-14). This procedure takes approximately 10 minutes, and three-dimensional images of the vasculature can

▶ **TABLE 1-6** A Comparison of Structure Appearances on Images

| | | MRI | |
Object	CT and Radiographs	T1	T2
Air	Black	Dark	Dark
Fat	Black	Very bright	Intermediate to dark
Muscles	Gray	Dark	Dark
Bone cortex	White	Dark	Dark
Bone marrow	Gray	Bright	Intermediate to dark
Gadolinium		Very bright	Bright

Remember: On MR images the words *dark, low-intensity signal,* and *black* are synonymous; *bright, high-intensity signal,* and *white* are synonymous; and *intermediate-intensity signal* and *gray* are synonymous.

be reconstructed with the digital information. MRA has been effective for imaging arteries and veins in the head and neck, abdomen, chest, and extremities.

Magnetic Resonance Spectroscopy (MRS)

MRS is useful for looking at disorders of metabolism, tumors, and inflammatory and ischemic diseases. In a con-ventional MRI, tomographic images are produced that reflect the magnitude of relaxation parameters at a specific frequency. One can also use MR technology to provide a spectral plot of the magnitude of chemical compounds in the acquisition volume as a function of frequency in the stimulating coils. This works because the resonant frequency of the protons is highly dependent on the local chemical environment where they are located.

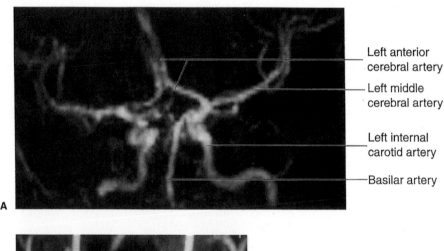

Left anterior cerebral artery

Left middle cerebral artery

Left internal carotid artery

Basilar artery

A

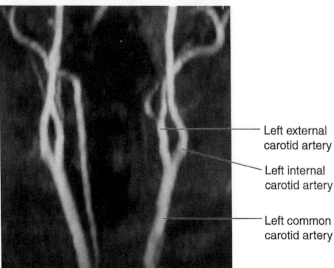

Left external carotid artery

Left internal carotid artery

Left common carotid artery

FIGURE 1-14. **A:** MRA axial image of the circle of Willis arteries (normal). **B:** MRA coronal image of the carotid arteries. Normal.

B

Magnetic Resonance Diffusion Weighted Imaging (MR DWI)

In MR DWI, the motion of water molecules in the brain is detected from the additional loss in the dephasing signal as the molecules diffuse through the tissues. Because free diffusion of protons is inhibited by cell membranes, MR DWI is particularly sensitive to cellular injuries. As a result, MR DWI is useful in the diagnosis of ischemic stroke and can detect it reliably within minutes of symptom onset.

ULTRASONOGRAPHY

Ultrasonography (US) is another useful diagnostic imaging tool that is noninvasive and does not use x-rays or radiation. US has significantly improved the diagnosis, treatment, and management of a number of diseases. Some common imaging applications of US are listed in Table 1-7. It has achieved excellent patient acceptance because it is safe, fast, painless, and inexpensive when compared to the other imaging modalities. The advantages and disadvantages of US are listed in Table 1-8.

Ultrasound technology produces sectional anatomy images or slices in multiple planes much like CT and MRI. An US machine consists of an ultrasound wave source, a computer, and a transducer (Fig. 1-15). The US machine emits high-frequency sound waves, ranging from 1 to 10 MHz, that are considerably above the human ear's audible range of 20 to 20,000 Hz. Short bursts of these high-frequency sound waves are alternately broadcast into the patient by a transducer, and some of the reflected sound waves from body tissues are intermittently received by the transducer (Fig. 1-16). The acoustic impedance *(Z)* of a structure determines the amount of sound energy transmitted and reflected at its boundary (Z = tissue density × sound velocity). When a sound wave encounters an acoustic interface or the boundary between two media of different acoustic impedance, the sound waves may be absorbed, deflected, or reflected (Fig. 1-17).

The analog sound waves that are reflected directly back to the transducer are subsequently digitized. Next, a computer converts this digital information to an image with

TABLE 1-7 Some Common Imaging Applications for Diagnostic US

Obstetrics
Pediatric brain
Testicle and prostate
Female pelvis
Chest for pleural fluid drainage
Abdomen (kidney, pancreas, liver, and gallbladder)
Vascular disease

TABLE 1-8 Advantages and Disadvantages of US Diagnostic Imaging

Advantages
Multiple plane imaging including obliques
Safe—no known biological harm at diagnostic sound frequency levels
Painless (noninvasive)
Less expensive than CT and MRI
Equipment cost is less than that of CT and MRI
Real time or cine is possible
Very portable
Disadvantages
Requires technical skill or is operator dependent
Not good for bone and lung imaging

shades of black, white, and gray. US, like MRI and CT, depends on computer technology to store digital information and subsequently convert it to an image.

Each organ and tissue has its own characteristic echo pattern. Solid organs have a homogeneous echo pattern, whereas fluid-filled organs and masses such as the urinary bladder, cysts, and the gallbladder have relatively fewer internal echoes.

The terminology used to describe the US image planes is slightly different from that used in describing CT and MR image planes. In US an axial view may be referred to as a *transverse* scan, and a sagittal view may be called a *longitudinal* scan or view (Fig. 1-18). As previously noted, a significant part of medicine is just learning the lingo.

While an US study is in progress, the images are viewed on a monitor. The monitor is analogous to a movie screen or television, and this viewing mode is called *real time*. This allows onlookers to observe a beating heart or the movements of an intrauterine fetus. Also, static images may be reproduced on film by a format camera.

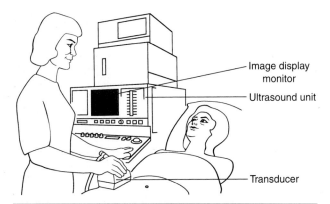

FIGURE 1-15. An US unit, an ultrasonographer, and the patient. The transducer is centered over the abdomen. The ultrasonographer moves the transducer with the right hand while making technical adjustments on the US unit with the left hand.

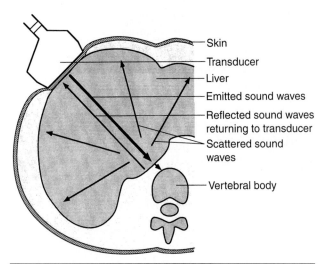

FIGURE 1-16. A transducer placed on the skin overlying the liver. The transducer broadcasts short bursts of high-frequency sound waves into the liver and deeper structures. Reflected sound waves are intermittently received by the transducer when it is not broadcasting sound waves. Note that some of the sound waves are deflected away from the transducer and are of no use for imaging.

TELERADIOLOGY

This term simply means the transmission of images from one site to another across telephone lines. This technology allows an image to be transferred to a radiologist's office or home for instant interpretation. Thus, a distant

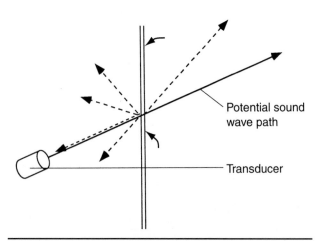

FIGURE 1-17. Illustration of what can happen to sound waves when they encounter an acoustic interface. An acoustic interface represents the intersection of two structures that possess different acoustic impedances or densities. When the sound waves are broadcast from the transducer (*solid black line*) and strike an acoustic interface (*curved arrows*), a number of things can happen to them such as the following: they can be reflected back to the transducer, be deflected away from the transducer, pass through the interface, or be absorbed at the interface.

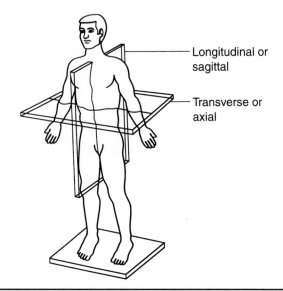

FIGURE 1-18. Clarification of some of the terminology used to describe sectional anatomy planes on US images.

site without a radiologist present can transfer images to a radiologist at another site.

PICTURE ARCHIVING SYSTEMS

The picture archive and computer system (PACS) is a comprehensive computer-based system designed to easily store and rapidly retrieve medical images. As one might expect, this is a challenging task as the size and number of images continue to grow rapidly. In recent years, the development of a standardized image format called Digital Imaging and Communications in Medicine (DICOM) has made the handling of medical images from a wide variety of modalities and manufacturers possible.

KEY POINTS

- There are four basic densities or appearances to observe on radiographs and CT images: *air,* which appears black; *fat,* which also appears black; *soft tissues and organs,* which appear gray; and *metal, calcium, and bone,* which appear white.
- Plain radiography images are produced by x-rays and radiographic film. CT images are produced by x-rays, detectors, and computers. MR images are produced by magnetic fields, radio-frequency waves, and computers. Ultrasound images are produced by high-frequency sound waves, transducers, and computers.
- Sectional anatomy is the imaging of anatomy in multiple planes, including the axial plane (transverse or cross-sectional), the sagittal plane, and the coronal plane.

- A key to distinguishing an MRI from a CT image is that the fat in an MRI appears white.
- T1 MR images tend to have excellent resolution and are therefore used to procure anatomic information. T2 MR images have better contrast than T1 images and cause water to light up; they are therefore frequently used when searching for pathology, which tends to contain a lot of water.
- The high resolution of CT makes it effective for imaging anatomy. MRI has high soft tissue contrast that makes it especially useful for soft tissue imaging.
- Commonly used contrast agents include barium sulfate, high and low osmolar iodinated compounds, ionic iodinated and nonionic (low osmolar) contrast media, air, and gadolinium. Images produced with water-soluble iodinated agents are generally less informative than barium studies because they are less dense and result in poorer contrast.

BIBLIOGRAPHY

Hashemi RH, Bradley WG. *MRI: the basics.* Baltimore: Williams & Wilkins, 1997.

Bushberg JT, Seibert JA, Leidholdt EM Jr, Boone JM. *Essential physics of medical imaging.* Philadelphia: Lippincott Williams & Wilkens, 2002.

SECTION II

Diagnostic Radiology

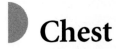

Chest

William E. Erkonen

Patients often complain of chest problems, and their symptoms might include shortness of breath, pain, cough, and hemoptysis or bloody sputum. The workup or investigation of these symptoms usually begins with a chest radiograph. Therefore, it is not surprising that the chest radiograph has become the most common imaging consultation requested by clinicians. The main purpose of this chapter is to demonstrate a simple way to approach chest radiographs.

TECHNIQUE

Fortunately, the amount of radiation required for a routine chest examination is extremely small and not a threat to the patient. The chest radiographic examination is usually accomplished in a radiology department, and a routine study consists of posteroanterior (PA) and lateral views.

When the patient is unable to tolerate these routine views, a portable anteroposterior (AP) view is obtained with the patient either standing, sitting, or supine. PA and lateral radiographs should be requested whenever possible because they are less expensive and give far more information than a portable study. Illustrations for these radiographic techniques have been previously demonstrated in Chapter 1 (Figs. 1-1 to 1-4).

Chest radiographs should not be requested to evaluate suspected problems in the ribs, shoulders, or the dorsal spine. When bone disease is suspected, the specific bone radiographs should be requested.

HOW TO VIEW THE PA AND AP CHEST RADIOGRAPH

Step 1 is to place the radiograph correctly on the viewbox, and the ability to do this is an immediate confidence

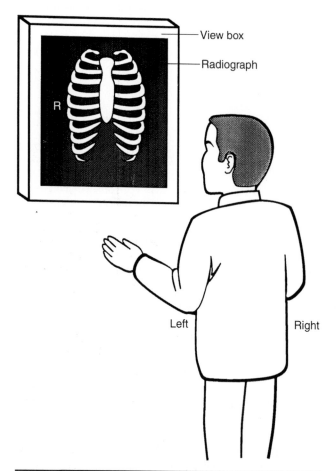

View box

Radiograph

R

Left   Right

FIGURE 2-1. The correct positioning of a chest radiograph on a viewbox. The patient's right side on the film should always be opposite the viewer's left side.

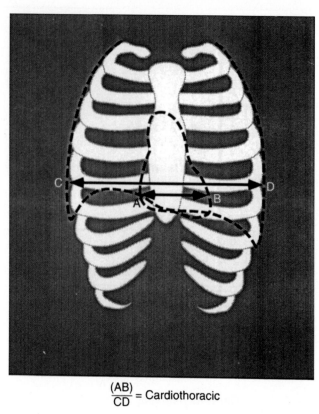

C   A   B   D

$$\frac{(AB)}{CD} = \text{Cardiothoracic}$$

FIGURE 2-3. Method for determining the cardiothoracic ratio.

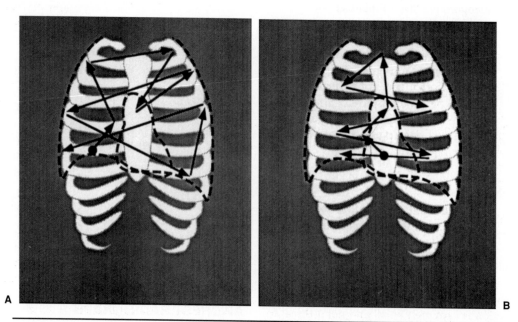

A   B

FIGURE 2-2. Illustration of a probable eye search pattern of a rookie **(A)** and by someone with a systematic approach **(B)** to a radiograph. Note that the rookie's search pattern is highly disorganized.

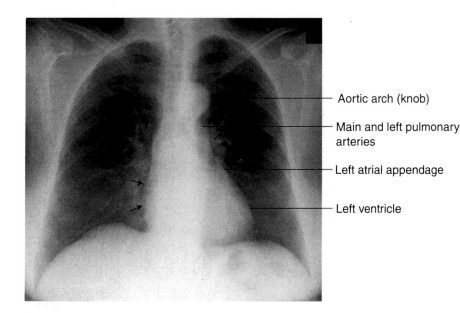

Aortic arch (knob)

Main and left pulmonary arteries

Left atrial appendage

Left ventricle

FIGURE 2-4. Chest posteroanterior (PA) radiograph. Normal. The convex right cardiac border is formed by the right atrium *(straight arrows)*, and the *curved arrows* indicate the location of the superior vena cava. The left cardiac and great vessels border might be considered as four skiing moguls. From cephalad to caudad the moguls are the aortic arch, the main and left pulmonary arteries, the left atrial appendage, and the left ventricle.

builder. There is nothing more pathetic, yet humorous, than watching somebody pontificate before a radiograph that is upside down or reversed side to side on the viewbox. *A significant part of the art and practice of medicine is just learning the jargon, lingo, routines, and rituals.*

Obviously, the R and L markers on the film indicate the patient's right and left side, respectively. Position the radiograph on the viewbox with the R film marker opposite your left side and the L film marker opposite your right side (Fig. 2-1). This routine applies to all AP and PA chest radiographs as well as nearly all other radiographs and images. Of course, the patient's head should be oriented to the top of the radiograph.

Step 2 is to approach and evaluate the radiograph by casually glancing at the entire image for any obvious abnormality that might jump out at you, such as a huge heart or a baseball-sized lung mass. *Remember always to look at all four corners of the image.*

Step 3 is to evaluate the radiograph systematically. Unfortunately, there is no single generally accepted or standardized system for evaluating a chest radiograph, so develop your own comfortable system. After all, even a veteran commercial pilot will use a checklist just prior to takeoff. The list might consist of such things as flaps down, brakes on, and check the fuel gauges. The pilot checklist is necessary, as it is virtually impossible to remember everything when preparing for takeoff.

Similarly, a mental checklist or system is needed to review a chest radiograph. So program your internal computer with a *systematic checklist* to avoid overlooking important areas or structures, as many of the errors made in medicine are errors of omission. The following suggested system can be used for a lifetime or until you develop your own system.

The arrows in Fig. 2-2A roughly approximate the haphazard visual pathway of a rookie viewing a chest radio-

graph. If you persist with this rookie approach, errors of omission are inevitable! The arrows in Fig. 2-2B demonstrate how someone with a system might approach a chest radiograph. On the other hand, a highly experienced radiologist generally views a radiograph in a more circumferential and peripheral manner.

After a general once-over glance at the entire image, use the water density cardiac silhouette as your starting point. First, determine the cardiac size. The transverse diameter of the cardiac silhouette should not exceed 50% of the transverse diameter of the thoracic cage measured or estimated at the same level. This is called the *cardiothoracic ratio* (Fig. 2-3). The exception to the cardiothoracic ratio is that the cardiac silhouette will appear larger on an AP view than on a PA view on the same patient. Because the heart is an anterior thoracic structure, it lies farther from the radiographic film on an AP radiograph than on a PA. Consequently, the heart casts a larger shadow on the AP view than on the PA. *The greater the distance between an anatomic structure and the radiographic film, the more the magnification.* Also, when the patient's inspiration is poor, the diaphragms will be elevated, causing the heart to appear larger than it is.

Cardiac contour and size are best evaluated by gross eyeballing, and generally a ruler is not needed. When you are waiting at the bus stop, you can instantly determine if a passerby is obese, tall, short, or acting strangely. Your visual-cerebral computer automatically concludes these facts based on prior experiences. After you have viewed many more chest radiographs, your evaluations of cardiac size and shape will become easier.

Next evaluate the cardiac shape. What actually determines the cardiac shape? The convex right cardiac border is formed by the water density right atrium, and just cephalad or superior to the right atrium is the straight-bordered superior vena cava (Figs. 2-4 and 2-38A). The cardiac apex

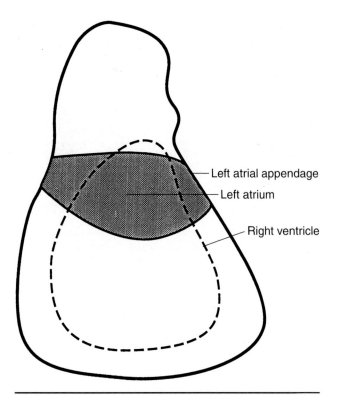

FIGURE 2-5. The approximate location of the left atrium and right ventricle on a normal PA or AP chest radiograph. These cardiac chambers cannot be delineated on normal studies. However, the left atrial appendage can occasionally be seen in normal hearts.

is formed primarily by the left ventricle, and the left atrium contributes to the superior left cardiac border (Fig. 2-4). The right ventricle is superimposed on the left ventricle and is not visualized as such on normal PA or AP radiographs. Also, a normal left atrium is not visible on the

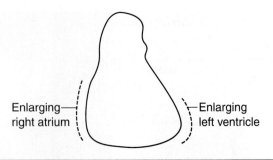

FIGURE 2-6. Cardiac silhouette changes during right atrium and left ventricle enlargement. As the right atrium enlarges, the convex right heart border enlarges to the patient's right. As the left ventricle enlarges, the cardiac apex moves to the patient's left and downward.

normal PA or AP radiograph (Fig. 2-5). As the left ventricle enlarges, the cardiac apex moves to the patient's left. As the right atrium enlarges, the cardiac silhouette enlarges to the patient's right (Fig. 2-6).

Next your visual pathway takes you to the aortic arch, pulmonary arteries, and the main stem bronchi. The left and right pulmonary arteries and the main stem bronchi form the hilar shadows (Fig. 2-7). On normal chest radiographs, the left hilum is more cephalad than the right hilum approximately 70% of the time and the hili are at the same level 30% of the time. The normal right hilum is rarely cephalad to the left hilum. The *aortopulmonary window* is the air density space between the water density aortic arch knob and the water density left pulmonary artery (Fig. 2-7). When the aortopulmonary window fills in with a water density, you should be suspicious of a mass such as a primary or secondary neoplasm occupying this space. The water density pulmonary arteries and their branches emanate outward from the hili. The main pulmonary artery

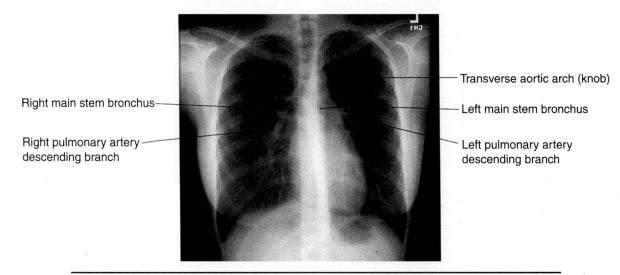

FIGURE 2-7. Chest PA radiograph. Normal. The air density aortopulmonary window *(straight arrow)* is situated between the water density aortic arch knob and the superior aspect of the water density left pulmonary artery. It is important to note that the air-filled main stem bronchi appear black, whereas the blood-filled pulmonary arteries appear white. See Table 1-1 in Chapter 1.

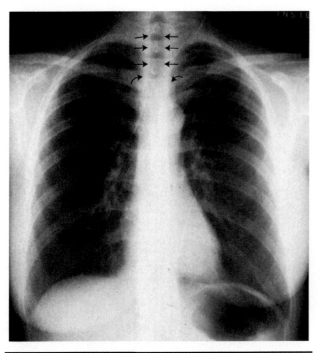

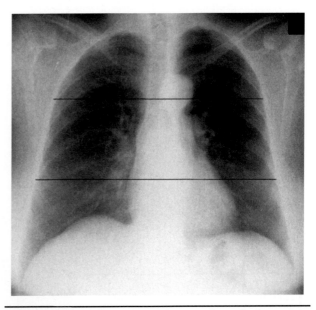

FIGURE 2-9. Chest PA radiograph. Normal. Divide the PA or AP chest radiograph into horizontal thirds and compare the right and left lung fields moving in a head-to-foot direction. Note the aortopulmonary window *(straight arrow)*.

FIGURE 2-8. Chest PA radiograph. Normal. The vertical air density trachea *(straight arrows)* should always be midline. The narrow mediastinum is water density *(curved arrows)*.

segment tends to be more prominent in the young and athletic, especially in females, and this prominence usually disappears with age. It is important to remember that in the elderly patient the aorta becomes tortuous, and this can be seen on frontal as well as lateral views. On frontal views a tortuous aorta often overrides or obliterates the superior vena cava.

Now your gaze should be directed to the water density mediastinum and evaluate it for widening, and again this is

based on experience. Most of the mediastinum water density is caused by the great vessels or the vascular pedicle. The vascular pedicle extends from the thoracic inlet cephalad to the base of the heart caudally. The right border of the pedicle is the superior vena cava, and the left border is the aortic knob near the origin of the subclavian artery. The air density or black trachea should be in the midline (Fig. 2-8). Now divide the lungs into horizontal thirds and compare the right and left lung fields (Fig. 2-9). Evaluate the domed curvilinear diaphragms, the costophrenic angles, and the gastric air bubble (Fig. 2-10).

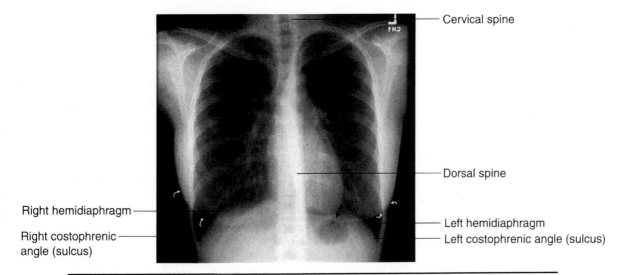

FIGURE 2-10. Chest PA radiograph. Normal. After comparing the lung fields, you next view the diaphragms, costophrenic angles, and lower dorsal spine. Note the close proximity of the gastric fundus air to the left hemidiaphragm *(arrow)*. Always remember to identify the breast shadows in female patients *(curved arrows)*.

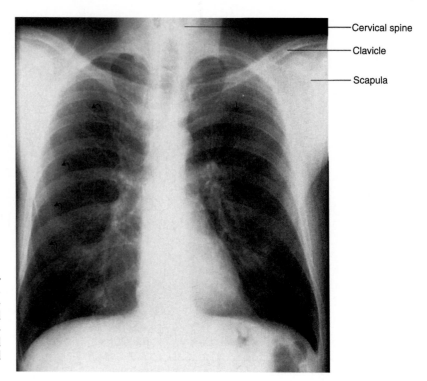

Cervical spine

Clavicle

Scapula

FIGURE 2-11. Chest PA radiograph. Normal. The posterior ribs *(straight arrows)* are horizontal and anterior ribs *(curved arrows)* are angled caudad or inferiorly. All of these osseous structures must be included in your checklist as well as the shoulder girdles and cervical and dorsal spine areas.

Next, examine the visible bones such as the cervical spine, dorsal spine, clavicles, shoulders, and ribs (Figs. 2-10 and 2-11). Ribs are difficult to evaluate, so you need to trace each one visually or use your fingertip. On a PA radiograph, the horizontal portions of the ribs are the posterior arcs and the anterior ribs are usually angled downward (see Fig. 2-11). As always, you should compare the right and left sides. The amount of cervical and dorsal spine visible on a radiograph is variable.

HOW TO VIEW THE LATERAL CHEST RADIOGRAPH

Now position the lateral chest radiograph on the viewbox with the patient's head oriented to the top of the film. There is no hard-and-fast rule about the direction that the patient should be facing, but we commonly have the patient facing to the viewer's left (Fig. 2-12). Once again, begin the radiograph evaluation by casually viewing the entire image so that something obvious can jump out at you. As on PA and AP radiographs, begin by estimating the size and shape of the anteriorly located heart. The right ventricle forms the anterior border of the cardiac silhouette. The left ventricle forms the major portion of the inferior-posterior cardiac border, and the left atrium forms the superior-posterior cardiac border (see Fig. 2-12). On most lateral chest radiographs, the inferior vena cava *(straight arrows)* can be seen as it enters the right atrium posteriorly and inferiorly

(Fig. 2-12). The left ventricle is considered enlarged if it is more than 2 cm posterior to the inferior vena cava. The right atrium is not visualized as such on the lateral view.

Now look at the hili structures and the trachea (Fig. 2-13). Then observe the sternum and search the retrosternal and retrocardiac spaces for abnormal or pathologic water and air densities (Fig. 2-14A). On the lateral view, the retrosternal lungs are primarily the upper lobes, whereas the right middle lobe and the lingular segments of the left upper lobe project over the cardiac silhouette. The lower lobes are located in the retrocardiac space (Fig. 2-14B). It is important to understand these pulmonary lobe spatial relationships to assist in locating pulmonary pathologic processes that usually are water density.

Finally, observe the contours of the diaphragms and the posterior costophrenic angles or sulci. Note that the right hemidiaphragm can be seen in its entirety because black air in the right lower lobe abuts the gray right hemidiaphragm and liver. However, the water density left hemidiaphragm abuts the water density heart anteriorly, and as a result the left hemidiaphragm disappears anteriorly (Fig. 2-15). *Whenever two abutting objects are of similar density, it is difficult to identify their boundaries or silhouettes.* This very important principle is called the *silhouette sign,* and it is a powerful and important radiologic tool. Because most pulmonary pathology is water density, the silhouette sign facilitates the detection and location of water density pathology. For example, if the left diaphragm cannot be seen on the PA view and it is obliterated posteriorly on the lateral view, then water density

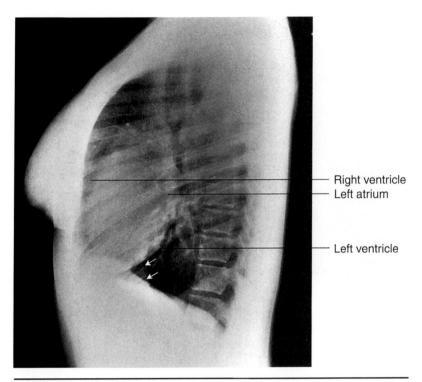

Right ventricle
Left atrium

Left ventricle

FIGURE 2-12. Chest lateral radiograph. Normal. The radiograph is positioned on the viewbox with the patient facing to either your left or right. Note that the cardiac silhouette is an anterior structure and makes an excellent starting point for your evaluation. The faint vertical water density line *(straight arrows)* represents the inferior vena cava.

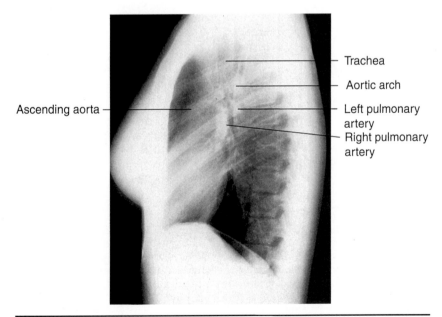

Ascending aorta

Trachea

Aortic arch

Left pulmonary artery

Right pulmonary artery

FIGURE 2-13. Chest lateral radiograph. Normal. Note that the oval-shaped right pulmonary artery lies anterior and inferior relative to the left pulmonary artery. The left pulmonary artery crosses cephalad over the left main stem bronchus and it lies inferior to the aortic arch.

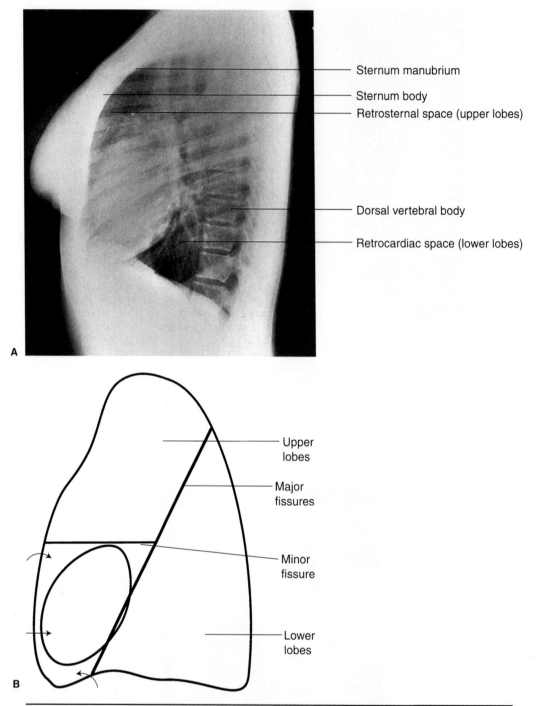

FIGURE 2-14. A: Chest lateral radiograph. Normal. The anterior and posterior osseous structures should always be routinely viewed. The spine appears darker or more dense as you proceed caudally as there is more air in the lower lungs. **B:** Illustration of the spatial relationships of the pulmonary lobes on the lateral view. Note that the right middle lobe and the lingular segments of the left upper lobe *(curved arrows)* project over the heart *(straight arrow)*. The lower lobes are primarily posterior structures. The major fissures extend up to approximately the T4 level.

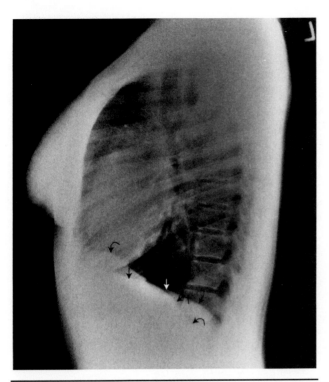

FIGURE 2-15. Chest lateral radiograph. Normal. Note that the left hemidiaphragm *(straight arrows)* is not visible anteriorly where it abuts the water density heart. On the other hand, the entire right hemidiaphragm *(curved arrows)* is visible. This is an excellent example of the silhouette sign.

pathology must be suspected in the left lower lobe (Fig. 2-48A, B). Furthermore, because the right middle lobe is situated anteriorly and adjacent to the right cardiac border, any water density pathologic process involving the right middle lobe will obliterate the anteriorly located right cardiac border on a PA or AP radiograph. Therefore, whenever the right cardiac border is obscured or indistinct on a PA or AP radiograph, a right middle lobe water density pathologic process such as pneumonia, atelectasis, tumor, blood, or infarction must be strongly suspected. Similarly, when the left cardiac border is obliterated on a PA or AP radiograph, pathology must be suspected in the anteriorly situated lingular segments of the left upper lobe.

AP LORDOTIC CHEST

There are occasions when disease is suspected in the pulmonary upper lobes; however, the ribs and clavicles may be obscuring the lesion. In these situations an AP lordotic radiograph (Fig. 2-16) is helpful for viewing the upper lobes without overlying clavicles. In general, the appearance of the lordotic AP radiograph is somewhat similar to that of a routine AP radiograph (Fig. 2-17).

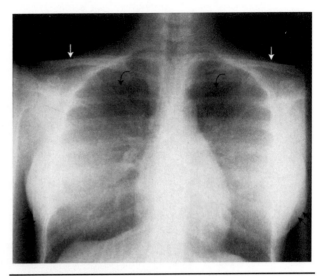

FIGURE 2-16. Chest AP lordotic radiograph. Normal. This view is obtained with the patient leaning backward a few degrees. Note how the clavicles *(straight arrows)* project cephalad to the pulmonary apices allowing an improved view of the upper lobes *(curved arrows)*. The scapulae project somewhat lower than on the standard AP or PA radiograph. The breasts are indicated by the *double straight arrows*.

NORMAL THORACIC SECTIONAL ANATOMY

The images in Figs. 2-18 through 2-26 demonstrate thoracic sectional anatomy in the axial, coronal, and sagittal planes. *The anatomy does not change, but the densities or the appearances of anatomic structures change, depending on the imaging modality used.*

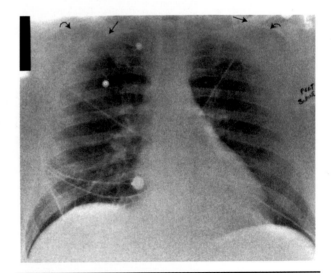

FIGURE 2-17. Chest AP portable supine radiograph. Normal. Compare the position of the clavicles *(straight arrows)* and scapulae *(curved arrows)* to those in the AP lordotic radiograph in Fig. 2-16. The white lines overlying the thorax are wires attached to external monitoring electrodes. The AP radiograph is similar in appearance to the PA radiographs shown earlier in this chapter. Although the cardiac silhouette may appear larger than normal, it is within normal limits for an AP view.

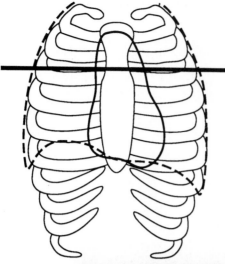

A

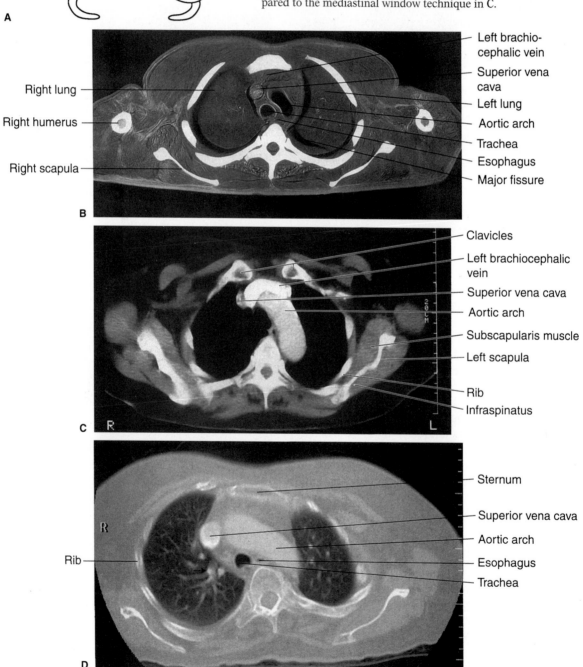

FIGURE 2-18. **A:** Approximate axial anatomic level through the aortic arch for B–D. **B:** Axial cadaver radiograph of the sectioned chest at the aortic arch level. Normal. A frozen cadaver was sectioned and then radiographed. **C, D:** Chest CT images at the aortic arch level with mediastinal windows (C) and parenchymal windows (D). Normal. The patient is scanned once, and the mediastinal windows and parenchymal windows are the result of technical adjustments. Note how well the pulmonary vessels *(straight arrow)* are visualized with the parenchymal or lung window technique compared to the mediastinal window technique in C.

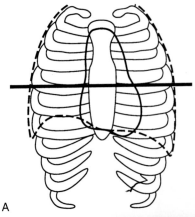

A

FIGURE 2-19. A: Approximate axial anatomic level through the pulmonary arteries for B–E. **B:** Axial cadaver radiograph of the sectioned chest at the level of the pulmonary arteries. Normal. **C, D:** Chest axial CT images at the level of the pulmonary arteries with mediastinal (C) and parenchymal windows (D). Normal.

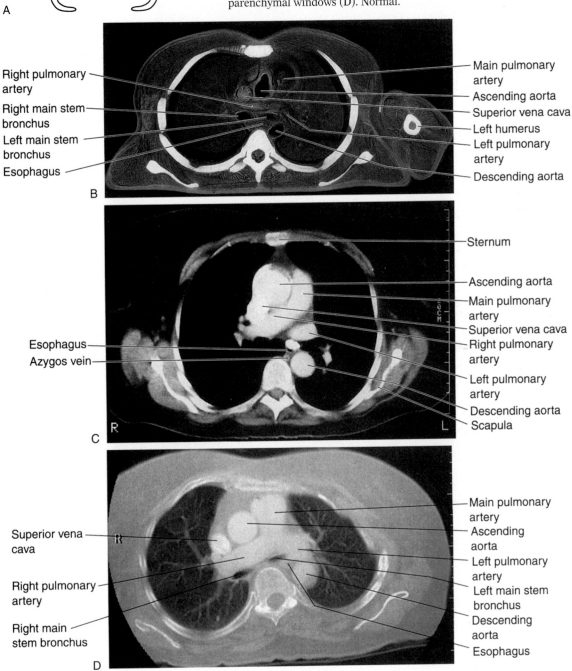

Right pulmonary artery

Right main stem bronchus

Left main stem bronchus

Esophagus

B

Main pulmonary artery

Ascending aorta

Superior vena cava

Left humerus

Left pulmonary artery

Descending aorta

Esophagus

Azygos vein

C

Sternum

Ascending aorta

Main pulmonary artery

Superior vena cava

Right pulmonary artery

Left pulmonary artery

Descending aorta

Scapula

Superior vena cava

Right pulmonary artery

Right main stem bronchus

D

Main pulmonary artery

Ascending aorta

Left pulmonary artery

Left main stem bronchus

Descending aorta

Esophagus

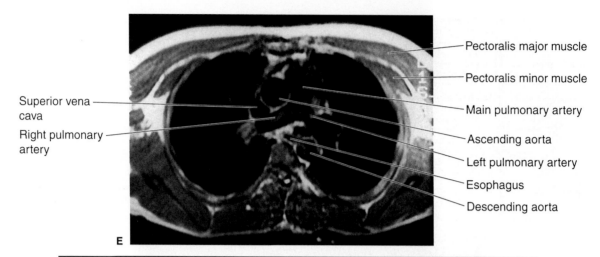

Superior vena cava

Right pulmonary artery

Pectoralis major muscle

Pectoralis minor muscle

Main pulmonary artery

Ascending aorta

Left pulmonary artery

Esophagus

Descending aorta

FIGURE 2-19. (*continued*) **E:** Chest axial MR image at the level of the pulmonary arteries. Normal.

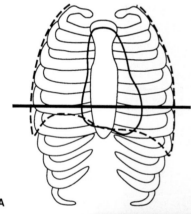

FIGURE 2-20. A: Approximate axial anatomic level through the right and left atria for B–E. **B:** Axial cadaver radiograph of the sectioned chest at the level of the right and left atria. Normal. **C, D:** Chest axial CT images at the level of the atria with mediastinal (C) and parenchymal (D) windows. Normal. **E:** Chest axial MR image at the level of the atria. Normal.

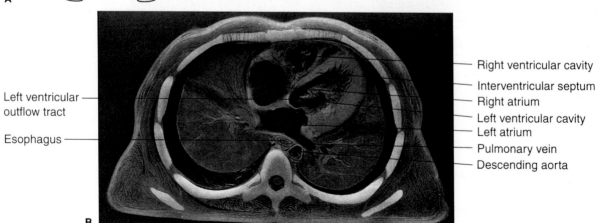

Left ventricular outflow tract

Esophagus

Right ventricular cavity

Interventricular septum

Right atrium

Left ventricular cavity

Left atrium

Pulmonary vein

Descending aorta

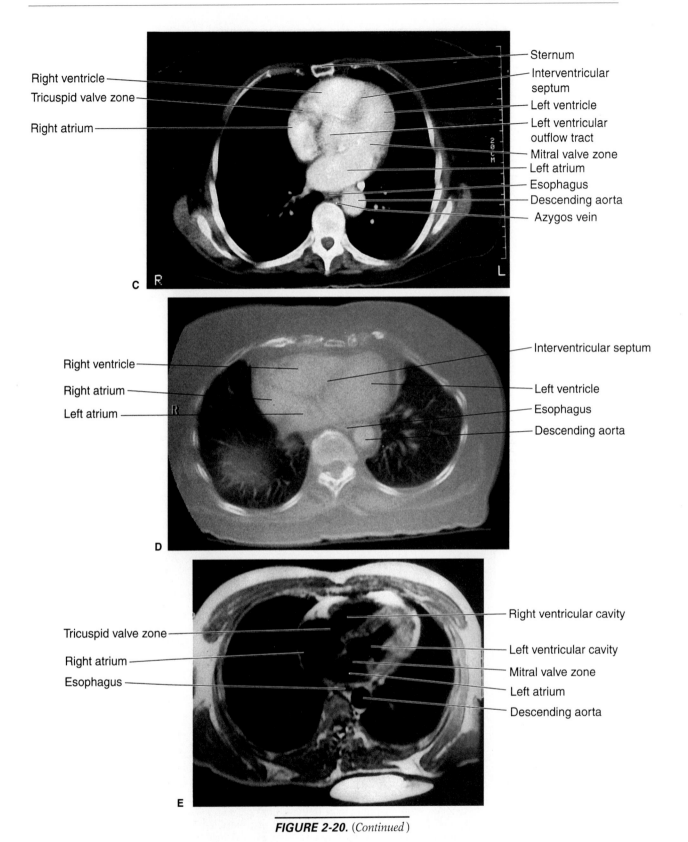

Right ventricle
Tricuspid valve zone
Right atrium

Sternum
Interventricular septum
Left ventricle
Left ventricular outflow tract
Mitral valve zone
Left atrium
Esophagus
Descending aorta
Azygos vein

C

Right ventricle
Right atrium
Left atrium

Interventricular septum
Left ventricle
Esophagus
Descending aorta

D

Tricuspid valve zone
Right atrium
Esophagus

Right ventricular cavity
Left ventricular cavity
Mitral valve zone
Left atrium
Descending aorta

E

FIGURE 2-20. (*Continued*)

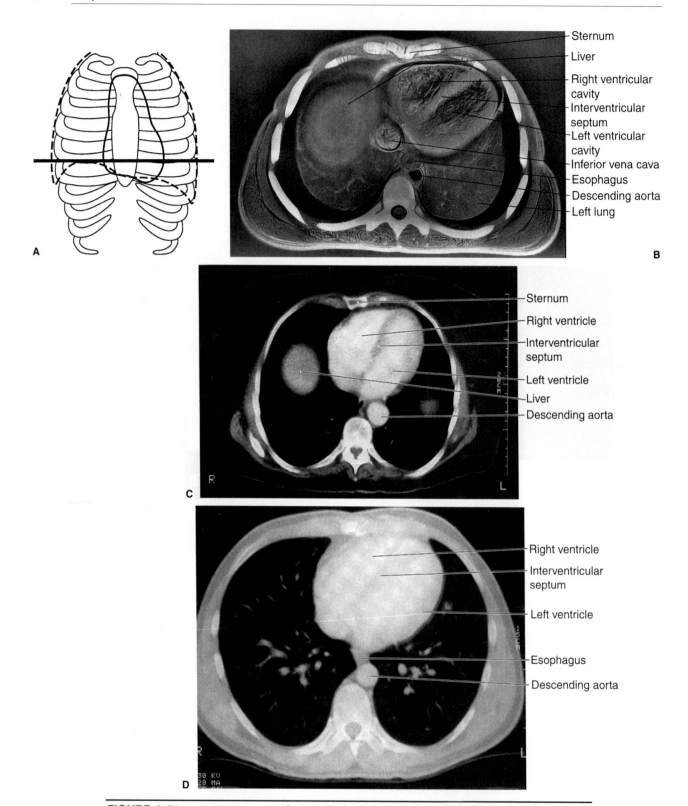

FIGURE 2-21. A: Approximate axial anatomic level through the right and left ventricles for B–E. **B:** Axial cadaver radiograph of the sectioned chest at the level of the ventricles. Normal. **C, D:** Chest axial CT image through the ventricles with both mediastinal (C) and parenchymal (D) windows. Normal. **E:** Chest axial MR image at the level of the ventricles. Normal.

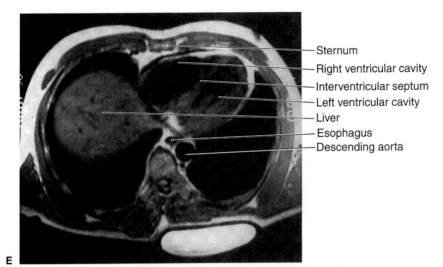

Sternum
Right ventricular cavity
Interventricular septum
Left ventricular cavity
Liver
Esophagus
Descending aorta

E

FIGURE 2-21. (*Continued*)

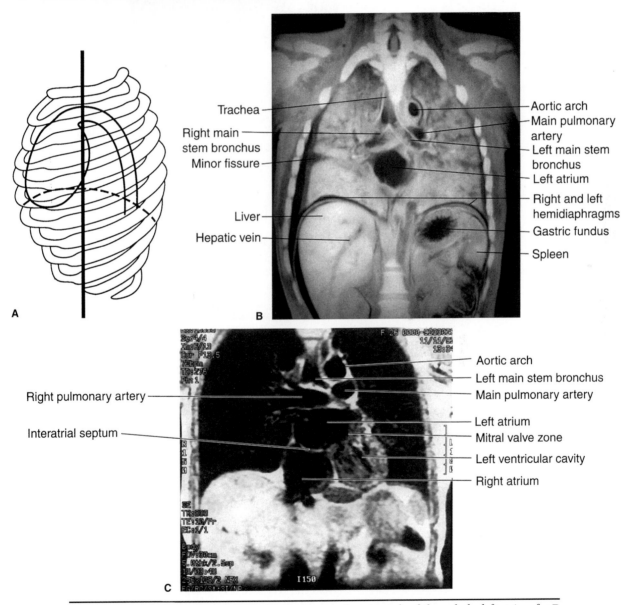

Trachea
Right main stem bronchus
Minor fissure
Liver
Hepatic vein

Aortic arch
Main pulmonary artery
Left main stem bronchus
Left atrium
Right and left hemidiaphragms
Gastric fundus
Spleen

A

B

Right pulmonary artery
Interatrial septum

Aortic arch
Left main stem bronchus
Main pulmonary artery
Left atrium
Mitral valve zone
Left ventricular cavity
Right atrium

C

FIGURE 2-22. A: Illustration of the approximate coronal anatomic level through the left atrium for B and C. **B:** Coronal cadaver radiograph of the sectioned chest through the level of the left atrium. Normal. **C:** Chest coronal MR image through the right and left atria. Normal.

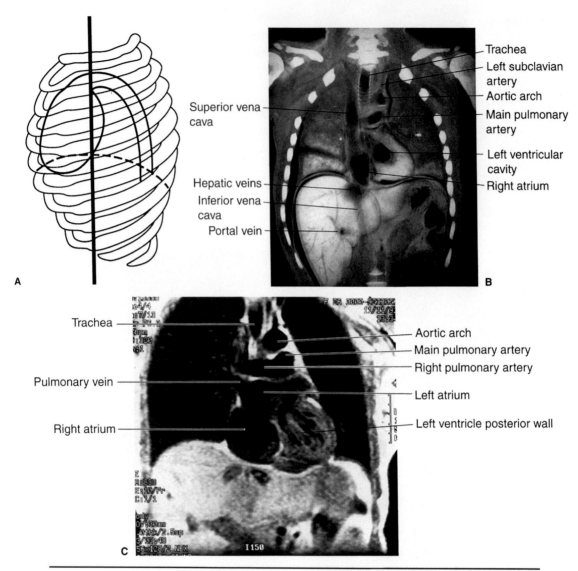

FIGURE 2-23. A: Approximate coronal anatomic level through the right atrium and left ventricle for B and C. **B:** Coronal cadaver radiograph of the sectioned chest through the level of the right atrium and left ventricle. Normal. **C:** Chest coronal MR image through the atria and left ventricle. Normal.

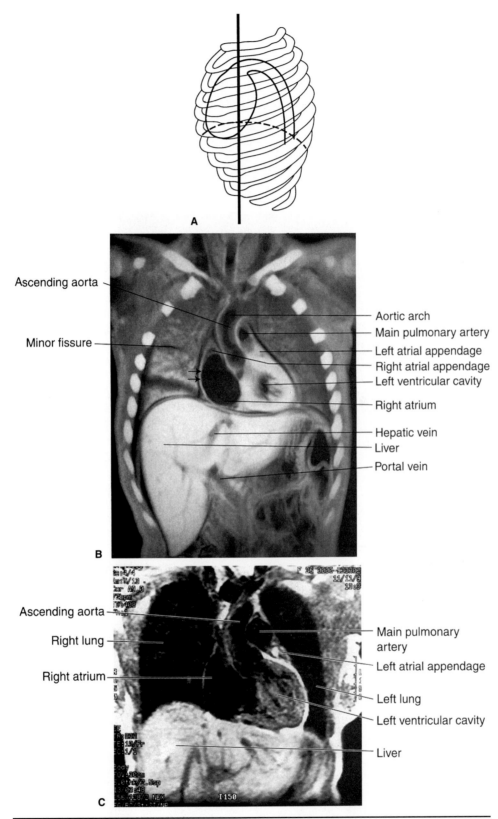

FIGURE 2-24. A: Illustration of the approximate coronal anatomic level through the left ventricle and the ascending aorta for B and C. **B:** Coronal cadaver radiograph of the sectioned chest through the left ventricle and the ascending aorta. Normal. Note that the convex right cardiac border is due to the right atrium *(straight arrows)*. **C:** Chest coronal MR image through the left ventricle and the ascending aorta. Normal.

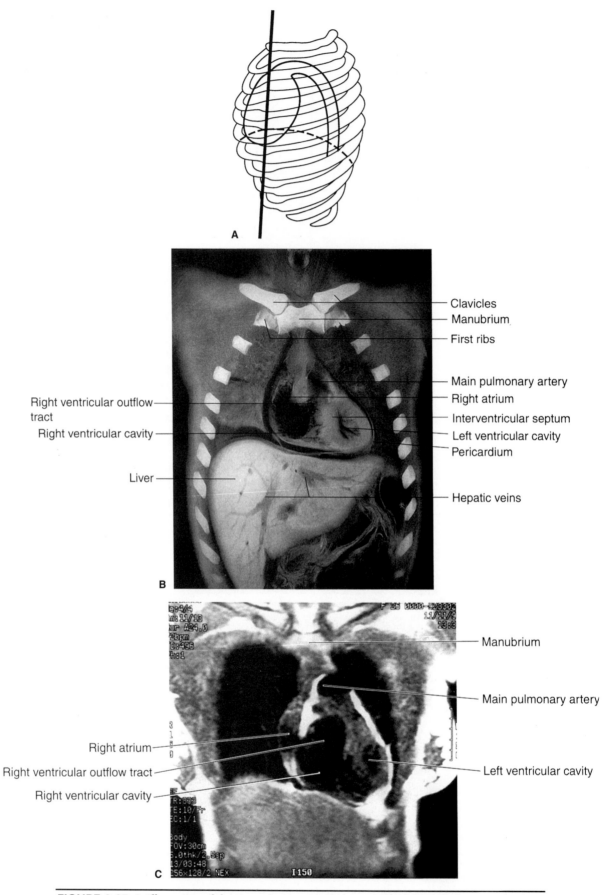

FIGURE 2-25. A: Illustration of the approximate coronal anatomic level through the ventricles for B and C. **B:** Coronal cadaver radiograph of the sectioned chest through the ventricles. Normal. **C:** Chest coronal MR image through the ventricles. Normal.

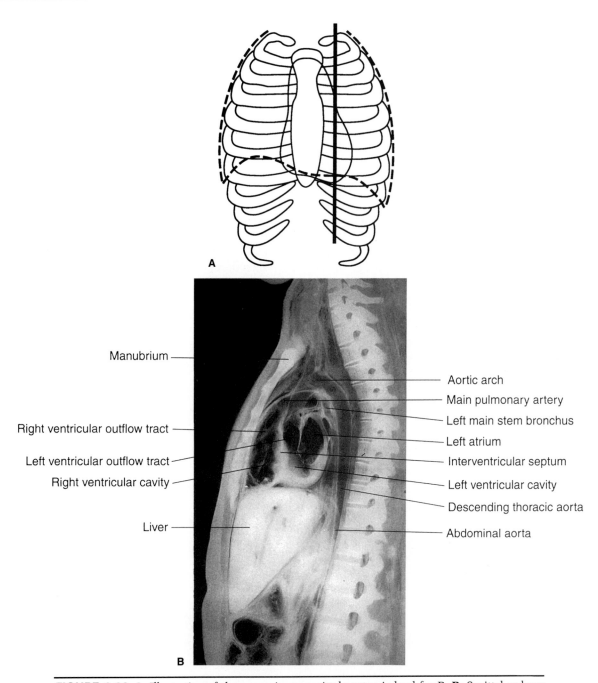

FIGURE 2-26. **A:** Illustration of the approximate sagittal anatomic level for B. **B:** Sagittal cadaver radiograph of the sectioned chest through the right ventricular outflow tract and the right ventricle. Normal.

CHEST ANGIOGRAPHY

Nearly all of the thoracic arteries and veins can be imaged via angiography. Examples of common thoracic angiographic images are shown in Fig. 2-27.

ANOMALIES

Numerous congenital anomalies involve the sternum, clavicles, bronchi, lungs, heart and great vessels, and diaphragms. There are many more, but only a few are demonstrated. The majority of thoracic congenital abnormalities are detected in infancy or early childhood.

Pectus excavatum, or funnel chest (Fig. 2-28), is a common and usually asymptomatic abnormality of the chest wall that may be associated with other congenital abnormalities such as Marfan's syndrome, scoliosis,

and Poland's syndrome (1). Therapy is usually not indicated. Pectus carinatum, or pigeon breast (Fig. 2-29), can be either a congenital or an acquired abnormality wherein the sternum projects more anterior than normal. The patients are usually asymptomatic, and therapy is usually not indicated (1). The acquired form may occur in patients with untreated congenital heart disease.

Another osseous abnormality is the congenital absence of the clavicles (Fig. 2-30). This abnormality is uncommon but very dramatic. It may be associated with cleidocranial dysostosis, which is a disease manifested by delayed or incomplete calvarial ossification, hypoplasia or aplasia of the clavicles, and many other associated osseous abnormalities (2).

When the azygos vein fails to migrate to its normal position just above the right main stem bronchus, the azygos fissure subtends a variable amount of the right upper lobe

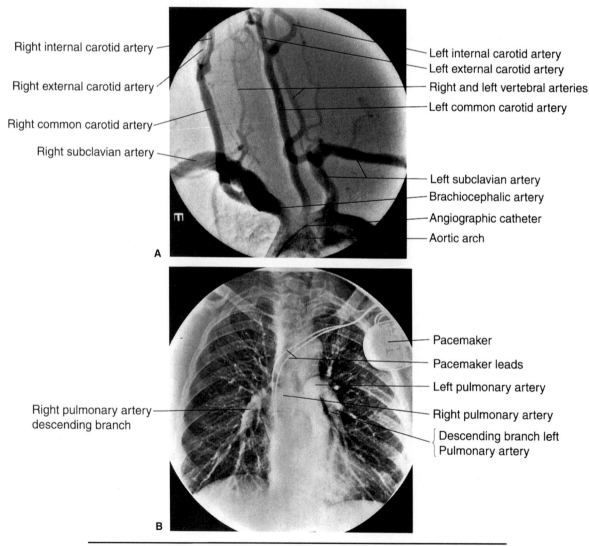

FIGURE 2-27. **A:** Aortic arch angiogram. Normal. **B:** Pulmonary arteriogram. Normal.

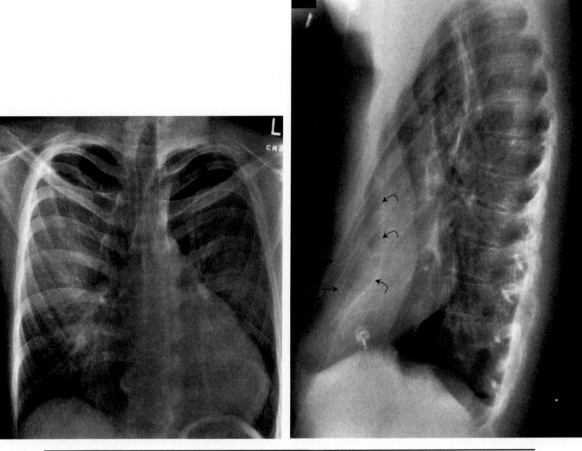

FIGURE 2-28. Chest PA **(A)** and lateral **(B)** radiographs. Pectus excavatum. Note that on the PA view the cardiac silhouette is rotated and displaced to the patient's left, and the left cardiac border is straight simulating mitral valve disease. There is mild deformity of the ribs bilaterally on the PA view. The extent of the defect is best appreciated on the lateral view where the anterior ribs *(straight arrows)* project anterior to the sternum *(curved arrows)*.

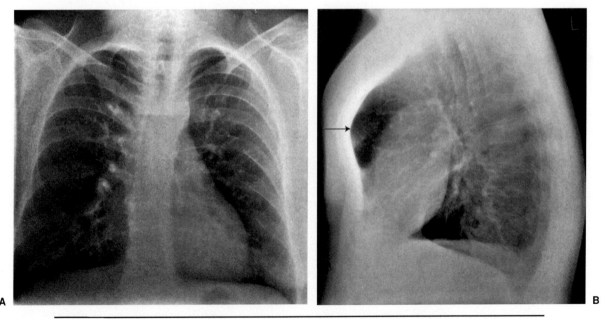

FIGURE 2-29. Chest PA **(A)** and lateral **(B)** radiographs. Pectus carinatum. The PA view is essentially normal with mild dorsal spine scoliosis. The exaggerated anterior projection of the sternum *(straight arrow)* is best appreciated on the lateral view.

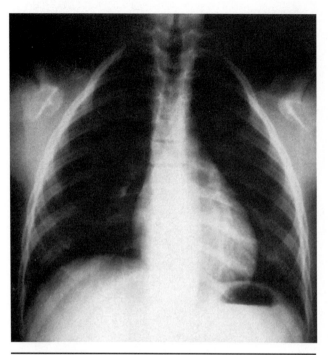

FIGURE 2-30. Chest AP radiograph. Cleidocranial dysostosis with bilateral absence of the clavicles. This was a routine chest radiograph in an asymptomatic 20-year-old woman.

to form the azygos lobe (Figs. 2-31 and 2-37B). The azygos fissure is best visualized on the PA radiograph as a thin curvilinear arc made up of two layers of visceral and two layers of parietal pleura. The azygos lobe is not particularly susceptible to disease.

The most common aortic arch anomaly is a right aortic arch with a left descending thoracic aorta wherein the aortic arch crosses the midline posterior to the esophagus to reach the left side (Fig. 2-32). There are five types of right aortic arch, and the classification is based on the arrangement of the arch vessels (3). Right-sided arches are also found in tetralogy of Fallot and other congenital heart problems. On the PA radiograph, the right-sided arch often appears more cephalad than a normal left-sided arch.

Another vascular anomaly is coarctation or stenosis of the proximal descending aorta. The degree of coarctation is variable, and the signs, symptoms, and physical findings vary with the location and degree of stenosis. Blood pressures in the upper body may be normal or above normal, whereas in the lower body they may be below normal. Even the upper extremities blood pressures may be unequal depending on the location of the stenosis relative to the left subclavian artery. Also, the presence of murmurs, cardiac enlargement, and aortic pre- and poststenotic dilatation depends on the location and severity of the stenosis. Often the site of stenosis can be identified on routine chest radiographs (see Fig. 2-33). Rib notching can occur along the inferior aspect of the ribs secondary to increased collateral flow through the intercostal arteries bypassing the aortic stenosis.

CONFUSING EXTRATHORACIC CONDITIONS

On occasion there are objects outside the thorax that can be confused with intrathoracic pathology (Figs. 2-34 to 2-36). It is important to keep such possibilities in mind at all times.

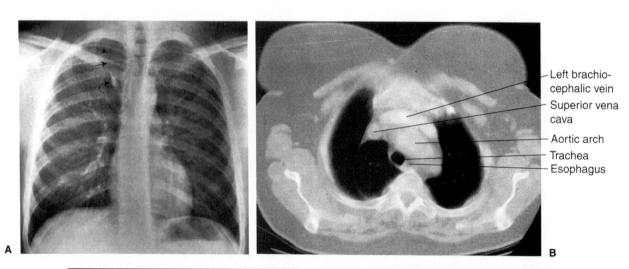

Left brachio-
cephalic vein
Superior vena
cava
Aortic arch
Trachea
Esophagus

FIGURE 2-31. A: Chest PA radiograph. Azygos lobe. The azygos lobe is outlined with *straight arrows.* The *curved arrow* indicates the azygos vein that is located more cephalad and lateral to its normal position near the right main stem bronchus. **B:** Chest axial CT image in a different patient. Azygos lobe. The image is through the level of the aortic arch and nicely demonstrates the azygos lobe fissure *(straight arrows)* and the azygos lobe *(curved arrow).*

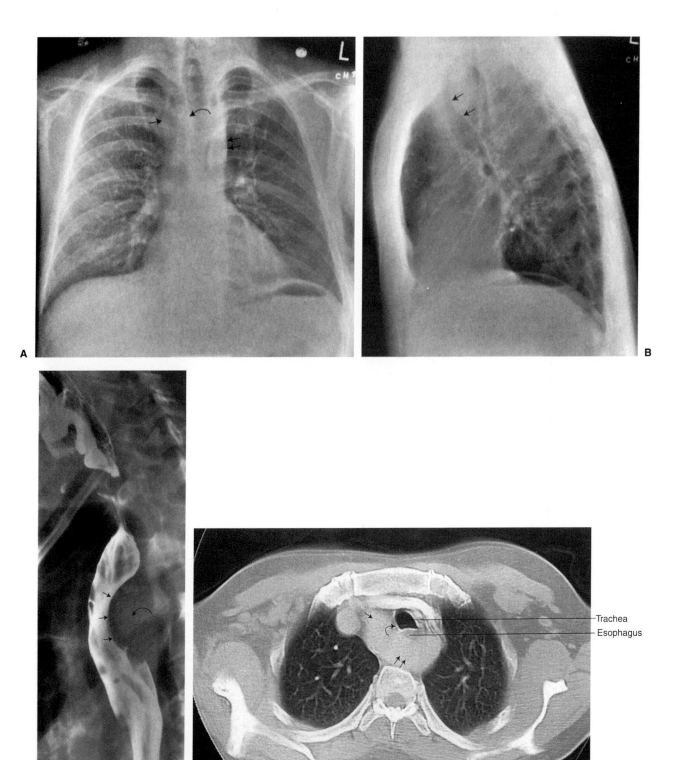

Trachea
Esophagus

FIGURE 2-32. Chest PA **(A)** and lateral **(B)** radiographs, barium swallow **(C)**, and chest CT **(D)**. Right-sided aortic arch and left descending thoracic aorta. This 42-year-old male smoker was suspected of having cancer of the lung. A neoplastic mass was suspected on the PA radiograph (A) but this proved to be an ill-defined aortic knob to the right of the midline *(straight arrow)*. The right aortic arch is indenting the right side of the trachea *(curved arrow)*. The *double straight arrows* are on the descending thoracic aorta that descends on the left side. The right-sided aortic arch indents the posterior aspect of the trachea *(straight arrows)* on the lateral radiograph (B). Barium swallow (C) confirms a significant indentation on the posterior aspect of the barium-filled esophagus *(straight arrows)* secondary to the crossing aortic arch *(curved arrow)*. The diagnosis is confirmed on chest CT (D) that shows the right-sided aorta *(single straight arrow)* passing posterior to the esophagus and trachea *(double straight arrows)* to reach the left side of the thorax. Again, note the indentation on the right side of the trachea *(curved arrow)* secondary to the right-sided aortic arch.

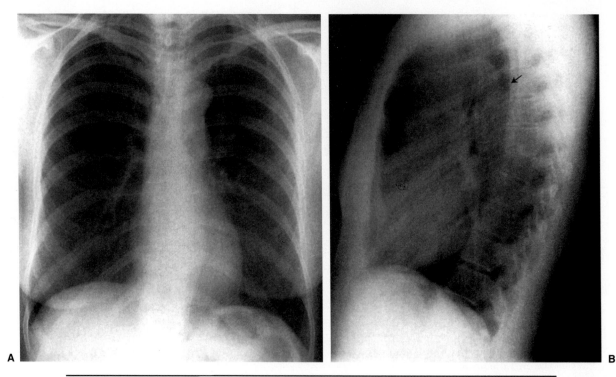

A

B

FIGURE 2-33. Chest PA **(A)** and lateral **(B)** radiographs. Coarctation of the aorta. The classical PA radiographic appearance is an indentation *(arrow)* involving the lateral aspect of the proximal descending aorta (A) and a posterior indentation *(arrow)* involving the posterior aspect of the proximal descending aorta on the lateral radiograph (B). These indentations represent the site of stenosis or coarctation in the proximal descending aorta. There is no evidence of rib notching, and the cardiac size is normal.

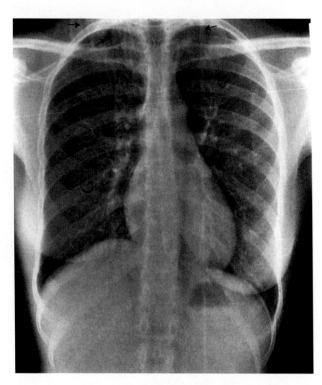

FIGURE 2-34. PA chest radiograph. Hair artifacts *(straight arrows)* projecting over the upper lobes. Hair, hair braids, ponytails, and ribbons can project over the upper lobes and should not be confused with a pathologic process.

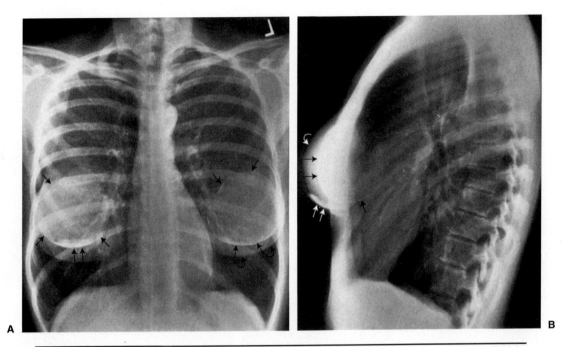

FIGURE 2-35. Chest PA **(A)** and lateral **(B)** radiographs. Bilateral breast augmentations or implants. The breast implants *(straight arrows)* are partially opaque, and the native breasts are indicated by the *curved arrows*. Note the benign postoperative calcification on both the PA and lateral views *(double straight arrows)* in the inferior aspect of the right breast. The hyperinflated lungs are probably within limits.

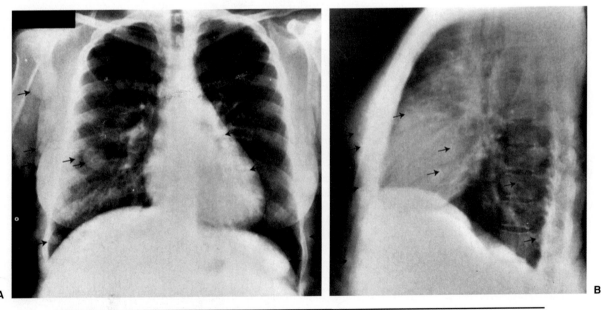

FIGURE 2-36. Chest PA **(A)** and lateral **(B)** radiographs. Multiple soft tissue nodules projecting over the thorax. Multiple subcutaneous soft tissue nodules *(arrows)* project over the thorax and must not be mistaken for pulmonary nodules.

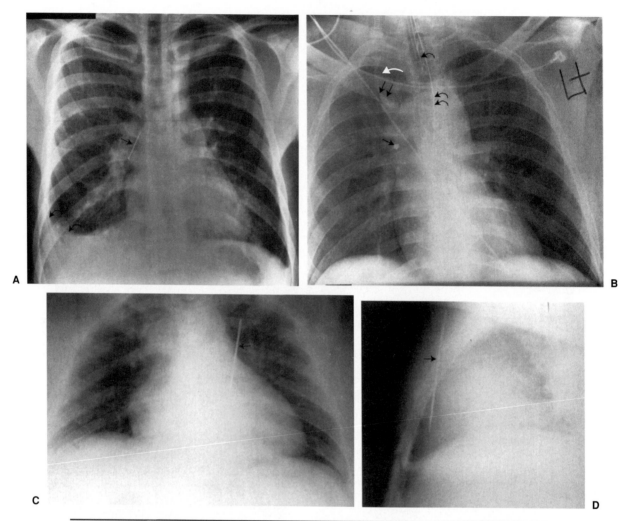

FIGURE 2-37. A: Chest PA radiograph. Straight pin *(straight arrow)* in the right intermediate bronchus. This 26-year-old mentally impaired male had a tendency to swallow everything in sight. He suddenly sneezed and apparently aspirated the pin into the bronchial tree. The pin was removed at bronchoscopy. Note the right pleural effusion *(curved arrows)*. It has been estimated that there must be at least 125 cc of pleural fluid before it is recognized on PA and AP views. **B:** Chest portable AP radiograph. Tooth fragment *(straight arrow)* in the right bronchial tree. The patient was involved in a motor vehicle accident, and a portion of a tooth was missing. The chest radiograph shows the tooth fragment projecting over the right upper bronchial tree. The tooth fragment was removed at bronchoscopy. Note that the endotracheal tube *(single curved arrow)* lies to the patient's right of the nasogastric tube *(double curved arrows)*. An azygos lobe is present, and the *double straight arrows* indicate the position of the azygos vein that is more lateral and cephalad than normal. The azygos fissure *(curved white arrow)* is visible. **C, D:** Chest AP (C) and lateral (D) radiographs. Darning needle lodged in the right ventricle. The child of this young mother accidentally stabbed her with a darning needle. Note that the needle *(straight arrows)* projects over the right ventricle region in both views. The needle was successfully removed at thoracotomy, and recovery was uneventful.

FOREIGN BODIES, LINES, AND TUBES

Another pitfall on chest radiographs that must be kept in mind is the presence of intrathoracic foreign bodies (see Fig. 2-37). Some foreign bodies such as lines and tubes are intentionally placed within the thorax. It is very important to recognize the typical appearances of these commonly used lines and tubes, especially when caring for patients in acute care areas. The normal and some ab-

normal locations of these lines and tubes are demonstrated in Fig. 2-38.

POSTOPERATIVE CHEST PROBLEMS

It is important to recognize some common radiographic findings that may be present on postoperative chest images (Fig. 2-39).

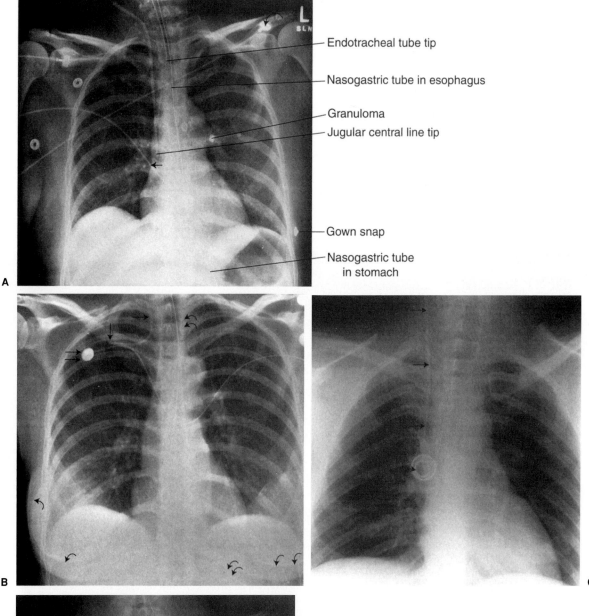

— Endotracheal tube tip

— Nasogastric tube in esophagus

— Granuloma
— Jugular central line tip

— Gown snap

— Nasogastric tube
  in stomach

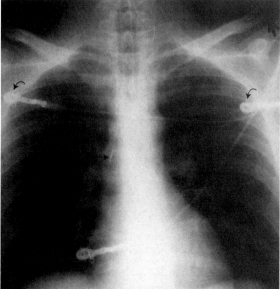

FIGURE 2-38. A: Chest AP radiograph. Normal tube and line positions. The tip of the central line via a right jugular vein approach projects over the superior vena cava. Note that the central line tip lies cephalad to the junction *(straight arrow)* of the straight bordered superior vena cava and the convex right atrium. The *curved arrow* points to a monitoring electrode that lies on the skin on the patient's left shoulder. **B:** Chest AP radiograph. Right jugular central line inadvertently passed into the right subclavian vein *(single straight arrow)*. Bilateral breast augmentations or implants are present *(single curved arrows)*. A monitoring electrode *(double straight arrows)* and a nasogastric tube *(double curved arrows)* are also present. **C:** Chest AP radiograph. A right jugular Hickman line passing cephalad. The Hickman line *(straight arrows)* with an infusaport *(curved arrow)* is directed cephalad in the jugular vein rather than caudad toward the superior vena cava. The tip of the line is beyond the edge of the radiograph. **D:** Chest AP radiograph. Endotracheal tube *(arrow)* inadvertently placed in right intermediate bronchus. External monitoring electrodes are present *(curved arrows)*.

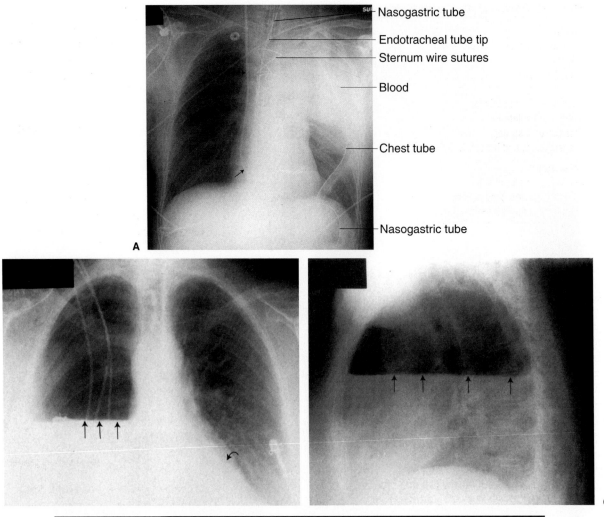

Nasogastric tube

Endotracheal tube tip

Sternum wire sutures

Blood

Chest tube

Nasogastric tube

FIGURE 2-39. A: Chest AP supine radiograph. Left thorax postoperative hemorrhage. The white homogeneous density in the region of the left upper lobe represents active bleeding in the thorax 2 hours following coronary artery bypass grafting. The patient was reoperated to evacuate the blood and control the bleeding. Infection, atelectasis, and tumor could give a similar appearance, but the history made the diagnosis obvious. The *straight arrows* indicate a right jugular Swan-Ganz catheter. **B, C:** Chest AP (B) and lateral (C) radiographs. Right pneumonectomy. The *straight arrows* indicate the presence of an air–fluid level that is a common finding following pneumonectomy. Gradually over a period of days the vacant right thorax will fill with fluid that will eventually fibrose. Left lower lobe atelectasis is manifested by the retrocardiac double density *(curved arrow)*. Left lower lobe atelectasis is common following thoracic surgery. There is obliteration of the right hemidiaphragm (silhouette sign) by the right pleural fluid.

TABLE 2-1 Partial List of Pneumothorax Etiologies

Traumatic
1. Accidents, e.g., motor vehicle
2. Iatrogenic
   a. Thoracoscopy
   b. Thoracentesis
   c. Placement of central line
   d. Artificial ventilation
   e. Postthoracic surgery
   f. Transthoracic and bronchoscopic biopsy

Spontaneous
1. Rupture of a bleb or bullae
2. Secondary to underlying pulmonary disease
3. Secondary to pneumomediastinum

Air in the Wrong Places

An important chest problem encountered in medicine is pneumothorax (air in the pleural space). Pneumothorax can be secondary to trauma or disease, or it may be spontaneous. Some of the etiologies are listed in Table 2-1. Spontaneous pneumothorax most commonly occurs in young male adults but does involve female patients as well. These patients typically present with a sudden onset of unilateral chest pain that can be accompanied by varying degrees of breathing difficulties. The radiographic diagnosis of pneumothorax is made by identifying the *visceral pleura line* (Fig. 2-40A), and varying degrees of pneumothorax are demonstrated in Fig. 2-40. A *tension pneumothorax* occurs when the pressure within the pneumothorax becomes elevated enough to cause cardiac and respiratory problems (see Fig. 2-40C). Tension pneumothorax requires immediate therapy in the form of a chest tube or syringe aspiration of the air.

Pneumomediastinum (Fig. 2-41) has a number of etiologies as shown in Table 2-2. It may be accompanied by thoracic and/or cervical subcutaneous emphysema.

When a patient has experienced chest trauma, lacerations of the lungs are generally unsuspected and con-

TABLE 2-2 Some Etiologies of Pneumomediastinum

Traumatic
1. Closed chest trauma
2. Secondary to chest and neck surgery
3. Esophageal perforation
4. Tracheobronchial perforation
5. Vigorous exercise
6. Asthma
7. Ventilator

Spontaneous
1. Bleb or bullae
2. No apparent etiology

sequently go undetected. Routine chest radiographs are usually negative or may show water density contusions. Nevertheless, lacerations of the lung should always be suspected when there has been chest trauma. Often pulmonary lacerations are incidental findings when chest CT imaging is performed for some other reason (Fig. 2-42).

Other Air Accumulations in and Around the Chest

Abnormal air accumulations may occur within the thorax secondary to esophageal hiatal hernias (Fig. 2-43). They represent a portion of the stomach herniated through or around the esophageal hiatus, and their size is variable. They may be asymptomatic or associated with mild to severe chest pain.

Abscesses can occur within the soft tissues surrounding the thorax, and they should be recognized as such (Fig. 2-44). Usually there is an air–fluid level that projects outside of the thorax on at least one of the views. If the air–fluid level projects over the lungs in both the PA and lateral view, then the abscess must by definition lie within the lungs (Fig. 2-55).

Pneumoperitoneum is a significant abnormal air accumulation in the abdomen that often can be identified on chest radiographs (Fig. 2-45). As little as a few cubic centimeters of air may be detected on up-right radiographs of the lower chest and upper abdomen.

Too Much Air in the Lungs

Chronic obstructive pulmonary disease (COPD; Fig. 2-46A, B) is a significant health problem. It is the fifth most common cause of death (1) and has become an important reason for work incapacity. The terminology surrounding lung disease is confusing and includes chronic bronchitis, emphysema, and COPD. COPD is airway obstruction without a specific known pathophysiology. Table 2-3 lists some of the COPD etiologies. Emphysema is enlargement of the airspaces distal to the terminal bronchioles without fibrosis (1).

On the other hand, idiopathic pulmonary fibrosis (Fig. 2-46C, D) is a disease characterized by normal inflation or hypoinflation (less than normal ventilation) with associated pulmonary fibrosis that is usually peripheral. It is fortunate the disease is not common because its etiology is unknown.

TABLE 2-3 Partial List of COPD Etiologies

1. Cigarette smoking
2. Air pollution
3. Childhood infections
4. Heredity

FIGURE 2-40. A: Chest PA radiograph. Mild to moderate right pneumothorax. A thoracentesis was performed to remove right pleural fluid *(straight arrow)*, but it resulted in a right pneumothorax. The visceral pleura is outlined by the *curved arrows*. There is air in the pleural space *(double straight arrows)* lying between the visceral pleura and the parietal pleura or chest wall. The result is a partially collapsed or atelectatic right lung. Note that the trachea (∗) is midline. **B:** Chest AP radiograph. Moderate right pneumothorax. While on the ventilator, this patient developed right chest pain and shortness of breath. There is a moderate-sized right pneumothorax. The right lateral costophrenic sulcus or angle is very deep and lucent compared to the left, and this is called the *deep sulcus sign*. A deep sulcus sign should always make you suspicious for pneumothorax. Note that the double density behind the cardiac silhouette *(straight arrows)* and the associated obliteration of the left hemidiaphragm medially *(curved arrow)* represent the atelectatic left lower lobe. **C:** Chest AP radiograph. Right tension pneumothorax. This patient was on the ventilator and developed right chest pain and hypotension. There is a large right pneumothorax with complete atelectasis of the right lung, and the *straight arrows* indicate the visceral pleural line. Note the right deep sulcus sign *(curved arrow)*. The heart is displaced to the left compatible with a tension pneumothorax.

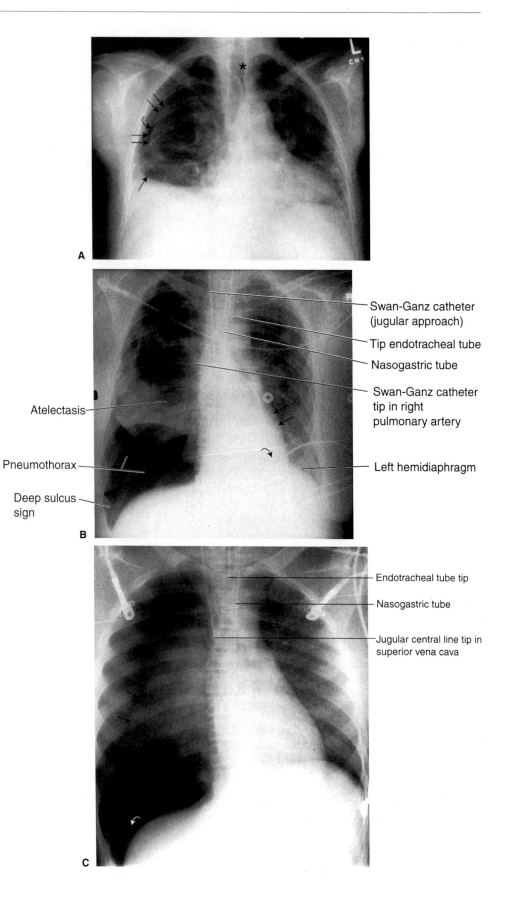

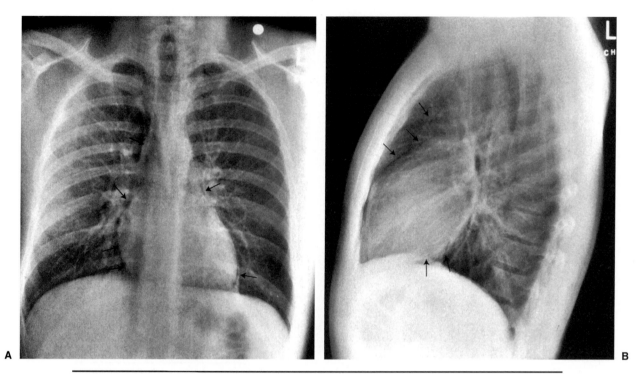

A   B

FIGURE 2-41. Chest PA **(A)** and lateral **(B)** radiographs. Pneumomediastinum. This patient had routine chest radiographs for vague chest pain, and surprisingly, the radiographs revealed mediastinal air *(straight arrows)*. The etiology was never found, and the air resolved spontaneously.

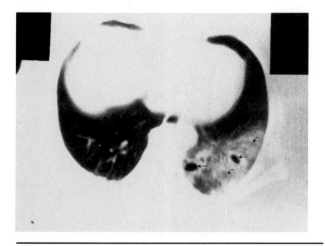

FIGURE 2-42. Chest axial CT through the lung bases. Lung parenchymal lacerations *(straight arrows)* in the left lower lobe. The lacerations are surrounded by water density contused lung parenchyma *(curved arrows)*.

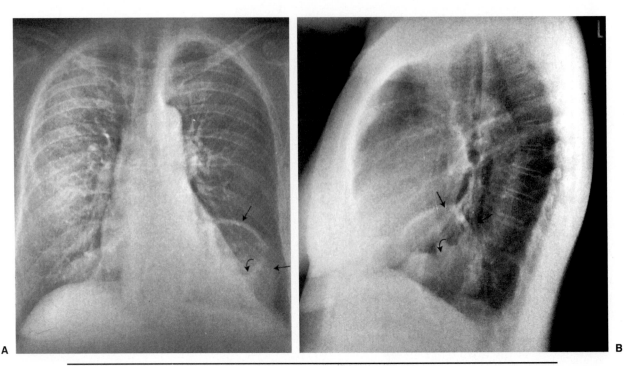

FIGURE 2-43. Chest PA **(A)** and lateral **(B)** radiographs. Esophageal hiatal hernia. The *straight arrows* indicate the large esophageal hiatal hernia that contains air–fluid levels *(curved arrows)*. The chest is otherwise normal.

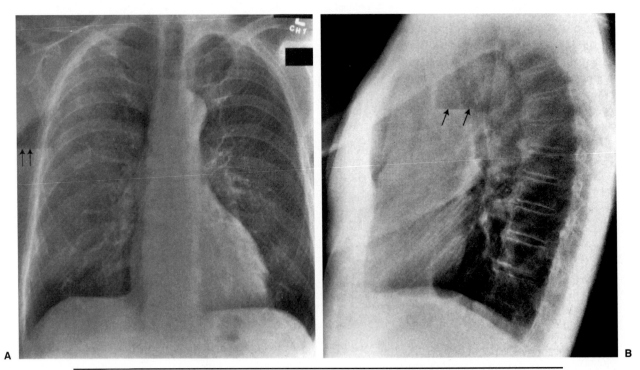

FIGURE 2-44. Chest PA **(A)** and lateral **(B)** radiographs. Right axillary abscess. This patient was postoperative following a right axillary node dissection. A right axillary air–fluid level *(straight arrows)* is well visualized on both the PA and lateral views. The abscess was subsequently drained.

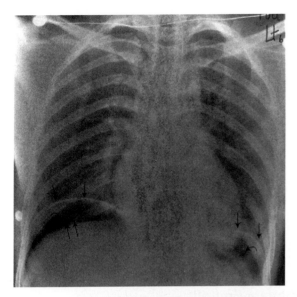

FIGURE 2-45. Chest AP radiograph. Pneumoperitoneum. The patient experienced sudden onset of severe abdominal pain, and physical examination revealed a boardlike rigidity of the abdomen. The patient proved to have a perforated duodenal ulcer at surgery. The *straight arrows* indicate the diaphragms bilaterally and the *curved arrows* delineate free subdiaphragmatic air secondary to the perforated ulcer. The dome of the liver is indicated by the *double straight arrows*, and the chest is otherwise normal.

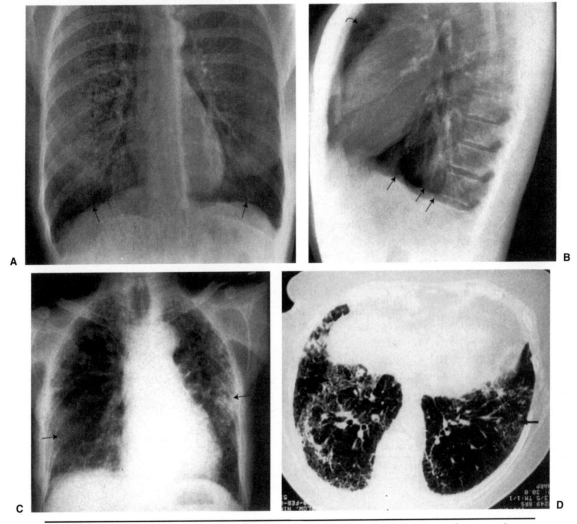

FIGURE 2-46. Chest PA **(A)** and lateral **(B)** radiographs. Chronic obstructive pulmonary disease (COPD). The lungs are hyperlucent and markedly overexpanded. The diaphragms are flat on the lateral view and nearly flat on the PA radiographs *(straight arrows)*. The retrosternal air space is overexpanded *(curved arrow)*, and the AP dimension of the chest is greater than normal. **C, D:** Chest PA radiograph (C) and axial prone chest CT (D). Idiopathic pulmonary fibrosis. This 79-year-old man had a long history of shortness of breath. On the PA chest radiograph (C), there are typical peripheral white linear streaks *(straight arrows)* that represent fibrosis. The lungs are normally inflated. On CT (D), the fibrosis is mainly peripheral *(straight arrow)* and there is an overall honeycomb appearance to the lung parenchyma.

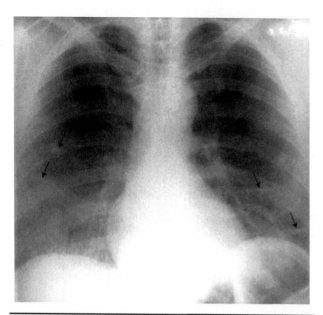

FIGURE 2-47. Chest PA radiograph. Bilateral discoid (platelike) atelectasis. The *straight arrows* indicate the typical appearance of this abnormality that is commonly found in postoperative, posttrauma, severely ill, and debilitated patients.

ATELECTASIS, PULMONARY EMBOLI, AND INFECTIONS

It is important to remember that most pathologic conditions such as pneumonia, tumor, infarct, and atelectasis will appear as water densities or shades of gray on radiographs. So think water density or gray when viewing radiographs and concentrate less on the black. After all, black densities in the lungs represent air.

Atelectasis

Atelectasis (Figs. 2-47 and 2-48) is the incomplete expansion or loss of volume of a portion of the lung that ranges from complete collapse of a lung to discoid or platelike atelectasis. Atelectasis is not a primary disease but a sign of disease or abnormality (3). The general etiologies are listed in Table 2-4 and the radiographic signs are listed in Table 2-5.

Discoid atelectasis (Fig. 2-47) is probably the most common linear opacity found on chest radiographs. It is generally believed that discoid atelectasis results from several factors including decreased diaphragmatic movement, cough-inhibiting factors, and the pooling of secretions. Radiographically discoid atelectasis appears as a horizontal linear density measuring a few millimeters in width and variable in length.

TABLE 2-4   General Etiologies of Atelectasis

1. Bronchial obstruction
   a. Tumor
   b. Foreign body
   c. Infection
2. Postoperative
3. Extrinsic pressure
   a. Pleural fluid
   b. Pneumothorax
4. Restrictive motion
   a. Trauma
   b. Neuromuscular diseases
   c. Infections

Pulmonary Emboli

Pulmonary emboli have a number of etiologies as shown in Table 2-6. For example, central lines can become infected and septic pulmonary emboli may result (Fig. 2-49A, B).

Pulmonary thromboembolus is an exceedingly common and important clinical problem that often occurs in hospitalized and inactive patients. The thrombus usually originates in the lower extremity and/or pelvic veins. Pulmonary thromboembolus is the presence of a thrombus or fragment of a thrombus in the pulmonary arterial tree, and the thromboembolus can result in infarction, atelectasis, hemorrhage, or increased pulmonary arterial pressure. The radiographic signs in these patients are highly variable and range from normal to grossly abnormal. Eventually some radiographic abnormality is usually present. A CT study (Fig. 2-49C) may make the diagnosis and eliminate the need for an invasive pulmonary angiogram. However, in some instances a pulmonary angiogram is necessary when radionuclide studies and CT imaging are indeterminate (Fig. 2-49D).

Pulmonary Infections

Pulmonary infections have many etiologies, some of which are listed in Table 2-7. These patients often present with

TABLE 2-5   Radiographic Signs of Atelectasis

Primary
1. Loss of volume of involved segment, lobe, or lung
2. White-appearing airless lung
3. Air bronchograms
4. Displaced bronchi and vessels

Secondary
1. Elevation of the hemidiaphragm
2. Mediastinal shift
3. Rib narrowing
4. Indistinct hilum and hilar displacement

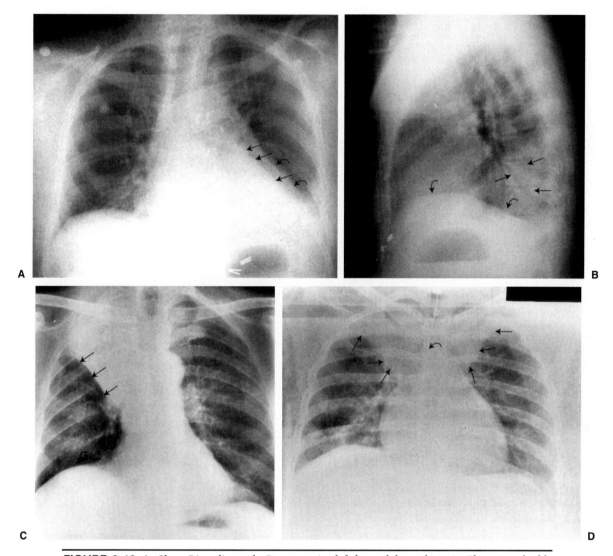

FIGURE 2-48. **A:** Chest PA radiograph. Postoperative left lower lobe atelectasis. There is a double density in the cardiac silhouette, and the *straight arrows* indicate the edge of the atelectatic left lower lobe whereas the *curved arrows* indicate the left cardiac border. The left hemidiaphragm is poorly visualized because the water density atelectatic left lower lobe is in juxtaposition to the left hemidiaphragm or a silhouette sign. **B:** Chest lateral radiograph. Same patient as in A. There is a positive spine sign *(straight arrows)*. Remember that on the lateral view, the spine should appear darker as you proceed caudad because there is more lung in the lower thorax. When a water density disease process like atelectasis or pneumonia is present in the lower lobes, the spine will appear whiter as you proceed caudad rather than darker (spine sign). The left hemidiaphragm cannot be seen as it is silhouetted by the atelectasis in the left lower lobe, but the entire right hemidiaphragm can be seen *(curved arrow)*. **C:** Chest AP radiograph. Right upper lobe atelectasis. There is a water density appearance to the atelectatic right upper lobe, the minor fissure is elevated *(straight arrows)*, the right pulmonary artery and the ascending aorta are silhouetted by the water density atelectasis, and the right hemidiaphragm *(curved arrow)* is elevated. **D:** Chest AP radiograph. Bilateral upper lobe atelectasis *(straight arrows)*. This 30-year-old woman developed bronchospasm in the operating room. Both upper lobes are airless and collapsed, and the mediastinum is silhouetted. The *curved arrow* indicates the tip of an endotracheal tube.

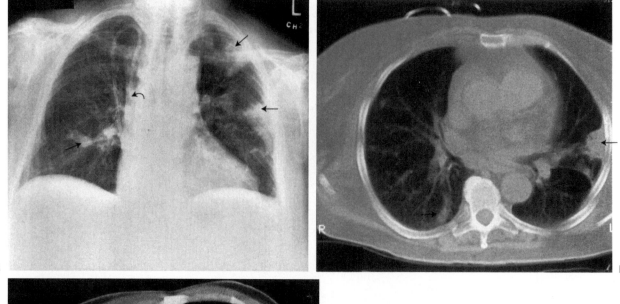

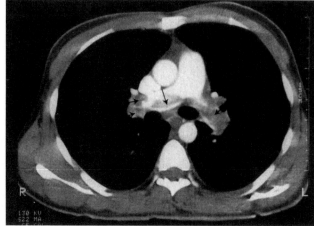

FIGURE 2-49. **A:** Chest PA radiograph. Bilateral septic emboli secondary to an infected Hickman catheter. The chest radiograph is grossly abnormal with multiple bilateral water densities *(straight arrows)* secondary to septic emboli, and the differential diagnosis would include pneumonia, emboli, atelectasis, and hemorrhage. The tip of the Hickman catheter *(curved arrow)* is in the superior vena cava. **B:** Chest axial CT through the level of the left atrium in the same patient as A. Bilateral pulmonary septic emboli from the infected Hickman catheter. The emboli *(straight arrows)* are commonly peripheral, wedge-shaped, homogeneous density, and pleural based. **C:** Chest axial CT through the pulmonary arteries in a different patient than A and B. Bilateral pulmonary artery thromboemboli secondary to lower extremity deep vein phlebothrombosis. This 30-year-old man developed bilateral lower extremity edema and shortness of breath following a long automobile trip. There are filling defects *(straight arrows)* in the right and left pulmonary arteries created by the thromboemboli. These findings necessitated pulmonary embolectomy, anticoagulation, and the placement of a Greenfield filter in his inferior vena cava. As a result of his pulmonary emboli, he had pulmonary hypertension. **D:** Left pulmonary arteriogram. Multiple left pulmonary artery embolic thrombi *(straight arrows)* within the left main pulmonary artery and its branches secondary to bilateral lower extremity deep vein phlebothrombosis. This 72-year-old woman was 72 hours postcoronary artery bypass grafting and developed shortness of breath and hypoxia. Radionuclide studies showed probable thromboemboli. The angiographic catheter *(curved arrows)* is visible in the left pulmonary artery.

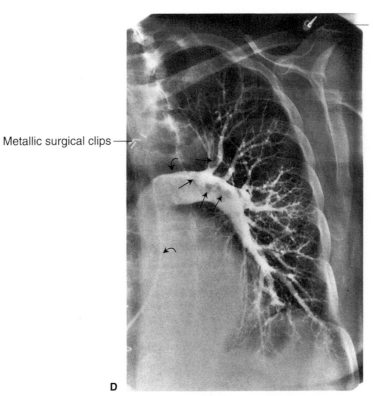

External monitoring electrode

Metallic surgical clips

D

FIGURE 2-49. (*Continued*)

fever and cough, and the cough may or may not be productive. If the cough is productive, the sputum may be colored and may even contain blood. Pleuritic and general chest pain may be present. If a pneumonia is mild, the patient may walk into your office, whereas other pneumonias can be severe enough to cause death. The radiographic appearances of pneumonia are highly variable, and often it is impossible to determine the etiology of a pneumonia based on the radiologic appearance alone. The radiographic findings vary from a small, ill-defined infiltrate to complete unilateral or bilateral opacification of the lungs (Figs. 2-50 to 2-54). Some pneumonias progress resulting in complications such as empyema, pleural fluid, and abscess formation (Fig. 2-55). Pneumonias can be easily confused with blood, fluid, atelectasis, and even tumor, as they are all water density.

Many patients are immune-suppressed secondary to disease or therapy, and they are susceptible to pulmonary tuberculosis (Fig. 2-56). Consequently, pulmonary tuberculosis continues to be a problem disease in spite of new therapies and improved public health measures. Tuberculosis should be considered in many pulmonary parenchymal differential diagnoses (Table 2-8).

▶ **TABLE 2-6 Common Etiologies of Pulmonary Embolic Disease**

1. Venous thromboembolism
   a. Postsurgical
   b. Bed rest
   c. Trauma
   d. Neoplasm
2. Foreign body
   a. Bone marrow post–long bone fracture
   b. Amniotic fluid
3. Septic emboli
4. Air

▶ **TABLE 2-7 Some General Etiologies of Pneumonia**

1. Infections
   a. Bacterial
   b. Viral
   c. Fungal
   d. Parasitic
2. Aspiration
3. Radiation
4. Chemical

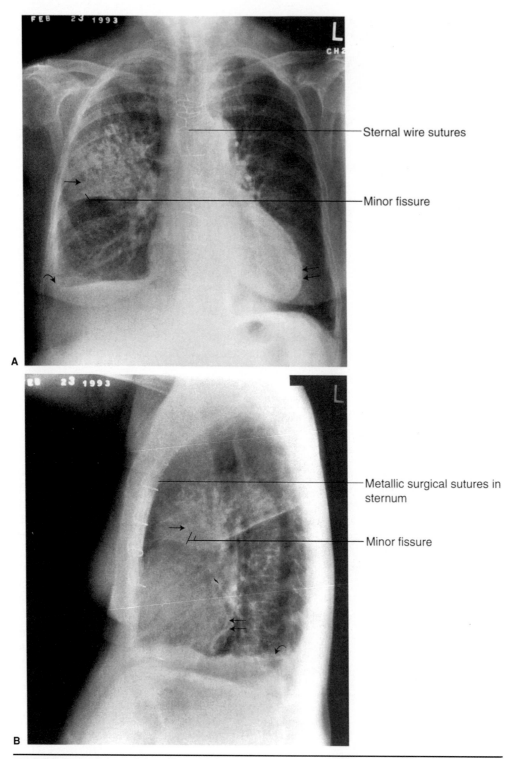

— Sternal wire sutures

— Minor fissure

— Metallic surgical sutures in sternum

— Minor fissure

A

B

FIGURE 2-50. Chest PA **(A)** and lateral **(B)** radiographs. Right upper lobe partially confluent pneumonia *(straight arrows)*. On the PA and lateral views, there is a small amount of right pleural fluid *(curved arrows)* and mild left ventricular enlargement *(double arrows)*. Note that the pneumonia is located in the upper lobe above the minor fissure.

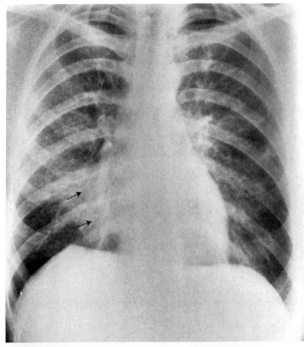

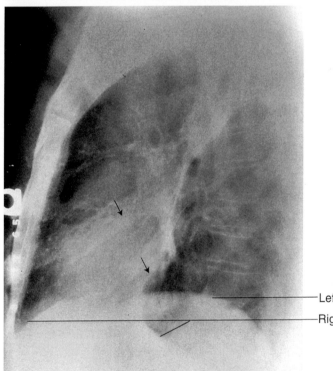

Left hemidiaphragm

Right hemidiaphragm

FIGURE 2-51. Chest PA **(A)** and lateral **(B)** radiographs. Right middle lobe pneumonia *(straight arrows)*. On the PA radiograph the right cardiac border is not visible (silhouette sign) as both the right middle lobe infiltrate and the right atrium are water density and anterior structures. Also, note that the right hemidiaphragm is clearly visible and not silhouetted on the PA view. On the lateral view, the pneumonia projects over the heart and partially silhouettes the right anterior hemidiaphragm.

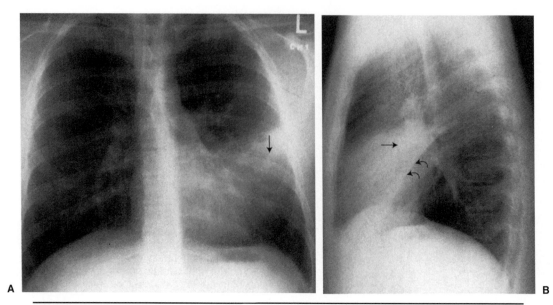

FIGURE 2-52. Chest PA **(A)** and lateral **(B)** radiographs. Left upper lobe lingular segments pneumonia *(straight arrows)*. On the PA radiograph the left cardiac border is not visible (silhouette sign) as both the left upper lobe lingular infiltrate and the heart are anterior water densities. Also, note that the left hemidiaphragm is clearly visible *(not silhouetted)* on the PA view. The *curved arrows* on the lateral view indicate the left major fissure, and note that the pneumonia projects over the heart.

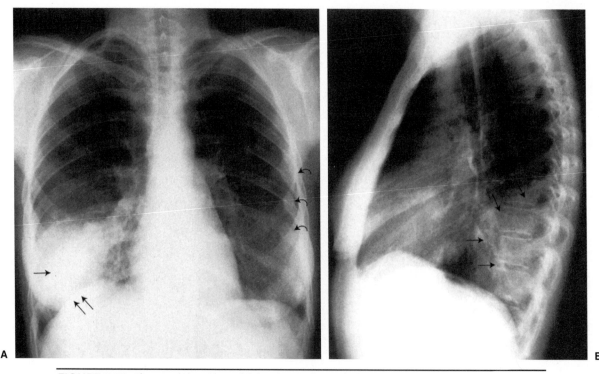

FIGURE 2-53. Chest PA **(A)** and lateral **(B)** radiographs. Right lower lobe pneumonia *(straight arrows)*. On the PA radiograph, the right cardiac border is clearly visible and the right hemidiaphragm is partially silhouetted *(double straight arrows)*. These findings indicate that the infiltrate is posterior or in the right lower lobe as confirmed on the lateral radiograph *(straight arrows)*. There is a positive spine sign on the lateral radiograph as the spine appears whiter as you proceed down the spine. Normally, the spine appears darker as you descend cephalad to caudad on the lateral view. Also, there are old healed left rib fracture deformities *(curved arrows)*.

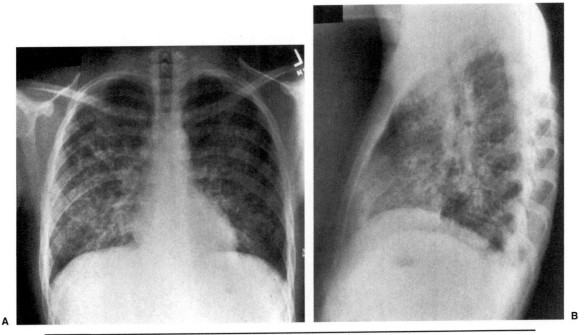

FIGURE 2-54. Chest PA **(A)** and lateral **(B)** radiographs. Bilateral varicella (chicken pox) pneumonia. There are diffuse nodular infiltrates throughout both lung fields. These patients are usually critically ill, and the skin lesions help to make the diagnosis.

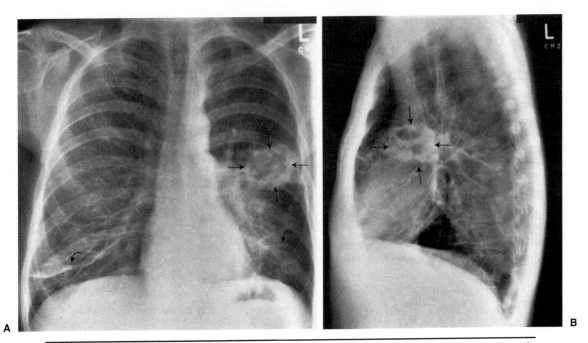

FIGURE 2-55. Chest PA **(A)** and lateral **(B)** radiographs. Left upper lobe lingular abscess *(straight arrows)*. There is air within the abscess cavity. Minimal infiltrates are present in the lower lung fields *(curved arrows)*.

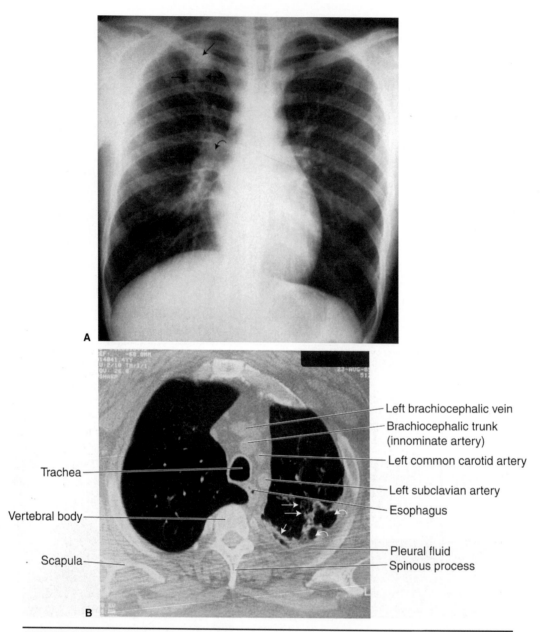

FIGURE 2-56. A: Chest PA radiograph. Right upper lobe tuberculosis. The tuberculous infiltrate in the right upper lobe *(straight arrows)* is partially obscured by the right clavicle. There is fullness in the right hilum compatible with hilar lymphadenopathy *(curved arrows)*. **B:** Chest axial CT through the upper thorax in a patient other than 56A. Cavitary tuberculosis of the left upper lobe with associated left pleural fluid. The cavitation *(curved arrows)* is surrounded by the tuberculous infiltrate *(straight arrows)*.

▶ **TABLE 2-8** Differential Diagnosis of Pulmonary Tuberculosis

1. All other pneumonias
2. Hemorrhage
3. Emboli
4. Tumor

Tuberculosis patients present with a variety of symptoms ranging from vague fatigue to fever, cough, weight loss, or hemoptysis. Also, the chest radiographic findings vary from a poorly defined infiltrate to obvious infiltrate with or without cavitation. *Remember that the diagnosis must be confirmed by laboratory findings.*

TUMORS

A wide variety of pulmonary nodules and/or tumor masses may be encountered on chest radiographs. These widely located lesions can be single or multiple, calcified or noncalcified, and poorly or well defined. One approach to their diagnosis is to divide them into benign and malignant categories (Table 2-9).

Multiple benign granulomas usually do not present much of a diagnostic problem. Solitary granulomas are easy to diagnose if they contain typical dense calcifications. These calcifications are variable in appearance including a diffusely homogeneous pattern, a centrally located nidus, multiple foci, or laminations. When such calcifications are present, a fairly confident diagnosis of benign granuloma can be made (Fig. 2-57). When the presence of calcification is not a certainty, CT imaging can be used to measure the density of the mass. When a pulmonary nodule measures

▶ **TABLE 2-9** A Partial List for the Differential Diagnosis of Pulmonary Masses

Benign
1. Granuloma (histoplasmoma, tuberculoma)
2. Adenoma
3. Hamartoma
4. Round pneumonia
5. Bronchogenic and pericardial cysts
6. Arteriovenous malformation
7. Pulmonary infarction
Malignant
1. Primary malignant tumors
a. Squamous cell carcinoma
b. Adenocarcinoma
c. Small cell carcinoma
d. Bronchoalveolar carcinoma
e. Carcinoid
2. Lymphoma
3. Metastatic neoplasm

greater than 200 Hounsfield units on a CT study, there is a very high probability that the lesion is a calcified benign granuloma or hamartoma and no further workup is necessary. A noncalcified mass does require further evaluation, and the workup varies with the clinical circumstances. A solitary noncalcified nodule that does not change in size or appearance in 2 years is probably benign. This rule should be applied with caution, as there are exceptions.

Approach to a Suspicious Pulmonary Nodule

In addition to noncalcification, a long history of cigarette smoking suggests the possibility of malignancy. Other factors that are suspicious for malignancy include poorly defined margins, rapid growth pattern, pleural fluid, atelectasis, and bone destruction. The workup of these suspicious masses ranges from obtaining old radiographs and follow-up radiographs to CT imaging, percutaneous biopsy, and actual thoracotomy (Fig. 2-58).

The location of a mass is sometimes useful in arriving at a diagnosis, especially if the mass is determined to be in the mediastinum. Classically, the mediastinum can be divided into three general areas, and the following is an easy and simplified method for remembering these mediastinal compartments. The anterior mediastinum lies between the sternum anteriorly and the anterior aspect of the pericardium and aorta. Tumor masses found in this area can be characterized by the letter *T*, and that represents a differential diagnosis of thyroid masses, teratoma, thymus masses, and tortuous or aneurysmal vessels (Fig. 2-59A, B). The middle mediastinum includes the heart, pericardium, the great vessels, and the proximal bronchi (Fig. 2-59C, D). The posterior mediastinum (Fig. 2-59E, F) extends from the posterior aspect of the pericardium to the dorsal spine vertebral bodies and includes the paravertebral gutters (1). A differential diagnosis can be made for a radiographic mass in each of these compartments (Table 2-10). Again, the silhouette sign will help to locate the mass depending on which structure borders are obscured by the mass. Notice that lymph nodes are found in all parts of the mediastinum, so that a lymphoma may occur in any thoracic location (Fig. 2-60).

Although some chest masses are difficult to detect, the visualization of most masses is fairly straightforward. A tumor mass can cause secondary signs that may be the first indication of a mass. Some secondary signs or complications suggesting the presence of tumor are atelectasis, malignant pleural effusions, cavitation of the tumor, hilar nodal enlargement, and local bone destruction (Figs. 2-61 to 2-63).

Detecting metastatic disease to the lungs is extremely important when caring for patients with primary neoplasms. Routine chest radiographs and CT imaging are used extensively to detect metastatic disease (Fig. 2-64).

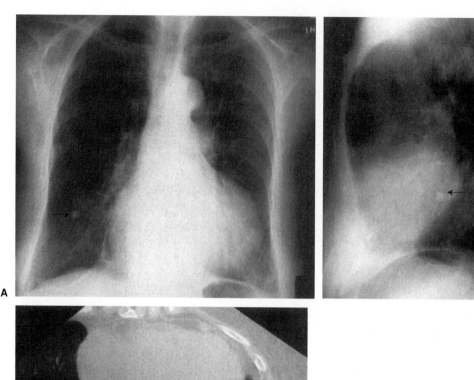

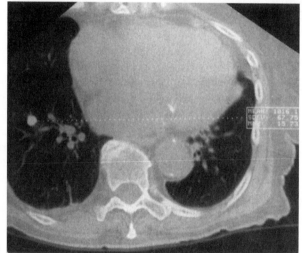

FIGURE 2-57. Chest PA **(A)** and lateral **(B)** radiographs. Calcified granuloma *(straight arrows)* in the right lower lobe. The homogeneous high-density appearance of this small nodule strongly suggests calcification, which makes the diagnosis of granuloma fairly certain, and no further workup was probably needed. Incidentally, there is mild cardiomegaly and hyperinflation of the lungs due to chronic obstructive pulmonary disease. **C:** Chest axial CT through the left atrium level. The lesion in the right lower lobe is very dense and calcific in appearance, and the lesion measures 1016 Hounsfield units. These findings indicate a high probability that it is a benign granuloma.

CARDIAC AND GREAT VESSELS

Unfortunately, the radiographic appearance of cardiac chambers does not correlate with their function. Echocardiography, magnetic resonance imaging, and cine CT allow not only improved cardiac anatomy visualization but physiologic and motion imaging such as ejection fractions and valve movement. However, this section is confined to static imaging.

Aneurysms, Enlarged Vessels, and Vascular Calcifications

An aneurysm of the thoracic aorta is a significant acquired abnormality. These aneurysms may present as a mass in any of the three mediastinal areas depending on their exact location (Fig. 2-65). Of course, aneurysms can occur in the pulmonary arteries or any other thoracic artery. On occasion, there are clinical situations wherein the central pulmonary arteries become markedly enlarged (Fig. 2-66), and a partial differential diagnosis is listed in Table 2-11. In addition, calcification of thoracic vessels does occur and should be recognized as such on radiographs and CT images (Fig. 2-67).

Pulmonary Edema

Pulmonary edema (Fig. 2-68) is a common and extremely important problem encountered by the primary physician and almost all health care providers. There are many etiologies for pulmonary edema (Table 2-12). The most common etiology is left-sided cardiac disease that results in an increased pulmonary venous pressure. These patients may complain of dyspnea on exertion, orthopnea, paroxysmal

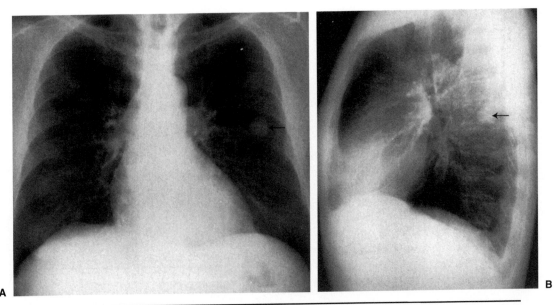

FIGURE 2-58. Chest PA **(A)** and lateral **(B)** radiographs. Histoplasmoma superior segment left lower lobe *(arrows)*. This noncalcified solitary nodule was seen on a routine chest radiograph on this 58-year-old asymptomatic man. The differential diagnosis of a solitary noncalcified pulmonary nodule was entertained, and malignancy could not be excluded. Thoracotomy and resection of the lesion resulted in the diagnosis of a benign histoplasmoma.

nocturnal respiratory distress, weight gain, lower extremity edema, cough, and, on occasion, hemoptysis.

It is important to appreciate and recognize the wide variety of radiographic presentations that may occur in this clinical problem (Table 2-13). The first radiographic

sign of pulmonary edema is generally considered to be a redistribution of the blood flow to the upper lobes. Normally the lower lobe vessels are three times larger than the upper lobe vessels. As the pulmonary venous pressure increases, patchy infiltrates appear representing fluid in the acini. These infiltrates may have a bat wing appearance around the hili and are usually more predominant in the lower lung fields because of a gravitational effect. Kerley B lines or thickening of the interlobular septa and pleural effusions eventually appear secondary to the increased venous and lymphatic pressures. As edema surrounds the pulmonary vessels, they tend to become indistinct with surrounding cuffs. Pleural effusions are common in pulmonary edema and have a variety of appearances as seen in Fig. 2-68. Occasionally chest decubitus views (the patient lies on his or her side) are obtained when pleural effusions are suspected or if it is important to know if the pleural fluid is free flowing (see Fig. 2-68E).

▶ **TABLE 2-10 Differential Diagnosis for Mediastinal Masses**

Anterior Mediastinum
1. Thyroid and parathyroid masses
2. Thymus masses (Fig. 2-59A, B)
3. Teratoma
4. Tortuous vessels such as aneurysm of ascending aorta (Fig. 2-59C, D)
5. Lymph nodes

Middle Mediastinum
1. Pericardial fat pad and pericardial cyst (Fig. 2-59C, D)
2. Bronchogenic cyst and bronchogenic carcinoma
3. Lymph nodes
4. Diaphragm hernia (Morgagni)
5. Dilated great vessels including aneurysms

Posterior Mediastinum
1. Neurogenic tumors
2. Duplication cysts
3. Lymph nodes
4. Esophageal lesions including esophageal hiatal hernia (Fig. 2-43A, B)

▶ **TABLE 2-11 Partial Differential Diagnosis of Enlarged Pulmonary Arteries**

High-volume Situations
1. Left-to-right shunts
2. High cardiac output situations (anemias, thyrotoxicosis)

Peripheral Arterial Narrowing and Occlusion
1. Thromboembolic disease
2. Idiopathic pulmonary hypertension

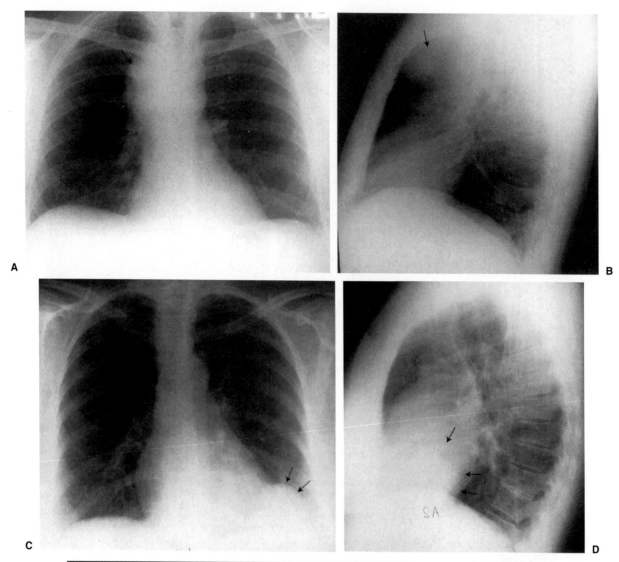

FIGURE 2-59. Chest PA **(A)** and lateral **(B)** radiographs. Thymoma *(straight arrows)*. The lesion clearly lies in the anterior mediastinum. **C, D:** Chest PA (C) and lateral (D) radiographs. Pericardial cyst *(straight arrows)*. This lesion was found on a routine chest radiograph in an asymptomatic 54-year-old female patient. These oval masses usually are on the right side at the cardiohepatic angle. This left-sided pericardial cyst lies near the apex of the cardiac silhouette on the PA view and projects over the heart on the lateral view. The differential diagnosis was left ventricle aneurysm, bronchogenic cyst, Morgagni hernia, and diaphragmatic tumor. The diagnosis can sometimes be made by ultrasound or CT imaging. In this case, the diagnosis was made at thoracotomy. **E, F:** Chest PA (E) and lateral (F) radiographs. Neuroblastoma. In the PA view, the mass can be seen through the cardiac shadow *(straight arrows)*. The lateral view shows the mass to be posterior as there is loss of distinction of the lower dorsal spine vertebral bodies or a positive spine sign.

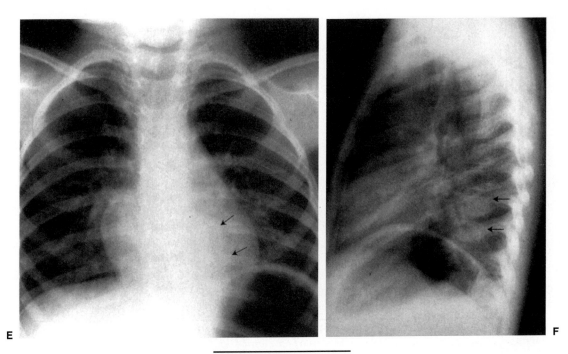

E   F

FIGURE 2-59. *(Continued)*

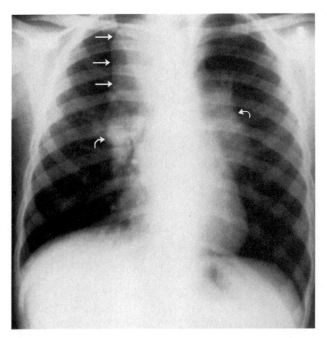

FIGURE 2-60. Chest PA radiograph. Lymphoma. This young adult male was admitted because of an abnormal white blood count. There is a large mediastinal mass *(straight arrows)* with associated bilateral hilar lymphadenopathy *(curved arrows)*. The mass resides within the anterior and middle mediastinum. This is a typical appearance of lymphoma of the chest.

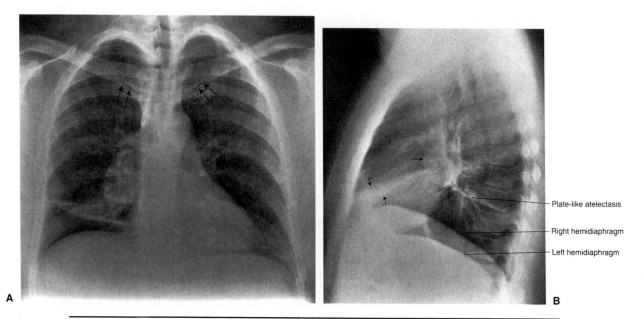

A

B

— Plate-like atelectasis

— Right hemidiaphragm

— Left hemidiaphragm

FIGURE 2-61. Chest PA **(A)** and lateral **(B)** radiographs. Right infrahilar primary neoplasm *(straight arrows)* causing right middle lobe atelectasis *(curved arrows)*. The right hemidiaphragm is mildly elevated secondary to the right middle lobe atelectasis. Note on the lateral view how nicely you can see the right and left hemidiaphragms. The right hemidiaphragm can be seen in its entirety whereas the left hemidiaphragm is silhouetted anteriorly by the heart. The *double arrows* indicate bilateral infraclavicular notching or rhomboid fossae. These fossae are a variation of normal, and they give origin to the costoclavicular or rhomboid ligaments. [1]

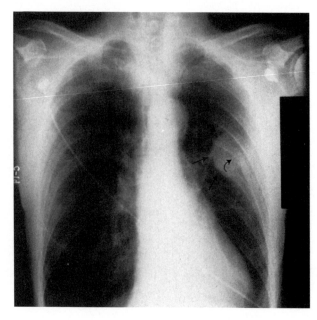

FIGURE 2-62. Chest AP radiograph. Carcinoma of the lung with rib destruction. The moderately sized primary carcinoma in the left upper lobe *(straight arrows)* has partially destroyed a left rib posteriorly *(curved arrow)*. Note that the lungs are overexpanded, probably secondary to chronic obstructive pulmonary disease. A monitoring electrode runs across the thorax from left to right.

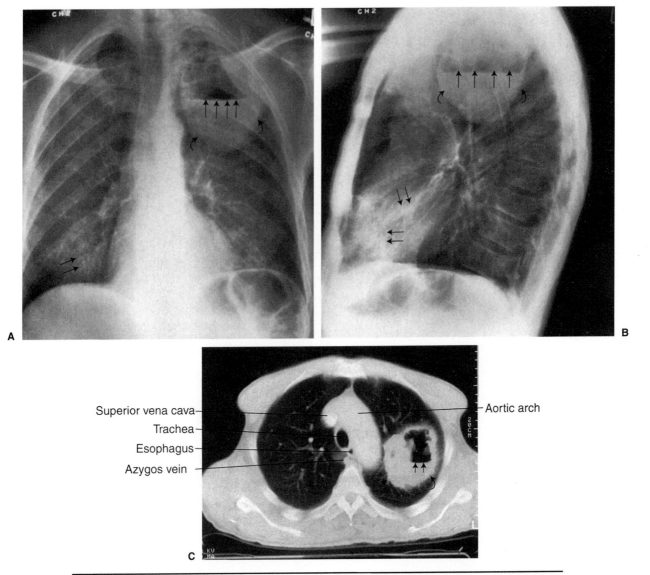

FIGURE 2-63. Chest PA **(A)** and lateral **(B)** radiographs and a chest axial CT image **(C)** through the level of the aortic arch. Cavitating primary squamous cell carcinoma of the left upper lobe. The large tumor mass *(curved arrows)* contains an air–fluid level *(straight arrows)* that is secondary to necrotizing tumor. There is a partially confluent pneumonia in the right middle lobe *(double straight arrows)*.

▶ **TABLE 2-12 Etiologies of Pulmonary Edema**

1. Cardiogenic
2. Neurogenic
3. Increased permeability
   a. Toxic inhalation
   b. High-altitude sickness
   c. Aspiration
   d. Contusion
   e. Fat embolism

▶ **TABLE 2-13 Radiographic Findings in Pulmonary Edema**

1. Redistribution (increase size of vessels to the upper lobes)
2. Patchy infiltrates (bat wing and gravitational)
3. Kerley B lines
4. Interlobar fissure thickening
5. Pleural fluid
6. Parahilar zone bronchial cuffing
7. Parahilar vessels less distinct

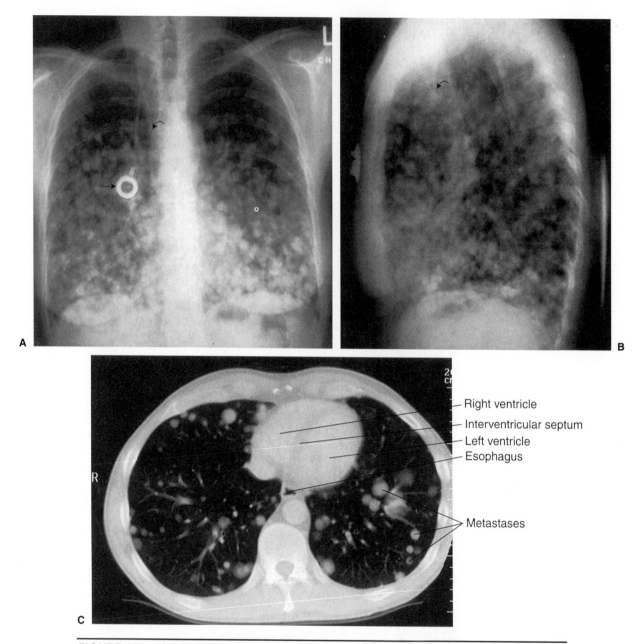

FIGURE 2-64. Chest PA **(A)** and lateral **(B)** radiographs. Diffuse bilateral metastases. The metastatic lesions are not calcified and typically are variable in size. The infusaport *(straight arrows)* is used to administer medications. The tip of the infusaport catheter *(curved arrows)* projects over the superior vena cava in both views. **C:** Chest axial chest CT through the level of the ventricles. The multiple widespread metastases are variable in size.

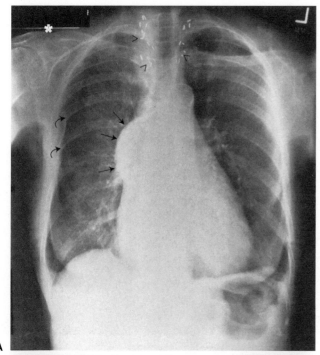

A

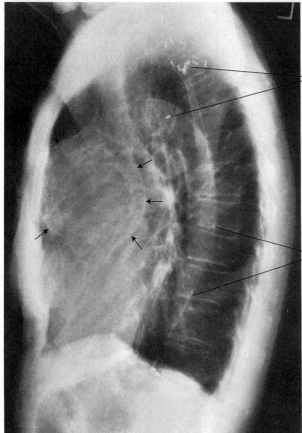

B

Surgical metallic
clips

Calcified descending
thoracic aorta

FIGURE 2-65. Chest PA **(A)** and lateral **(B)** radiographs. Large calcified ascending thoracic aorta aneurysm *(straight arrows)*. The aneurysmal calcification is faint on both views. On the PA radiograph, the heart appears enlarged but on the lateral view it is within normal limits. Note the old healed right rib fracture deformities *(curved arrows)*. The lungs are hyperinflated. Note the surgical clips *(arrowheads)* and the artifact (∗) appearing on the right shoulder.

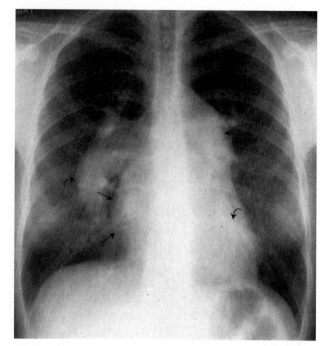

FIGURE 2-66. Chest PA radiograph. Right atrial enlargement and large pulmonary arteries. The right atrium is enlarging to the patient's right side *(straight arrows)*, and the pulmonary arteries are larger than normal *(curved arrows)*. The etiology in this patient is unknown.

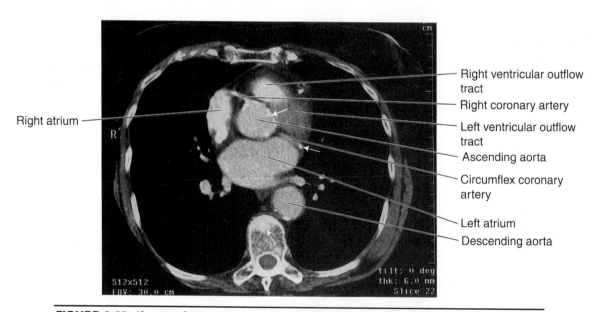

Right atrium

Right ventricular outflow tract

Right coronary artery

Left ventricular outflow tract

Ascending aorta

Circumflex coronary artery

Left atrium

Descending aorta

FIGURE 2-67. Chest axial CT image through the level of the left atrium. The right coronary artery, the circumflex coronary artery, and ascending and descending aorta all contain calcifications *(straight arrows)*.

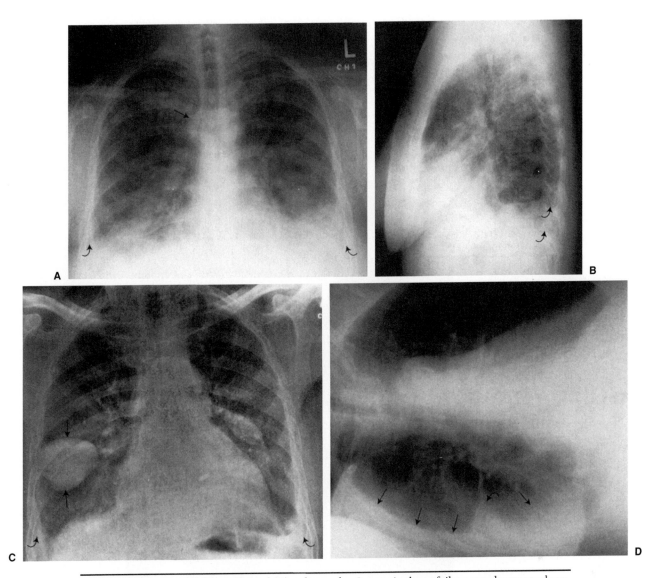

FIGURE 2-68. Chest PA **(A)** and lateral **(B)** radiographs. Congestive heart failure or pulmonary edema. The azygos vein *(straight arrow)* is enlarged. The pulmonary vasculature is increased on both views, especially toward the bases (gravitational). The pulmonary vessels are indistinct, and there are bilateral pleural effusions *(curved arrows)*. It is interesting to note that the cardiac size is within normal limits, suggesting a sudden onset of pulmonary edema. **C:** Chest PA radiograph. Pseudotumor sign and congestive heart failure. There is moderate cardiomegaly and mild bilateral pleural effusions *(curved arrows)*. Some of the pleural fluid secondary to the pulmonary edema flowed into the minor fissure *(straight arrows)* mimicking a tumor, hence the term pseudotumor. This nicely demonstrates that the fissures are contiguous with the pleural space. **D:** Chest right lateral decubitus radiograph. Moderate amount of free-flowing right pleural fluid. The free-flowing pleural fluid *(straight arrows)* flows cephalad in the dependent right pleural space. Some of the pleural fluid flows into the minor fissure *(curved arrow)*.

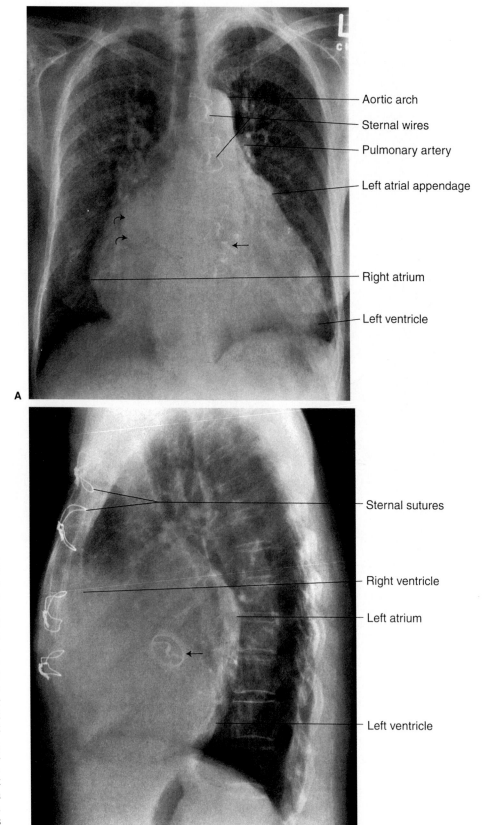

Aortic arch

Sternal wires

Pulmonary artery

Left atrial appendage

Right atrium

Left ventricle

Sternal sutures

Right ventricle

Left atrium

Left ventricle

FIGURE 2-69. Chest PA **(A)** and lateral **(B)** radiographs. Severe cardiomegaly and a prosthetic mitral valve *(straight arrows)*. The patient had mitral valve stenosis and regurgitation that necessitated a prosthetic mitral valve. All of the cardiac chambers are enlarged. On the PA view, the enlarged left atrium creates the double density indicated by the *curved arrows*, and the left atrial appendage is prominent along the left cardiac border. Also, on the PA view, there is right atrial and left ventricular enlargement. On the lateral view, enlargement of the right ventricle results in fullness of the retrosternal space. Also, on the lateral view, there is enlargement of the left atrium and ventricle.

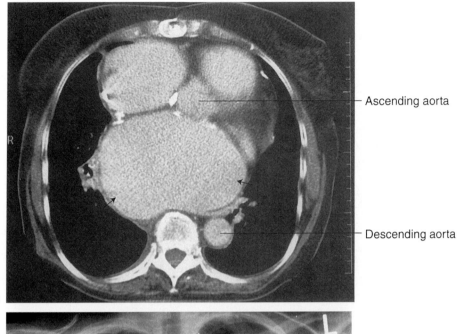

— Ascending aorta

— Descending aorta

C

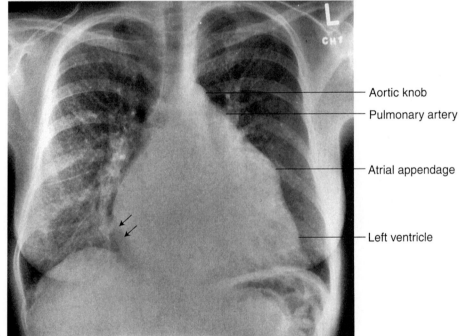

— Aortic knob
— Pulmonary artery

— Atrial appendage

— Left ventricle

D

FIGURE 2-69. (*continued*) **C:** Chest axial CT image through the atrium level. Left atrial enlargement (*straight arrows*). This is a different patient from that in A and B. This patient also had mitral stenosis resulting in left atrial enlargement. **D:** Chest PA radiograph. Mitral stenosis and cardiomegaly. There is a nice demonstration of the classic moguls in mitral stenosis that are visible along the left cardiac border consisting of the aortic knob, a prominent left pulmonary artery, the enlarged left atrial appendage, and the left ventricle. Also, the double density of an enlarged left atrium (*straight arrows*) can be identified.

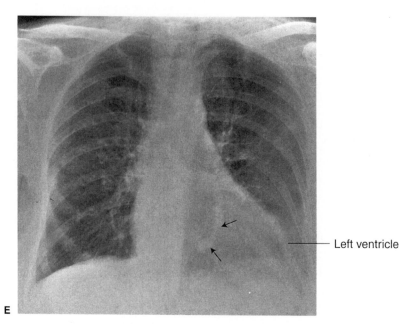

Left ventricle

FIGURE 2-69. (*continued*) **E:** Chest PA radiograph. Mitral annulus calcification (*straight arrows*). This patient was asymptomatic, and the calcified mitral annulus was an incidental finding on a routine chest study. There is mild cardiomegaly with mild enlargement of the left ventricle.

E

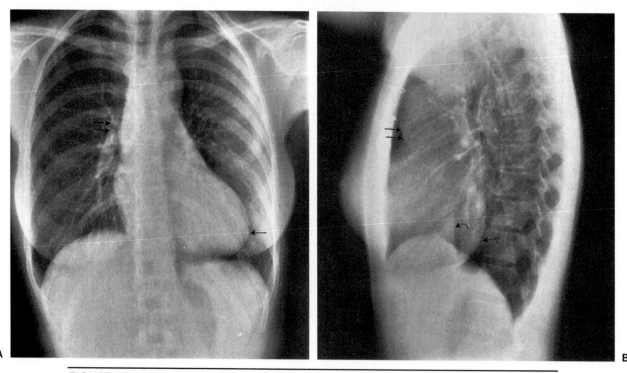

A

B

FIGURE 2-70. Chest PA (**A**) and lateral (**B**) radiographs. Aortic valve stenosis and regurgitation. Systolic and diastolic aortic valve murmurs were discovered during a routine physical examination. There is left ventricular enlargement (*straight arrows*) manifested by rounding of the cardiac apex on the PA view, and on the lateral view the enlarged left ventricle projects more than 2 cm posterior to the inferior vena cava (*curved arrow*). The latter finding is a fairly reliable sign for left ventricular enlargement. The ascending aorta shows poststenotic dilatation (*double straight arrows*), and this is often found in aortic stenosis.

Widening of the vascular pedicle can occur when there is too much fluid and salt circulating as in fluid overload and pulmonary edema. The vascular pedicle width is measured from the lateral aspect of the superior vena cava as it crosses the right main stem bronchus to the aortic arch where approximately the subclavian artery arises. The azygos vein lies lateral to the right main stem bronchus and tends to enlarge in similar situations. In situations characterized by increased capillary permeability as in adult respiratory distress syndrome, the edematous pattern is more diffuse and more patchy and *tends to change very slowly.*

Valvular Heart Disease

Acquired and congenital cardiac valve diseases have the potential to cause chamber enlargement and pulmonary edema. Valve disease can obstruct the flow of blood out of a chamber (stenosis) or the valve may allow retrograde flow (regurgitation). Either situation can result in increased pressure and size in the involved cardiac chamber. Two good examples of this type of problem are found in diseases of the mitral valve (Fig. 2-69) and the aortic valve (Fig. 2-70).

As the left atrium enlarges, it can create a double density along the right heart border as the enlarged left atrium projects through the right atrium. Also, the enlarging left atrium may widen the tracheal bifurcation and elevate the left main stem bronchus. As the left atrium and/or atrial appendage enlarge, they create a bulge along the left upper cardiac border (Fig. 2-69A).

KEY POINTS

- PA and lateral views are the routine standard chest radiographs.
- AP is the standard portable chest radiograph.

- If thoracic bone imaging is necessary, it is best to order the specific radiographs such as ribs, shoulders, or dorsal spine.
- Position chest radiographs on the viewbox with the patient's labeled right side opposite the viewer's left hand, and this generally applies to almost all other images.
- Develop a simple systematic approach for viewing chest radiographs to avoid errors of omission.
- The cardiac transverse diameter should not exceed 50% of thoracic cage transverse diameter. This is called the *cardiothoracic ratio.*
- Cardiac size estimation is most generally accomplished by gross eyeballing and becomes easier with experience.
- Cardiac size appears larger on the AP than the PA view because of magnification.
- The right atrium forms the convex right cardiac border, and the left ventricle forms the cardiac apex on AP or PA radiographs.
- On a chest radiograph, look for water densities as most chest radiographic pathology is water density.
- Excessive black density on a chest radiograph generally indicates too much air, and its location will help make the diagnosis.
- When two similar densities abut each other, it is virtually impossible to differentiate their borders on a radiograph. This is called the *silhouette sign.*

REFERENCES

1. Fraser RS, Pare JA, Fraser RG, Pare PD. *Synopsis of diseases of the chest,* 2nd ed. Philadelphia: WB Saunders, 1994.
2. Edeiken J. *Roentgen diagnosis of diseases of bone,* 4th ed. Baltimore: Williams & Wilkins, 1990.
3. Juhl JH, Crummy AB. *Paul and Juhl's essentials of radiologic imaging,* 7th ed. Philadelphia: JB Lippincott Co, 1993.

FURTHER SUGGESTED READINGS

El-Khoury GY, Bergman RA, Montgomery WJ. *Sectional anatomy by MRI,* 2nd ed. New York: Churchill Livingstone, 1995.

Abdomen

Edmund A. Franken, Jr., MD

Careful history and physical examination allow diagnosis of most abdominal complaints. When diagnosis remains uncertain following these procedures, an abdominal radiograph is often the first diagnostic imaging procedure requested. Recall that in women of childbearing age, consideration of possible pregnancy should precede a radiograph.

The anteroposterior (AP) radiograph, the most frequently performed abdominal imaging study, is performed with the patient supine (Fig. 3-1A). An upright radiograph (Fig. 3-1B) is useful in searching for free intraperitoneal air and/or intestinal air–fluid levels. If the patient cannot stand, a decubitus radiograph obtained with the patient lying on either the right or, preferably, the left side (Fig. 3-1C) can be substituted.

VIEWING ABDOMINAL RADIOGRAPHS

Step 1 is to position the radiograph correctly on the viewbox, with the film R (right side) marker opposite the viewer's left side and the patient's head toward the top of the film (Fig. 3-2). On the AP upright radiograph, there should be a sign indicating an upright view, usually an arrow near the R or L marker, pointing toward the patient's head. Similarly, decubitus radiographs should be clearly labeled as such and should note which side is up or down.

Step 2 is to glance at the entire radiograph in a relaxed manner to allow an obvious abnormality to jump out at you. When you do discover an abnormality, do not terminate your subsequent search.

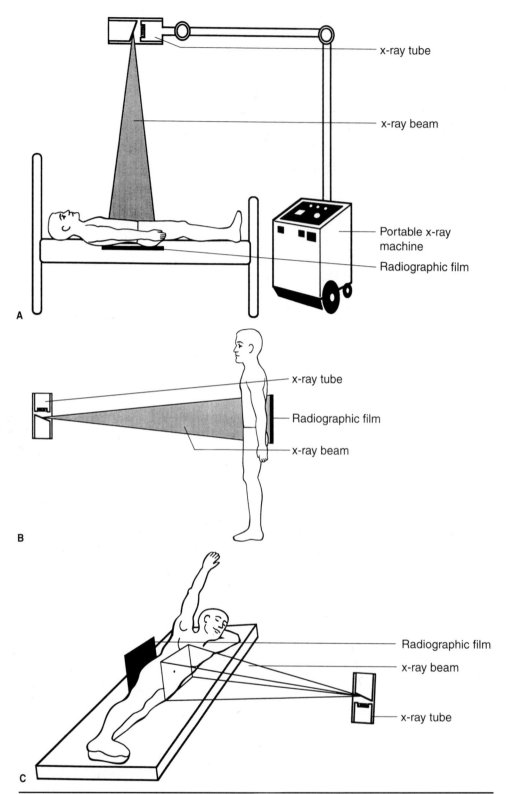

FIGURE 3-1. A: Patient positioning for an AP supine abdomen radiograph. This examination is performed with the patient supine, either on a radiographic table or in bed (using a portable x-ray unit). **B:** Patient positioning for an AP upright abdomen radiograph. This examination is usually accomplished in the radiology department, with the patient standing. **C:** Patient positioning for a left lateral decubitus abdomen radiograph. The patient's arms are positioned comfortably out of the way.

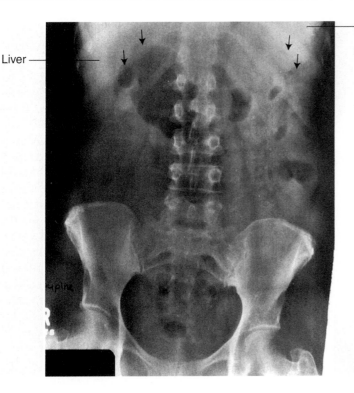

Liver —

Spleen

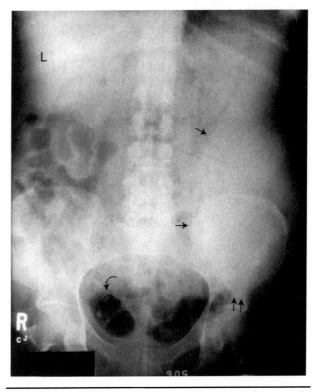

FIGURE 3-2. Abdomen AP supine radiograph. Normal-sized liver and spleen. The intestinal gas (*straight arrows*) demarcates the inferior liver and spleen margins.

Step 3 is to evaluate the radiograph systematically. Any system or checklist will suffice. Table 3-1 will work, until you develop your own. First, locate the water density liver and spleen silhouettes. One clue to locating liver and spleen edges is the presence of bowel gas in the right and left upper abdominal quadrants. Such bowel gas permits an indirect estimate of the location of the hepatic and splenic borders, because it is located at the lower edges of the liver and spleen.

With a little experience, you will automatically recognize a normal-sized liver. When the liver shadow extends to the iliac crest, it is usually enlarged. Also with more experience, you will readily detect an enlarged spleen (splenomegaly; Fig. 3-3). Medicine is an apprenticeship and requires practice and repetition.

In the normal radiograph, psoas muscle margins are usually visible (Fig. 3-4). A nonvisible psoas margin should alert you to a possible abnormality. As your eyes drift toward the renal shadows, evaluate their size, shape,

▶ **TABLE 3-1 Routine for Evaluating Abdominal Radiographs**

1. Once-over glance
2. Liver and spleen
3. Psoas shadows
4. Renal contours and position
5. Abdominal calcifications
6. Intestinal gas pattern
7. Bones

FIGURE 3-3. Abdomen AP supine radiograph. Splenomegaly. The water density spleen is enlarged (*straight arrows*), and the inferior margin projects just above the left hip (*double straight arrows*). The large spleen has displaced the intestinal gas into the right abdomen. The liver size is normal (*L*, liver). Incidentally noted are phleboliths (*curved arrows*), small intravenous stones secondary to calcified thrombi.

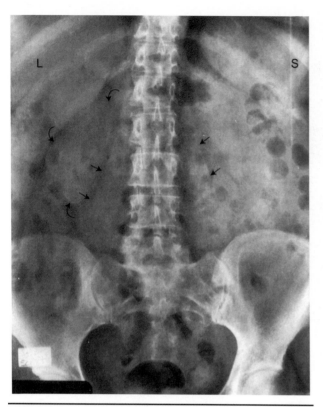

FIGURE 3-4. Abdomen AP supine radiograph. Normal. The psoas muscles (*straight arrows*) and the right kidney (*curved arrows*) are visible. The left renal silhouette is obliterated by intestinal gas. It is common to have intestinal gas and contents obliterating the renal shadows. (*L*, liver; *S*, spleen).

and position. Renal shadows are visible because they are water density structures (gray) surrounded by variable amounts of fat (black). Identifying renal outlines is about as easy for the rookie as visualizing the bottom of the muddy Mississippi River. You should attempt to locate the upper and lower renal poles, as well as their medial and lateral borders. If the renal long axis is not parallel with the psoas muscle margin, you should consider a mass or other water density abnormality in the kidney or the retroperitoneum. Always look for calcifications (white) in the abdomen, especially in the region of the kidneys, ureters, urinary bladder, and the gallbladder (discussed later).

The term *Aunt Minnie*, coined by the late Dr. Ben Felson, refers to the unmistakable and unforgettable appearance of your Aunt Minnie, or Uncle Al, or any other family character. A radiologic Aunt Minnie describes an image appearance so classic that, once you see it, you never forget it. The following abdominal radiographic Aunt Minnies (Figs. 3-5 to 3-10) are commonly encountered. File them away in your visual-cerebral computer, and your ability to recognize them will make you a star in the eyes of your colleagues, teachers, and patients.

Now, evaluate the bowel gas pattern (see the next section). Last but not least, look at the bones systematically, beginning with the visible ribs and spine (Fig. 3-11). Study the pedicles of the lower dorsal and lumbar spine, proceeding from head to foot. They resemble automobile headlights on an AP radiograph; a missing pedicle indicates a destructive process, such as metastatic disease. Evaluate

FIGURE 3-5. Abdomen AP supine radiograph. Classic appearance of tablets or pills (*straight arrows*) in the GI tract. All the tablets are the same size and shape with homogeneous density. (Not all tablets or pills can be visualized on a radiograph.)

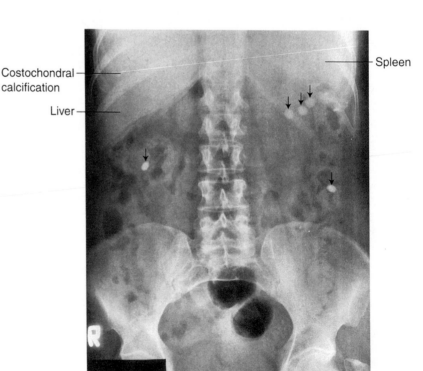

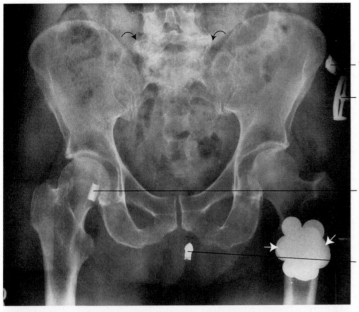

— Trouser clasp

— Belt buckle

— Trouser clasp

— Zipper pull

FIGURE 3-6. Abdomen AP supine radiograph. Metal coins (*straight arrows*) in the left trouser pocket. The patient was not completely disrobed prior to obtaining the radiographs. Note the degenerative or osteoarthritic changes in the lower lumbar spine (*curved arrows*).

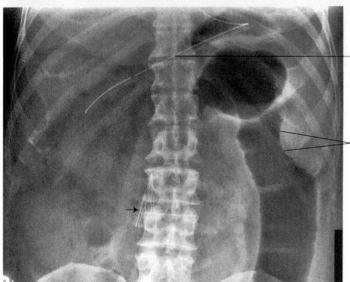

— Nasogastric tube

— Splenic impression on descending colon

FIGURE 3-7. Abdomen AP supine radiograph. An umbrella-shaped inferior vena cava filter (*straight arrow*), placed in the inferior vena cava by angiographic technique, entraps venous thromboemboli originating in the lower extremities and pelvis.

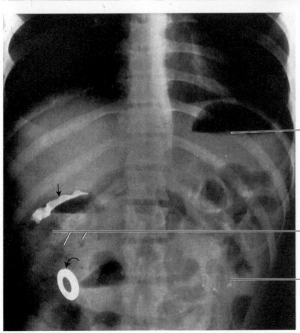

— Gastric air–fluid level

— Air trapped in laparotomy pad

— Opaque sutures

FIGURE 3-8. Abdomen AP upright radiograph. Surgical laparotomy pad in a postoperative abdomen. The radiograph was obtained when the patient experienced severe postoperative abdominal pain and distention. The *straight arrow* indicates the opaque strip in the laparotomy pad, and the *curved arrow* indicates the metallic ring attached to the laparotomy pad. Note the mottled black appearance of the air trapped in the laparotomy pad. The air–fluid level in the gastric fundus gives a clue to the upright position of the patient.

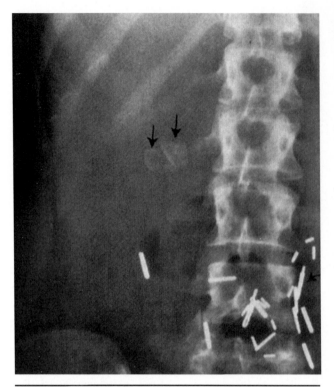

FIGURE 3-9. Abdomen AP supine radiograph. Cholelithiasis (gallstones). The calcified calculi (*straight arrows*) are faceted. Surgical metallic clips (*curved arrows*) are secondary to previous abdominal surgery.

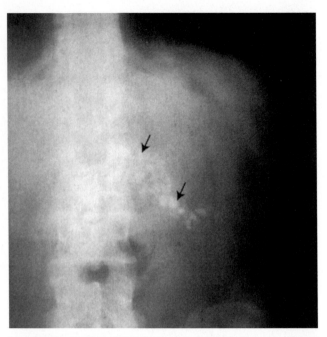

FIGURE 3-10. Abdomen AP supine radiograph. Calcifications (*straight arrows*) in the body and tail of the pancreas, owing to chronic pancreatitis.

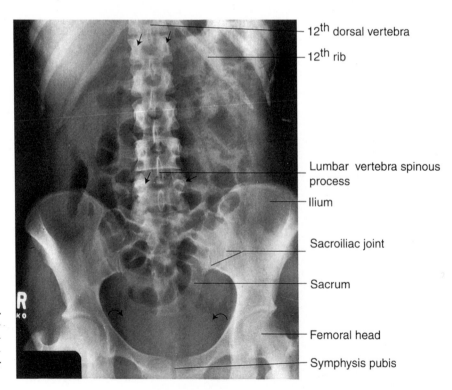

FIGURE 3-11. Abdomen AP supine radiograph. Normal. Representative vertebral pedicles are shown by *straight arrows*. The water density urinary bladder is shown by *curved arrows*.

12th dorsal vertebra

12th rib

Lumbar vertebra spinous process

Ilium

Sacroiliac joint

Sacrum

Femoral head

Symphysis pubis

all visible bones, including the pelvis, hips, and femurs, for their overall density and any abnormalities.

Use a similar search system for the AP upright abdominal radiograph while being especially alert for free air beneath the diaphragms. Free intraperitoneal air is usually visualized only on an upright radiograph, because only this position allows free air to rise to the subdiaphragmatic regions.

EVALUATING THE INTESTINAL AIR OR GAS PATTERN

Intestinal gas (black) provides a natural contrast media that can be useful for detecting abdominal disease. When evaluating the intestinal gas pattern, you should ask yourself several important questions. Is the bowel gas pattern normal? Remember that there is normally some air or gas in the stomach, small intestine, colon, and rectum. With experience, you will begin to recognize abnormal amounts of air in the gastrointestinal (GI) tract. This is similar to recognizing a normal heart on a chest radiograph. If the gas pattern is not normal, ask more questions. Is there too much or too little air? Is the air in the wrong place?

Too Much Bowel Gas

Here, where differential diagnosis includes adynamic ileus and bowel obstruction, we need a systematic approach to arrive at the correct diagnosis. In adynamic ileus (also referred to as *paralytic ileus* or just *ileus*), there is too much bowel gas in the entire GI tract, including the small and large intestines (Fig. 3-12A, B). Adynamic ileus may arise from intraabdominal cases or as a reflex phenomenon from disease elsewhere. The multiple etiologies are listed in Table 3-2. If you identify comparable amounts of gas in the small and large intestines and in the rectum, this generally indicates adynamic ileus. Air in the rectum may be a key differential point; however, be careful, as small amounts of air can be introduced into the rectum by a rectal thermometer, enema, or digital rectal examination.

▶ **TABLE 3-2 Adynamic Ileus—Major Causes**

Intraabdominal
- Postoperative or posttraumatic
- Postinflammatory: pancreatitis, enteritis, colitis
- Pain-related: renal colic, epidural disease

Extraabdominal
- Septicemia
- Metabolic disease: hyperkalemia, uremia
- Medications (especially narcotics)
- Prolonged bedrest

In intestinal obstruction, another reason for too much bowel gas, there is usually air-filled, dilated intestine proximal to the point of obstruction and little or no air distal to the obstruction (Fig. 3-13A, B). In both ileus and obstruction, often the dilated small and large bowel containing too much air will have air–fluid levels noted on upright and decubitus radiographs.

If a diagnosis of obstruction versus adynamic ileus is not readily apparent, it may be necessary to obtain additional studies to arrive at the correct diagnosis. These include barium studies, CT (Fig. 3-14), or occasionally, ultrasound.

If you diagnose obstruction, you next need to determine the location of the obstruction. Is the obstruction in the small or large intestine? In small bowel obstruction, there are loops of dilated small bowel proximal to the obstruction site and little or no gas in the colon or the rectum. In large bowel obstruction, there is dilated colon proximal to the obstruction site, but little or no air distally and minimal air in the rectum.

Sometimes it is difficult to differentiate dilated small or large bowel. One way is to identify the valvulae conniventes and colon haustra. *Valvulae conniventes* are regularly spaced, thin mucosal folds that extend across the entire small bowel lumen (Fig. 3-13). On the other hand, the colon can usually be identified by the somewhat irregularly spaced transverse bands, called *colon septa* or *haustral folds*, that do not extend completely across the colon lumen (Fig. 3-12).

Sigmoid volvulus is a dramatic clinical event that occurs predominantly in elderly patients with a long history of constipation. The chronic constipation results in a redundant sigmoid mesentery that has the potential to twist on itself like a garden hose. If twisting occurs, there is complete or partial obstruction, and an abdominal radiograph shows a dramatically dilated sigmoid colon. Barium enema is confirmatory, with complete obstruction to the retrograde flow of barium at the site of the twist (Fig. 3-15). The obstruction can often be relieved by gently passing a sigmoidoscope past the point of the obstruction or twist.

Too Little Bowel Gas

When the abdominal radiographs show a paucity or absence of bowel gas, the differential diagnosis listed in Table 3-3 should be entertained.

Gas in the Wrong Places

There are several situations in which air is found outside of the intestinal lumen (Table 3-4). Free air in the peritoneal cavity results from any process that perforates the intestinal tract. AP supine and upright abdominal radiographs (*text continues on page 88*)

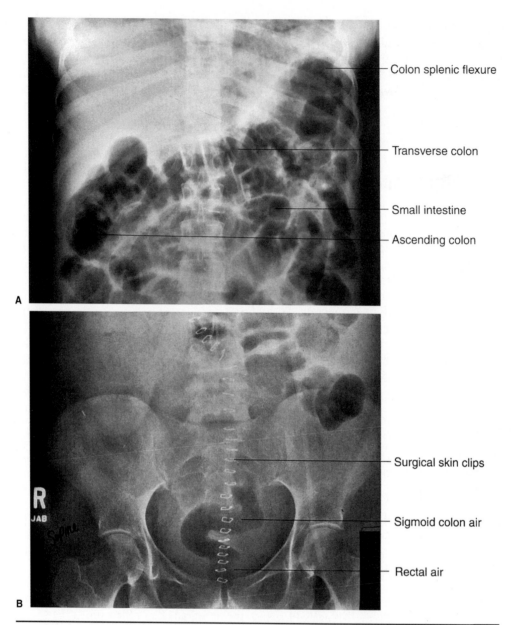

Colon splenic flexure

Transverse colon

Small intestine

Ascending colon

Surgical skin clips

Sigmoid colon air

Rectal air

FIGURE 3-12. **A:** Abdomen AP supine radiograph. Postoperative adynamic ileus. Air is present throughout the entire GI tract, including the rectum (not shown). Note the haustrations in the transverse colon. **B:** Lower abdomen AP supine radiograph 24 hours later in the same patient. A considerable amount of intestinal air has moved into the rectum and sigmoid colon, confirming the diagnosis of adynamic ileus.

▶ **TABLE 3-3 Too Little Bowel Gas**

- Enlarged abdominal organs
- Intraabdominal tumor
- Fluid-filled intestines
- Gastroenteritis
- Neurological deficit (with reduced swallowing)

▶ **TABLE 3-4 Abdominal Air or Gas in the Wrong Place**

- Pneumoperitoneum from ruptured intestines: ulcer, trauma, cancer, enteritis
- Abscess
- Pneumatosis intestinalis

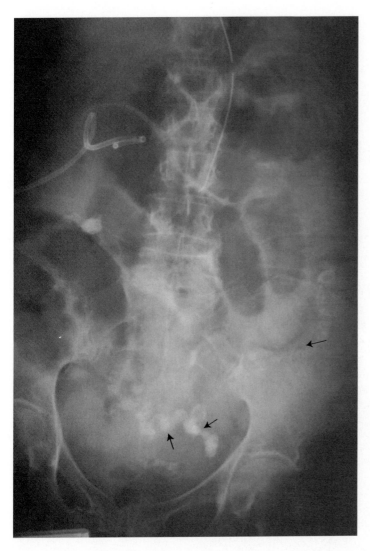

FIGURE 3-13. Abdominal radiograph. Small bowel obstruction. There are many dilated loops of small bowel in the midabdomen. They are identified as small bowel by their position, semihorizontal orientation, and valvulae conniventes traversing the entire transverse diameter. There is a small amount of residual barium in a collapsed descending colon (*arrows*). Incidentally noted are the nasogastric and abdominal drainage tubes. (Courtesy of Bruce Brown, M.D.)

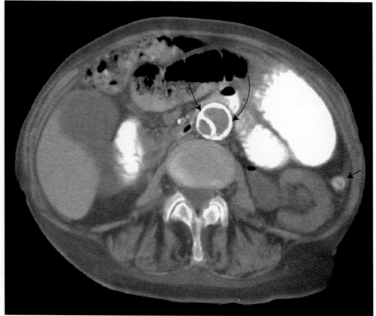

A

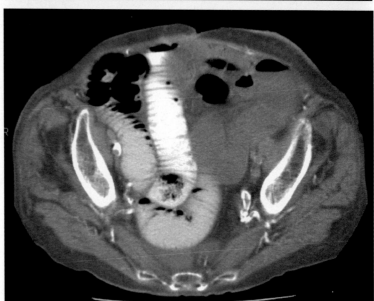

B

FIGURE 3-14. Abdominal axial CT. Small bowel obstruction. **A:** Here are many dilated loops of small bowel, some of which contain barium. The only colon visualized (*arrow*) in the left lower abdomen is tiny. (The aortic image (*curved arrows*) shows a segment of calcified intima, indicating previous aortic dissection.) **B:** CT at the level of the pelvis confirms the dilated small bowel extending into the pelvis (the rectum is surgically absent). (Courtesy of Gerald Decker, M.D.)

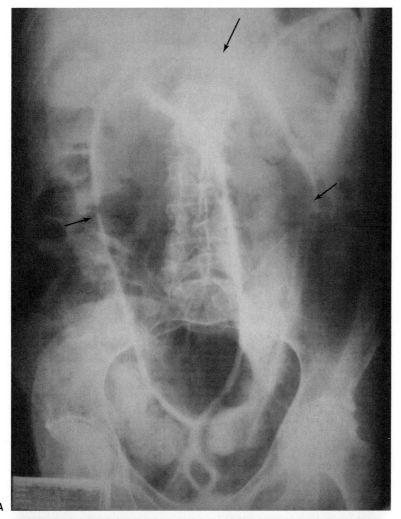

A

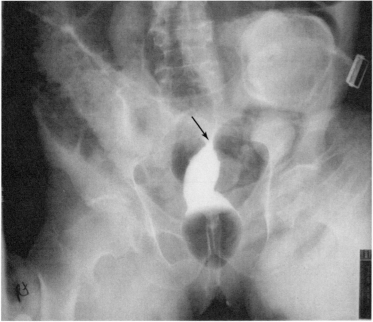

B

FIGURE 3-15. Sigmoid Volvulus **A:** Abdominal radiograph. The air-filled, obstructed sigmoid colon (*arrows*) arises from the pelvis. **B:** Barium enema. Contrast introduced per rectum shows obstruction and a twist (*arrow*) at the sigmoid colon. (Courtesy of Bruce Brown, M.D.)

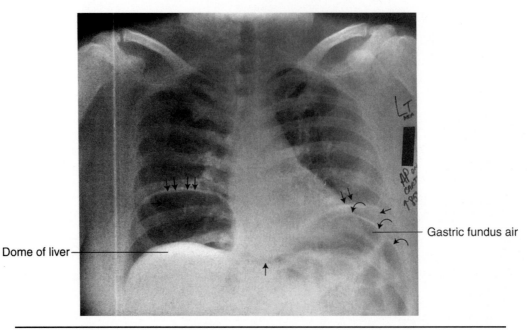

Dome of liver—

Gastric fundus air

FIGURE 3-16. Chest AP upright radiograph. Free intraperitoneal air. The right and left hemidiaphragms (*double arrows*) are elevated, owing to bilateral subdiaphragmatic air (*single straight arrows*). The black zone between the right hemidiaphragm and the dome of the liver represents free intraperitoneal air. On the left, there is air in the gastric fundus as well as free air surrounding the gastric fundus, allowing visualization of both sides of the stomach wall (*curved arrows*). When you see both sides of the gut wall, this represents free intraperitoneal air (Rigler's sign).

should be performed if there is clinical suspicion of gut perforation. The upright position allows free intraperitoneal air to rise to the subdiaphragmatic regions of the abdomen (Fig. 3-16). If the upright view is not possible owing to the patient's condition, a decubitus radiograph will suffice. On a decubitus radiograph, the air rises to the nondependent portion of the peritoneal cavity (Fig. 3-17). Either technique has the potential to identify as little as 2 cc of free intraperitoneal air, as long as the patient is in the upright or decubitus position approximately 5 minutes prior to the radiograph.

Another example of air in the wrong place is pneumatosis intestinalis (Fig. 3-18). Causes of this are listed in Table 3-5. Gas-filled abscesses can be found in any location, including the abdomen (Fig. 3-19).

GASTROINTESTINAL CONTRAST STUDIES

For inspection of the mucosal surface of the esophagus, stomach, and duodenum, endoscopy is often performed. Traditional radiologic GI contrast studies are accurate, safe, and less expensive than the endoscopic studies and enjoy excellent patient acceptance. These studies consist of fluoroscopy and radiographs obtained following introduction of barium sulfate (metallic density or white) and/or air (black) into the GI tract.

Upper GI Series

For an upper GI series, the patient swallows liquid barium, often with gas-producing crystals, under fluoroscopy to visualize the esophagus, stomach, and small intestine (Fig. 3-20). When both barium and air are used, the process is referred to as a double-contrast study. When barium is used alone, it is a single-contrast study. Preparation for an upper GI series consists simply of nothing by mouth (NPO) for 8 to 12 hours prior to the study. When perforation of the upper GI tract is suspected, water-soluble contrast media is used.

▶ TABLE 3-5 Pneumatosis Intestinalis

- Bowel ischemia
- Steroid and immunosuppressive therapy
- Proximal to intestinal obstruction
- Collagen diseases
- Neonatal necrotizing enterocolitis
- Benign idiopathic pneumatosis

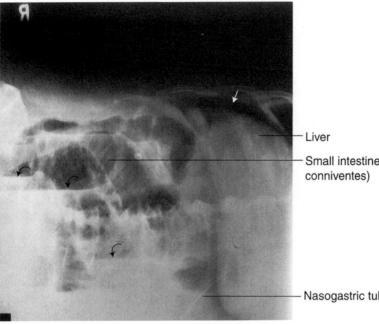

— Liver

— Small intestine (valvulae
 conniventes)

— Nasogastric tube

FIGURE 3-17. Abdomen left lateral decubitus radiograph (left side down). Free intraperitoneal air in a patient with small bowel obstruction and perforation. The free intraperitoneal air (*straight arrow*) is between the right rib cage and the liver. The dilated small bowel contains multiple air–fluid levels (*curved arrows*).

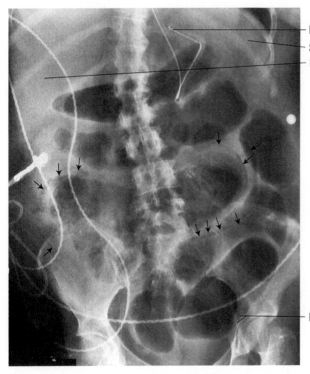

— Nasogastric tube
— Spleen
— Liver

— Femoral line

FIGURE 3-18. Abdomen AP supine radiograph. Pneumatosis intestinalis (air in the bowel wall). There is widespread bubbly air within the small intestine walls (*arrows*).

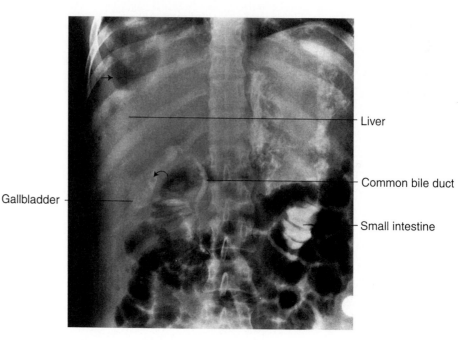

FIGURE 3-19. Abdomen AP supine radiograph. Right subdiaphragmatic abscess. The black areas along the right lateral aspect of the liver represent air in the abscess cavity (*straight arrows*). Incidentally noted is contrast material in the common bile duct, gallbladder, and small bowel, injected during an endoscopic retrograde cholangiopancreatography (ERCP). Some of the contrast spilled into the small intestine. The filling defect (*curved arrow*) in the gallbladder is probably a calculus.

Antegrade Small Bowel Examination

The usual small bowel examination is performed after an upper GI series by having the patient drink additional barium. Serial radiographs of the abdomen are performed at 15- to 30-minute intervals thereafter to evaluate the small bowel as barium passes through (Fig. 3-21). Fluoroscopy is commonly used as a supplement to study the terminal ileum when barium begins to enter the colon or to further investigate abnormalities seen on the serial radiographs.

Enteroclysis

Enteroclysis is a focused examination of the small intestine, wherein air and barium sulfate are introduced directly into the small intestine via a nasointestinal tube. Under fluoroscopy, the tip of the tube is placed just beyond the duodenal–jejunal junction and contrast is injected (Fig. 3-22). Advantages of this procedure are that the small bowel can be distended and the stomach and duodenum do not obstruct visualization. The main disadvantages are the discomfort associated with a nasal tube and the radiation exposure.

Retrograde Small Bowel Examination

On occasion, especially when disease of the terminal ileum is suspected and previous examinations are nondiagnostic, barium can be refluxed from a filled colon into the ileum. Although the procedure is useful, there is considerable patient discomfort, alleviated slightly by antispasmodic agents.

Barium Enema

Introduction of barium sulfate and/or air into the colon via a rectal tube is called a lower GI series or barium enema. For this study, it is important to have a clean colon; this is best accomplished with laxatives and large amounts of orally ingested fluids. Barium and often air are administered via a rectal tube under fluoroscopic observation. When both air and barium are used, it is called a double-contrast study (Fig. 3-23), whereas barium alone is a single-contrast study. A properly performed barium study of the colon has minimal associated discomfort. The double-contrast study is preferred to evaluate intraluminal and mucosal diseases, such as small ulcers and polyps. Again, if colon perforation is suspected, a water-soluble contrast medium is used.

Colonoscopy, an expensive alternative to colon barium studies, can directly visualize the mucosa. However, it requires conscious sedation because of patient discomfort.

STUDY OF GALLBLADDER AND BILIARY TRACT

The oral cholecystogram visualizes the gallbladder following the oral ingestion of special iodinated compounds that are excreted into the biliary system and subsequently concentrated in the gallbladder. The study is seldom performed now, because of the greater accuracy of ultrasound. With ultrasound, one can examine the liver and biliary tract as well as the gallbladder. CT and MRI are needed in certain situations to complement ultrasound.

(*text continues on page 94*)

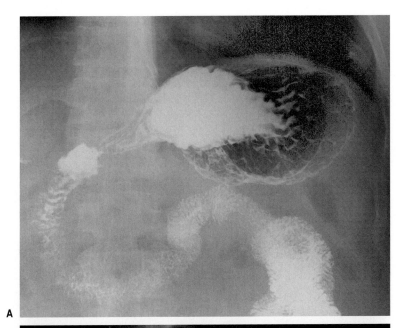

A

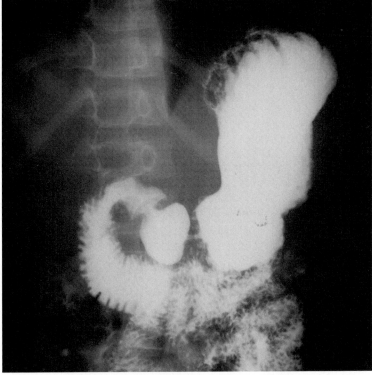

B

FIGURE 3-20. Normal upper gastrointestinal series **A:** Barium and air fill the stomach and duodenum. The transverse position of the stomach is owing to the patient's obesity. (Courtesy of Charles Jacoby, M.D.) **B:** Barium-filled stomach and duodenum in another patient.

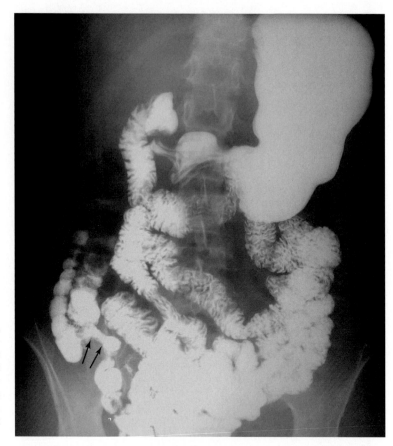

FIGURE 3-21. Normal antegrade small bowel examination. Barium was administered by mouth, and this radiograph was done about 30 minutes later. Note the barium-filled stomach, duodenal C-loop, feathered jejunum in the upper abdomen, and relatively formless mucosa of the ileum in the lower and right abdomen. The terminal ileum (*arrows*) entering the cecum can be identified. (Courtesy of Bruce Brown, M.D.)

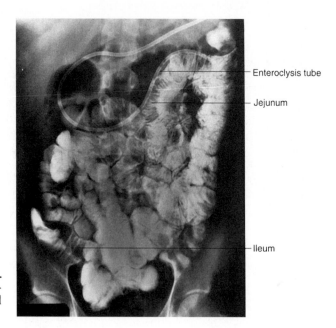

Enteroclysis tube

Jejunum

Ileum

FIGURE 3-22. Small bowel enteroclysis. Normal. The nasointestinal tube has been positioned just beyond the duodenal–jejunal junction. Barium fills the entire small bowel.

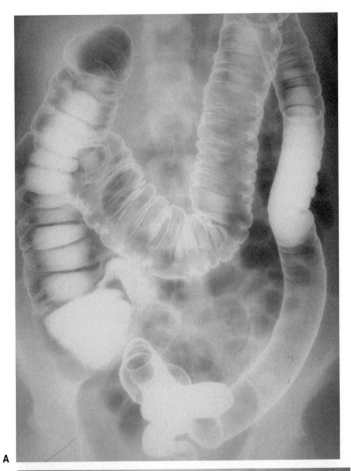

A

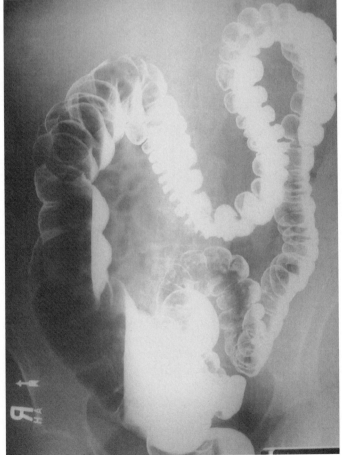

B

FIGURE 3-23. Barium–air contrast colon examination. Note the shift of barium and air in the colon in the supine **(A)** and left lateral decubitus **(B)** radiographs, so that different parts of the colon are visualized with the air-contrast technique. The opposite positions (prone and right lateral decubitus) and several additional radiographs are needed for a complete examination. (Courtesy of Bruce Brown, M.D.)

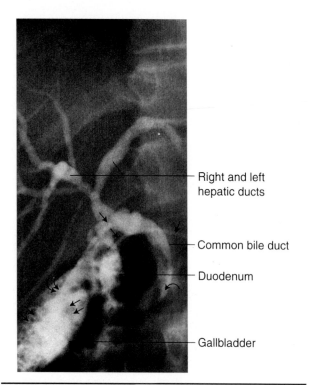

Right and left
hepatic ducts

Common bile duct

Duodenum

Gallbladder

FIGURE 3-24. Endoscopic retrograde cholangiopancreatography (ERCP). Cholelithiasis and choledocholithiasis. The gallbladder is filled with calculi (*double straight arrows*), and there is a large calculus in the distal common bile duct (*curved arrow*). A nasobiliary drain (*straight single arrows*) is in place with the tip (*double curved arrows*) in the gallbladder.

In endoscopic retrograde cholangiopancreatography (ERCP), an endoscopist passes a fiberoptic scope under fluoroscopic control antegrade through the esophagus, stomach, and duodenum and retrograde into the common bile duct. The pancreatic ducts can also be cannulated. Contrast media can be injected into any of these structures and appropriate radiographs obtained (Fig. 3-24). ERCP is usually performed when less-invasive studies (computed tomography, ultrasound, magnetic resonance imaging, or contrast studies) are indeterminate or nondiagnostic, or as part of a therapeutic endoscopic procedure.

URINARY TRACT EXAMINATIONS

In the early twentieth century, the only methodology to examine the urinary tract directly was to inject radiopaque material directly into the bladder or other urinary structures (retrograde cystography or pyelography). About 70 years ago, it was discovered that intravenous contrast material that is excreted by the kidneys could be given with relative safety. Excretory urography (EU) was developed shortly thereafter. With the advent of ultrasonography, CT,

and MRI, we now have a multifaceted radiologic approach to genitourinary problems.

EU, although still a useful technique, is performed much less frequently in the investigation of genitourinary disease than are ultrasound, CT, and MRI. In general, EU is used in those circumstances where delineation of the calyces, renal pelvis, and ureters is deemed most important. Cross-sectional modalities are of greater value in assessing the renal parenchyma. Other names given for the EU are intravenous urogram (IVU) and intravenous pyelogram (IVP).

Excretory Urography

Excretory urography (EU) does not require special patient preparation. The patient abstains from food and liquids for several hours before contrast administration; this lessens the risk of vomiting.

The timing of EU radiographs varies, depending both on local practice and the patient's clinical problems. Delayed films can be obtained for hours, or even days, in situations such as obstruction or renal failure.

How to View an Excretory Urogram

An EU study begins with a preliminary or scout radiograph that includes the entire abdomen. You can evaluate this preliminary radiograph using the same system as described previously.

The radiographs obtained immediately following intravenous contrast media demonstrate the nephrogram phase wherein the contrast media is located in the renal capillaries, glomeruli, and proximal convoluted tubules (Fig. 3-25). Compare the nephrograms for symmetry, as size discrepancy is suspicious for unilateral renal disease.

Next, evaluate the later, postcontrast injection radiographs, at which times the contrast media is normally present in the calyces, renal pelves, ureters, and urinary bladder (Fig. 3-26). Normal calyces are sharp in outline, with various numbers and geometry. The distance from the tip of the calyces to the renal border (calyceal–cortical distance, 2.5 to 3 cm) is a good indicator of renal cortex thickness. This distance decreases with age as our renal cortex thins, so that by the time a person becomes a professor, his or her renal (and cerebral) cortices may be much thinner than that of the students. When the ureters are dilated, there may be distal obstruction.

If the bladder empties incompletely on the postvoid radiograph, there may be obstruction at the bladder neck (e.g., prostatic enlargement; Fig. 3-27) or neurologic disease. Oblique, prone, and abdominal-compression radiographs are occasionally obtained to better display portions of the urinary tract.

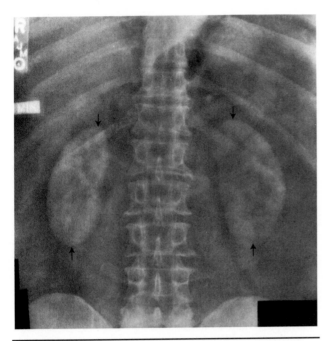

FIGURE 3-25. Abdomen AP EU. Normal. There are symmetric nephrograms one minute postinjection of contrast media. The renal outlines (*straight arrows*) are clearly defined, owing to the presence of the contrast media within the kidneys.

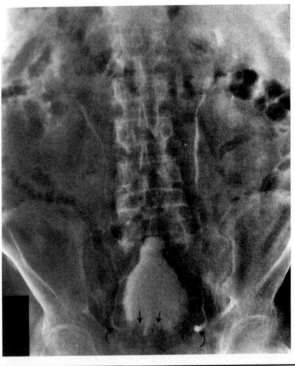

FIGURE 3-27. Abdomen postvoid EU. Partial bladder outlet obstruction, owing to benign prostatic hypertrophy. The enlarged prostate has created a filling defect and elevation of the floor of the bladder (*straight arrows*) with hooking of the distal ureters (*curved arrows*).

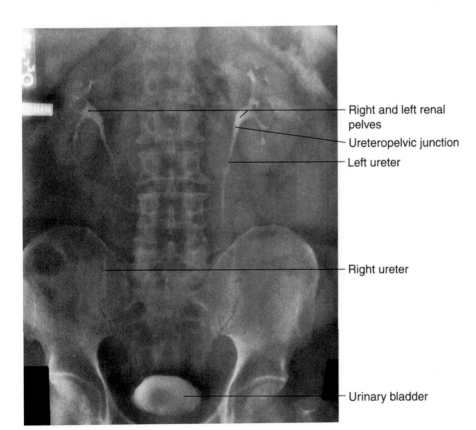

Right and left renal pelves

Ureteropelvic junction

Left ureter

Right ureter

Urinary bladder

FIGURE 3-26. Abdomen AP EU. Normal. Note that it is possible to see the calyces, infundibula, renal pelves, portions of ureters, and urinary bladder on this 15-minute radiograph.

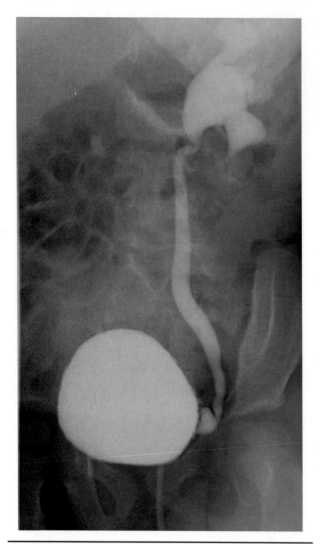

FIGURE 3-28. Cystourethrogram. Vesicoureteral reflux. Contrast introduced via urethral catheter into the bladder fills the bladder and refluxes into the left ureter.

Other Urinary Tract Examinations

Direct injection of contrast material into the bladder or ureter (retrograde pyelogram) is of value when a detailed view of a portion of the ureter or pelvocalyceal system is necessary. It is often an adjunct to endoscopy.

Vesicoureteral reflux, a condition in which bladder urine refluxes in retrograde fashion into the ureters, is a common phenomenon in children and infrequent in adults. It can be accompanied by urinary tract infection. With the voiding cystourethrogram (VCUG), contrast medium is introduced via urethral catheter into the bladder. Subsequent fluoroscopy and filming allow one to identify and quantitate vesicoureteral reflux if present (Fig. 3-28). At the completion of the study, the patient voids, with the voiding sequence recorded in some imaging form. This allows detection of urethral abnormalities, which can

produce bladder obstruction and secondary vesicoureteral reflux. Cystography and retrograde urethrography are examinations usually performed to detect urinary extravasation in trauma cases.

ABDOMINAL ULTRASOUND

Ultrasound (US), being a different modality from x-rays, shows abdominal organs in a different fashion. There are roughly three patterns of reflected US:

1. No reflection of the sound wave. Almost all of the sound passes through the area. This is termed sonolucent and is traditionally viewed as black on images. Fluid, such as in ascites or abdominal cysts, is sonolucent.
2. Reflection of some and transmission of some sound. Solid organs, such as the kidney or liver, are examples. US waves are reflected, particularly at boundaries of organs of differing echogenicity, such as the boundary between the liver and kidney.
3. Reflection of all sound. Bone, other calcifications, and air in the gut are examples. One can make use of this by noting shadowing and the absence of echoes distal to a lesion to help diagnose gallstones and like abnormalities.

There are two major problems in learning to read US images:

1. It requires one to think differently. You are looking at differences in transmission and reflection of US rather than transmitted x-rays.
2. Orientation of the image. This is the chief stumbling block. One may think of US images as representing a roughly pie-shaped wedge of tissues, less than 1 cm thick, below the US transducer.

Even experienced radiologists and clinicians have considerable difficulty figuring out the nature of the US image if they did not perform the study. Orientation must be provided by the person who performed the scan. In most situations, there is a relatively fixed method of performing abdominal US. In general, one evaluates each area of interest in at least two dimensions, typically axial (transverse) and longitudinal (sagittal). For technical reasons, the direction of the scan beam shows the anatomy best if it is parallel to the organ of interest. As few abdominal organs are 100% oriented anterior-posterior or medial-lateral, the scanned images are, to some degree, oblique.

Probably the best method to be introduced to US is to attend an imaging session with a knowledgeable mentor who discusses the anatomy as it is being scanned. Combined with this, learn the usual routines for US scanning in your institution and try to figure out how each image was performed. Conventionally, images are labeled as to

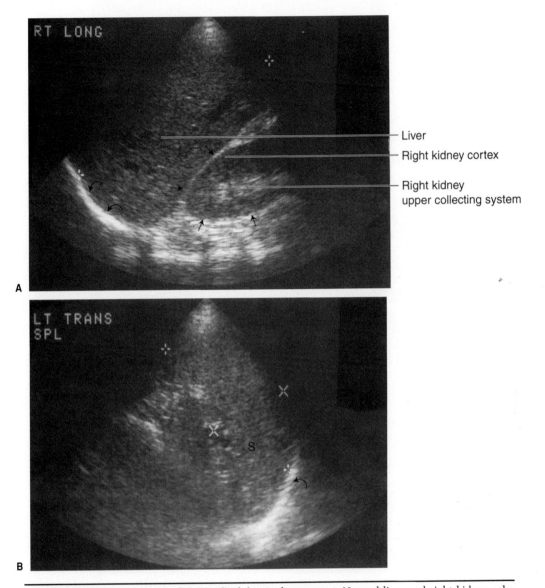

Liver
Right kidney cortex
Right kidney
upper collecting system

FIGURE 3-29. A: Longitudinal (sagittal) abdominal sonogram. Normal liver and right kidney echo patterns. The *cross marks* indicate the longitudinal (sagittal) liver dimension. The right kidney borders are demarcated by the *straight arrows* and the right hemidiaphragm by the *curved arrows*. **B:** Transverse (axial) abdominal sonogram. Normal spleen echo pattern. The side-to-side spleen dimension lies between the *X marks*, and the cephalocaudal dimension lies between the *crosses*. The left hemidiaphragm is indicated by the *curved arrow* (S, spleen). Note the labels on the images (A, Rt long; B, Lt trans spl). Such labels are helpful in orienting the images for the observer.

the method by which they are done; for example, kidney—transverse.

There are many abdominal applications of US related to its widespread availability and cost (it is about half the cost of CT and about one-third that of MRI). Ultrasonography is valuable in the workup of diseases involving the liver, biliary tract, kidneys, abdominal aorta, and abdominal masses. It is particularly useful in defining fluid versus solid (e.g., cyst versus solid mass), as well as in imaging fluid-filled structures, such as the gallbladder, urinary bladder, and renal pelvis. The various abdominal organs and

pathologic processes have their own characteristic echo patterns, as shown in Fig 3-29.

Obstetric and gynecologic US is particularly important because of the absence of significant biological risk to the fetus or maternal genital structures. In obstetric US, the fetus is surrounded by amniotic fluid, making visualization easier (Fig. 3-30). In addition, one can use real-time US images to evaluate the beating heart. For gynecological examinations, both transabdominal (Fig. 3-31) and transvaginal techniques are used. Transvaginal imaging has the technical advantage of eliminating echoes from the abdominal
(*text continues on page 100*)

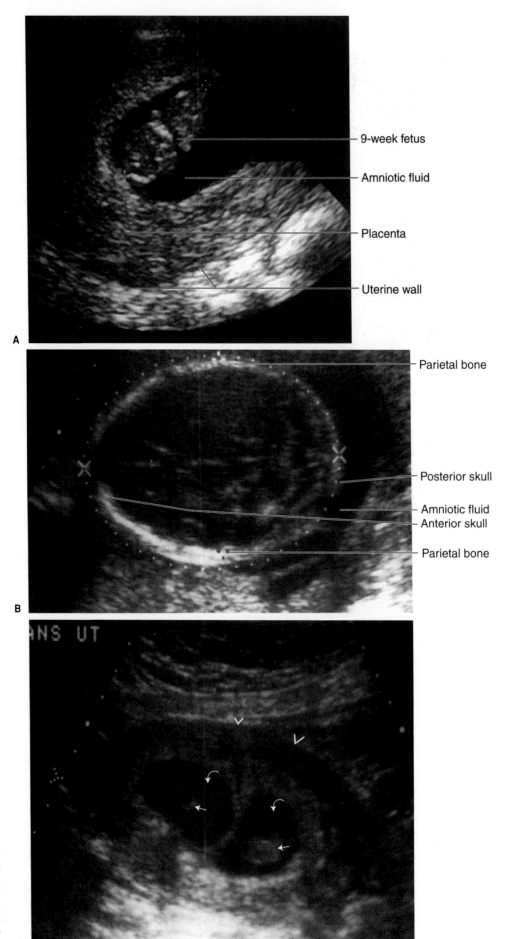

— 9-week fetus

— Amniotic fluid

— Placenta

— Uterine wall

A

— Parietal bone

— Posterior skull

— Amniotic fluid
— Anterior skull

— Parietal bone

B

C

FIGURE 3-30. Obstetric sonograms **A:** Study in a 9-week fetus. The *caliper markers* indicating crown to rump distance confirm the 9-week gestation. **B:** Skull of a fetus near term. The *white dotted lines* outline the skull, and the biparietal diameter confirms the fetal age. The cerebral ventricles are vaguely seen within the skull. **C:** Twin pregnancy. The uterine wall is marked by the *arrowheads*. Each fetus (*straight arrows*) is surrounded by amniotic fluid (*curved arrows*). These are separate sacs.

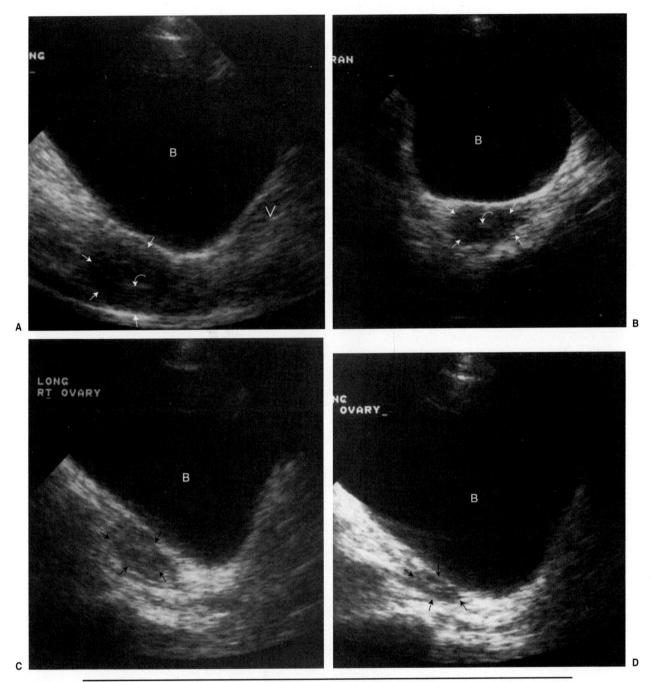

FIGURE 3-31. A: Transabdominal midline longitudinal (sagittal) sonogram. Normal uterus (*straight arrows*). The urine-filled bladder is essentially echo free and thus serves as an acoustic window to the pelvis. Notice the characteristic homogeneous echo pattern of the normal uterus. The endometrial stripe (*curved arrow*) represents the layers that line the endometrial cavity. The presence of the endometrial stripe indicates the absence of an intrauterine pregnancy or other intrauterine mass (*B*, urinary bladder; *V*, vagina). **B:** Transabdominal transverse (axial) sonogram. Normal uterus. The uterine fundus is outlined by the *straight arrows*; the endometrial stripe (*curved arrow*) appears smaller on the transverse image. **C:** Transabdominal right longitudinal (sagittal) sonogram. Normal right ovary (*straight arrows*). **D:** Transabdominal left longitudinal (sagittal) sonogram. Normal left ovary (*straight arrows*).

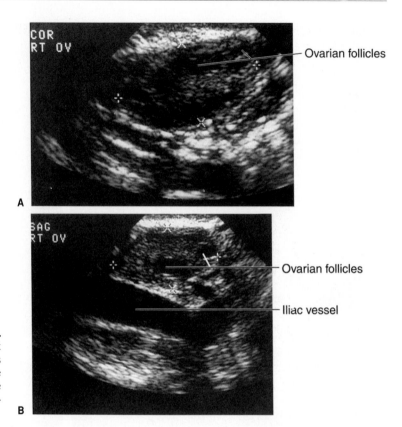

Ovarian follicles

A

Ovarian follicles

Iliac vessel

B

FIGURE 3-32. Transvaginal sonograms of the right (**A**) and left (**B**) ovaries. The dimensions of the ovaries are indicated by the *X marks* and *crosses*. Note the better definition of the ovaries, so that follicles are visible, when compared with the transabdominal images (Fig. 3-31).

wall from the area of interest, allowing better definition of genital organs (Fig. 3-32).

US evaluation of the prostate has been disappointing, as it is relatively insensitive to identifying abnormalities of this organ. In the scrotum, US is superb. It localizes the site of disease (e.g., testis versus epididymis), and often allows specific diagnosis of the abnormality present (Fig. 3-33). Correct diagnosis of epididymitis versus testicular torsion versus orchitis is possible, separating those who need surgery from those who require only medical treatment. Hydrocele and varicocele are easily identified with

US. Identification of testicular tumors is good, although identifying tumor type is less reliable.

COMPUTED TOMOGRAPHY AND MAGNETIC RESONANCE IMAGING OF THE ABDOMEN

Both CT and MRI are useful in the diagnosis and management of abdominal disease. CT is usually the favored procedure because of its wide availability and lower cost.

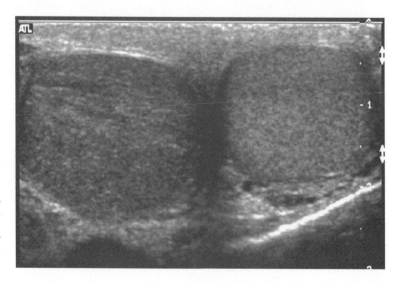

FIGURE 3-33. Transverse scrotal sonogram. The left testis is normal. The right testis is enlarged, has reduced echogenicity, and shows streaky, black linear echodensities. These findings indicate orchitis. (Courtesy of Monzer Abu-Yousef, M.D.)

Patient motion is seldom a problem in CT, but is a frequent occurrence in MRI. Both techniques have the ability to perform axial studies of the abdomen. MRI can, in fact, produce images in any dimension (axial, sagittal, coronal, or oblique).

Except in emergencies, the patient for CT has usually fasted for several hours. In most cases (suspected renal disease is the usual exception), a dilute contrast material is given orally before the study begins to demarcate the GI tract. This allows one to identify bowel loops, distinguishing them from masses and solid organs.

Immediately before (or sometimes during) abdominal CT, contrast material is injected intravenously to allow identification of arteries and veins (the enhanced CT). The intravenous contrast is excreted by the kidneys, so that the kidneys (and later the urinary collecting systems and bladder) will be opacified.

The abdominal MRI examination is tailored to the suspected abnormality, the technical details being beyond the scope of this discussion. Intravenous contrast agents, such as gadolinium, which can change the MR signal in many organs and diseases, are frequently given as part of the MR study.

How to Read Abdominal Computed Tomography and Magnetic Resonance Imaging

Reading axial images of the abdomen is not particularly difficult for the neophyte radiologist *if* one's anatomical knowledge is adequate. You will find the system described herein to be time-consuming but rewarding. First, arrange the images in order, from top (toward the head) to bottom. In many circumstances, that is already done for you electronically. Next, look at all the images in Gestalt fashion to discover any obvious abnormalities. Then, look at each organ individually, from top to bottom (i.e., all CT slices containing the organ of interest). In each organ, evaluate the size and shape of each area of reduced or increased density. Do this for visible lung, liver, gallbladder, spleen, pancreas, adrenals, both kidneys and ureters, the bladder, and genitals. Evaluate the stomach, duodenum, small bowel mesentery, and colon/appendix. Study the retroperitoneum from top to bottom—aorta, vena cava, and mesenteric vessels, also looking for adenopathy or other masses. Check the peritoneal cavity for fluid or masses. Look at the vertebrae (and spinal cord within) and bony pelvis. Finally, concentrate on the abdominal wall, hips, and adjacent soft tissues. Thoroughness leads to success in reading abdominal CT scans.

The same system can be applied to abdominal MRI, but—unfortunately for the nonradiologist—there are usually many more images, with sagittal and coronal planes and several pulse sequences, often later supplemented with intravenous magnetic contrast material. Normal abdominal CT and MRI anatomy is illustrated in Fig. 3-34 to 3-45.

ANGIOGRAPHY

Aortography (catheter injection into the abdominal aorta) and selective arteriography of individual vessels in the abdomen are sometimes performed for diagnostic reasons, particularly in trauma or with gastrointestinal hemorrhage. With rapid CT imaging, visualization of the arteries and/or veins can be obtained using this modality after intravenous contrast material, thus avoiding the necessity for placing an intraaortic catheter.

Recall that moving tissue, such as intravascular blood, has less MRI signal than surrounding tissue. Various technical manipulations are possible using this phenomenon, with or without the addition of magnetic contrast material, to allow excellent visualization of almost all of the major abdominal vessels without aortic catheterization (Figs. 3-46 and 3-47). The choice of CT angiography versus MR angiography is largely dependent on the expertise of the radiologist and the type of equipment available at individual institutions.

Conventional angiography was used in the past to delineate tumors of the solid organs. CT and MRI are now more effective and less invasive methods for characterizing masses.

IMAGING FEATURES OF GASTROINTESTINAL ABNORMALITIES

The gut, being a hollow organ extending from the mouth to the anus, has a basic structure and radiographic appearance throughout. If contrast material (barium) fills the gut, one obtains information about the lumen and gut wall. Visualization of the mucosal surface is improved by double-contrast techniques, as barium coating the mucosal surface contrasts with the intraluminal air. Thus, there are only a few basic patterns that are much alike within the esophagus, stomach, and small or large bowel (Fig. 3-48). They are the following:

1. Intraluminal lesion. Examples include a polyp, foreign body, or exophytic tumor.
2. Mucosal diseases. Examples include inflammation of the mucosa and adjacent musculature, indicative of enteritis.
3. Mural lesion. The abnormality is in the bowel wall (with or without concomitant mucosal involvement). Examples include tumor, transmucosal inflammation, and edema. If the abnormality encircles the bowel wall (as is often seen in colon cancer), a napkin-ring appearance results.
4. Extrinsic lesions. Here, both the bowel wall and lumen are displaced by an extrinsic force. Examples include enlarged mesenteric nodes adjacent to the gut.
5. Extraluminal projections beyond the bowel lumen. Typical abnormalities are ulcerations and diverticula.

(*text continues on page 112*)

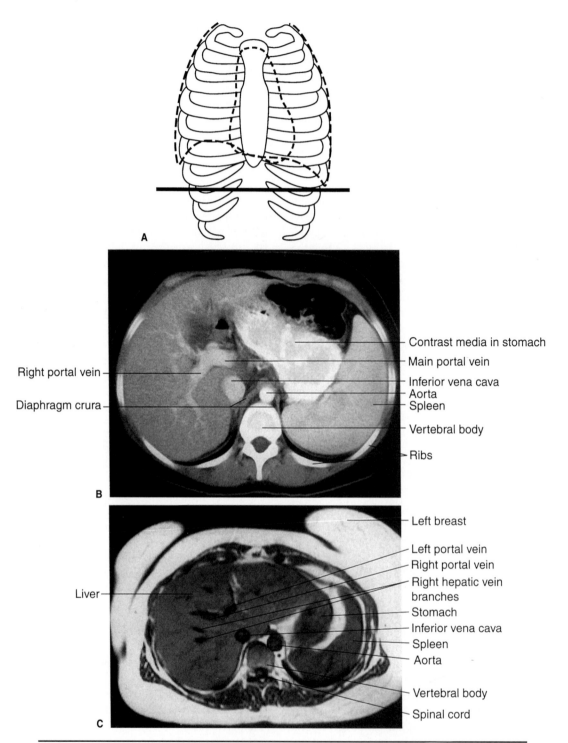

FIGURE 3-34. A: Illustration of the approximate axial anatomic level through the liver and spleen for B and C. **B:** Abdomen axial CT image through the liver and spleen. Normal. **C:** Abdomen axial MR image through the liver and spleen. Normal.

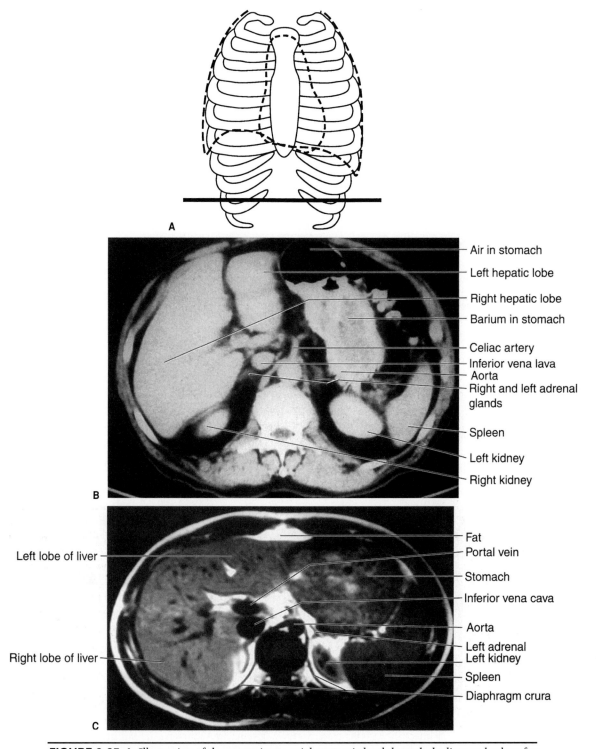

FIGURE 3-35. **A:** Illustration of the approximate axial anatomic level through the liver and spleen for B and C. This level is just caudad to the level in Fig. 3-34. **B:** Abdomen axial CT image through the liver and spleen. Normal. **C:** Abdomen axial MR image through the liver and spleen. Normal.

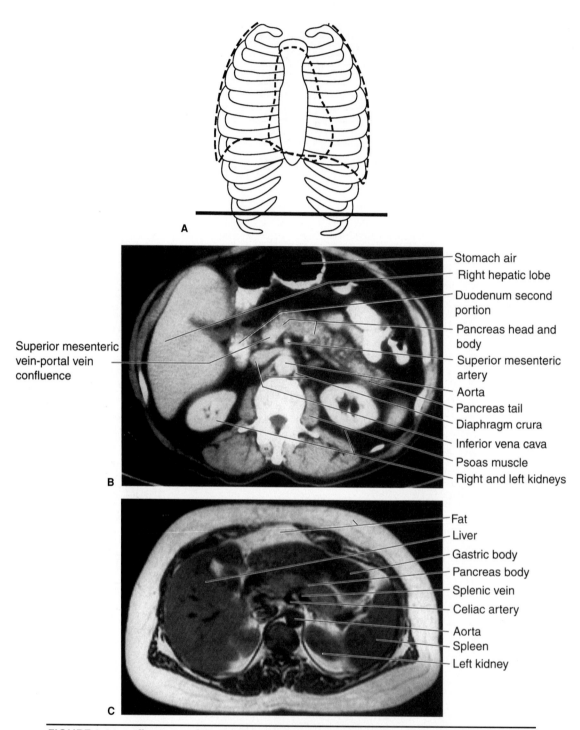

Stomach air

Right hepatic lobe

Duodenum second portion

Pancreas head and body

Superior mesenteric vein-portal vein confluence

Superior mesenteric artery

Aorta

Pancreas tail

Diaphragm crura

Inferior vena cava

Psoas muscle

Right and left kidneys

Fat

Liver

Gastric body

Pancreas body

Splenic vein

Celiac artery

Aorta

Spleen

Left kidney

FIGURE 3-36. A: Illustration of the approximate axial anatomic level through the pancreas for B and C. **B:** Abdomen axial CT image through the pancreas level. Normal. **C:** Abdomen axial MR image through the pancreas level. Normal.

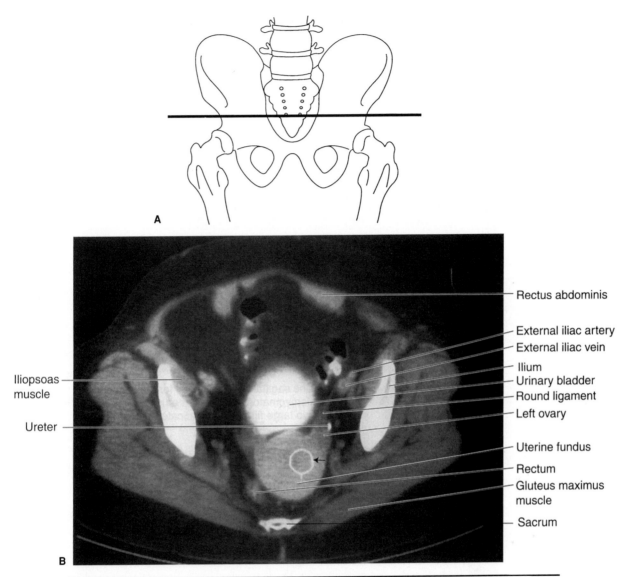

A

B

Iliopsoas muscle

Ureter

Rectus abdominis

External iliac artery
External iliac vein

Ilium
Urinary bladder
Round ligament
Left ovary

Uterine fundus

Rectum
Gluteus maximus muscle

Sacrum

FIGURE 3-37. A: Illustration of the approximate axial anatomic level for B. **B:** Female pelvis axial CT image through the uterus after intravenous contrast media. Normal. The white metallic density ring (*straight arrow*) that projects over the uterus is merely a region of interest (ROI) cursor for measuring tissue density.

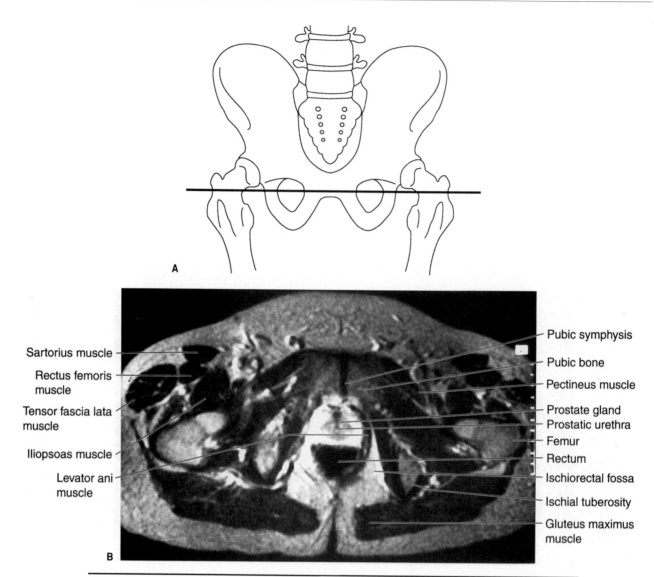

A

Sartorius muscle

Rectus femoris muscle

Tensor fascia lata muscle

Iliopsoas muscle

Levator ani muscle

B

Pubic symphysis

Pubic bone

Pectineus muscle

Prostate gland

Prostatic urethra

Femur

Rectum

Ischiorectal fossa

Ischial tuberosity

Gluteus maximus muscle

FIGURE 3-38. **A:** Illustration of the approximate axial anatomic level for B. **B:** Male pelvis axial T2 MR image at the level of the pubic symphysis and prostate. Normal.

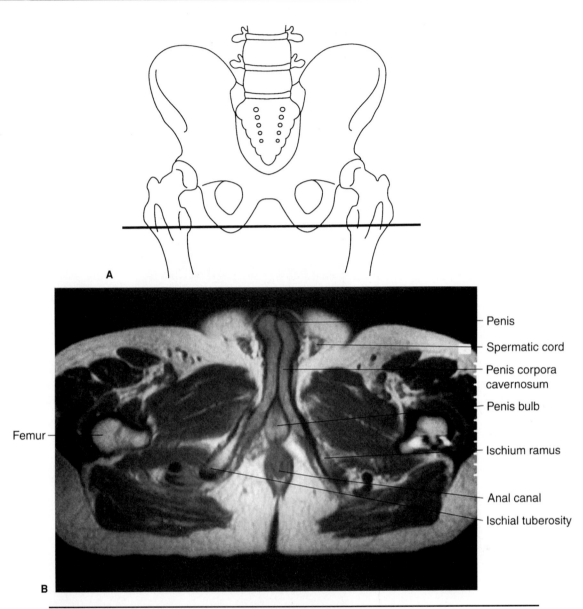

FIGURE 3-39. **A:** Illustration of the approximate axial anatomic level for B. **B:** Male pelvis axial T2 MR image at the level of the penile structures. Normal.

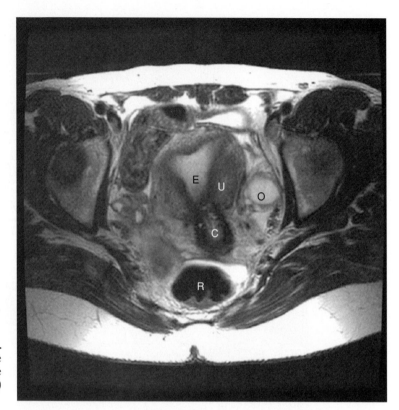

FIGURE 3-40. Female pelvis axial T2 MR. Same anatomic level as Fig. 3-38 (R, rectum; U, uterine wall; E, endometrial cavity; C, cervix; O, ovary.) (Courtesy of Alan Stolpen, M.D.)

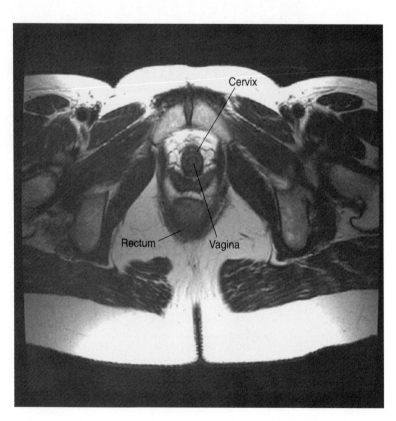

FIGURE 3-41. Female pelvis axial T2 MR. Same anatomic level as Fig. 3-39. (Courtesy of Alan Stolpen, M.D.)

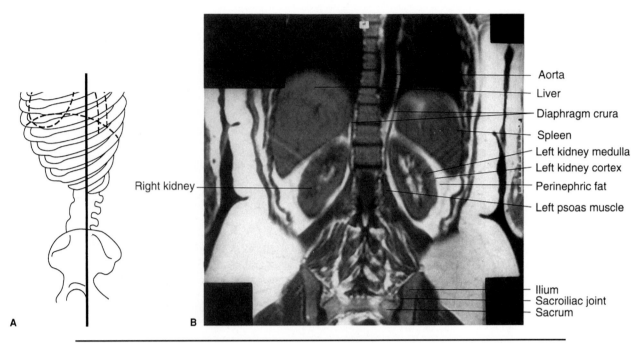

FIGURE 3-42. A: Illustration of the approximate coronal anatomic level through the kidneys for B. **B:** Abdomen coronal MR image through the kidneys. Normal.

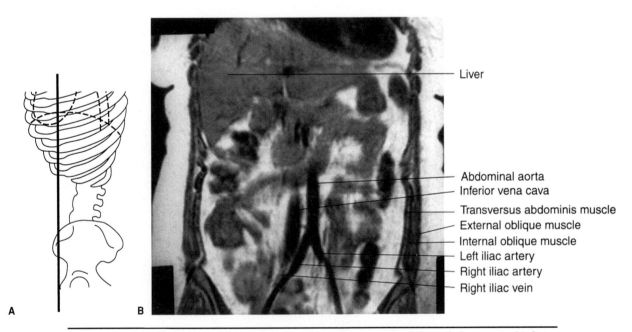

FIGURE 3-43. A: Illustration of the approximate coronal anatomic level through the aorta and inferior vena cava for B. **B:** Abdomen coronal MR image through the abdominal aorta and inferior vena cava. Normal.

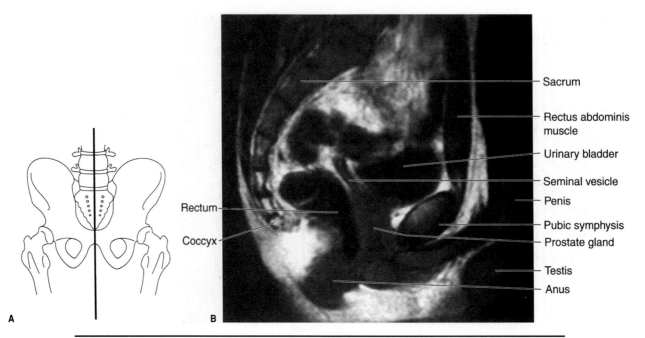

FIGURE 3-44. A: Illustration of the approximate midline sagittal anatomic level for B. **B:** Male pelvis midline sagittal T2 MR image at the level of the urinary bladder and pubic symphysis. Normal.

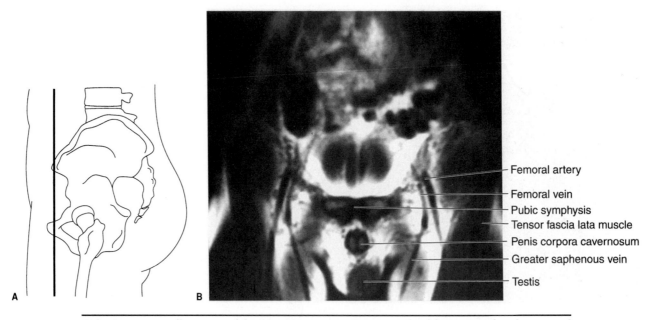

FIGURE 3-45. A: Illustration of the approximate coronal anatomic level for B. **B:** Male pelvis coronal T1 MR image through the pubic symphysis. Normal.

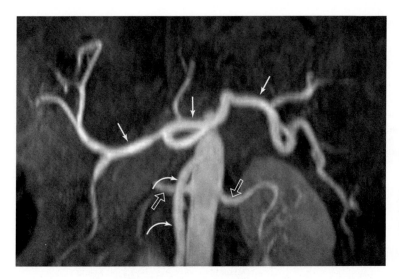

FIGURE 3-46. Magnetic resonance angiography of the upper abdomen. This MR image clearly defines the celiac (*straight arrows*) and superior mesenteric (*curved arrows*) arteries and their branches. The origins of the renal arteries (*open arrows*) from the aorta are noted. (Courtesy of Alan Stolpen, M.D.)

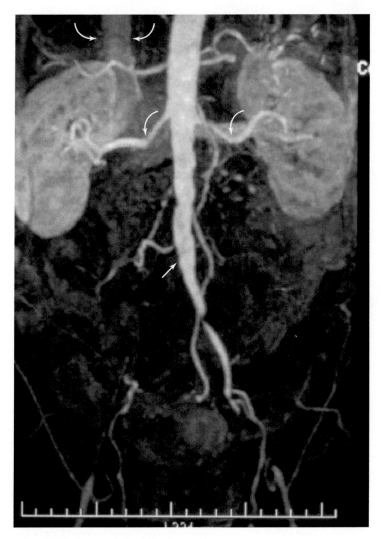

FIGURE 3-47. Magnetic resonance angiography of the aorta and its branches in a patient with arteriosclerosis. The right iliac artery is occluded at its origin (*arrow*). Both renal arteries (*curved arrows*) are intact. The inferior vena cava (*curved arrows*) can be seen. (Courtesy of Alan Stolpen, M.D.)

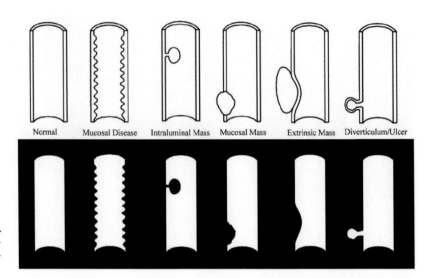

FIGURE 3-48. Types of gastrointestinal abnormalities (**above**) and their radiographic appearance (**below**).

Symptoms arising from esophageal disease include heartburn and dysphagia (difficulty swallowing). In gastroesophageal reflux disease, common in elderly patients, heartburn and later dysphagia occur, owing to reflux of gastric contents into the esophagus, with resultant esophagitis and eventual stricture. Hiatal hernias often accompany gastroesophageal reflux. The barium esophagram easily detects hiatal hernia and stricture (Fig. 3-49). The esophagram is less sensitive in the diagnosis of esophagitis alone when compared with endoscopy. Esophageal cancer typically has an intraluminal and an intramural component with abnormal mucosa and narrowing of the esophageal lumen (Fig. 3-50). Esophagography is also useful in studying motility disorders of the esophagus.

The majority of upper GI series are performed to detect peptic ulcer disease in either the stomach or duodenum. Clearly protruding from the lumen, ulcers are most easily seen on double-contrast examinations (Fig. 3-51). If seen *en face*, the ulcer crater appears as a glob of increased density as barium fills the ulcer crater and the lumen is filled with air (Fig. 3-52). Often, mucosal folds radiate toward the ulcer crater, aiding in its detection. With recurrent disease, deformity of the adjacent bowel, particularly in the duodenum, accompanies the ulcer.

Gastric tumors are uncommon in North America. Polyps (Fig. 3-53) are seen in the elderly. Stomach cancer usually appears as an ulcerated, irregular mucosal mass, often accompanied by concentric narrowing of the adjacent stomach.

Localized small bowel disease in North America is most often Crohn's disease, which produces inflammation with mucosal ulcerations and thickening of the bowel wall (Fig. 3-54). Other localized lesions and primary small bowel tumors are rare.

A wide variety of metabolic, immune, and other disorders can involve the entire small bowel. The classic example is sprue (gluten hypersensitivity) with associated small bowel dilatation. Dilution of barium and prominence of the mucosal folds are also noted.

Barium enema studies are useful in the workup of inflammatory colon disease. Ulcerative colitis begins in the rectum and extends a variable distance proximally

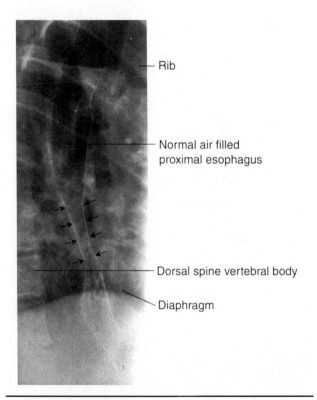

FIGURE 3-49. Double-contrast esophagram. Distal esophageal stricture. The smooth, long, tapered appearance of the narrowed distal esophagus (*straight arrows*) is typical of a benign stricture, owing to reflux of gastric contents into the esophagus.

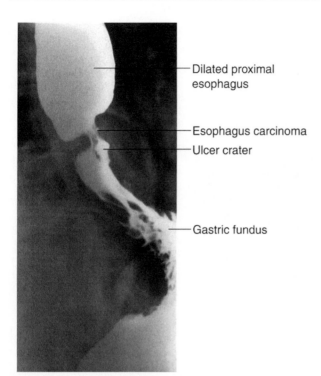

Dilated proximal esophagus

Esophagus carcinoma
Ulcer crater

Gastric fundus

FIGURE 3-50. Barium contrast esophagram. Carcinoma of the esophagus. The cancer produces a narrowed segment with irregular mucosa and ulceration. The proximal esophagus is dilated but otherwise normal.

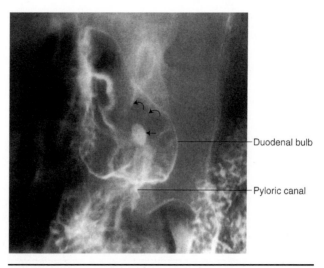

Duodenal bulb

Pyloric canal

FIGURE 3-52. Double-contrast upper GI series. Central duodenal bulb ulcer (*arrow*). The duodenal mucosal folds (*curved arrows*) radiate toward the ulcer crater.

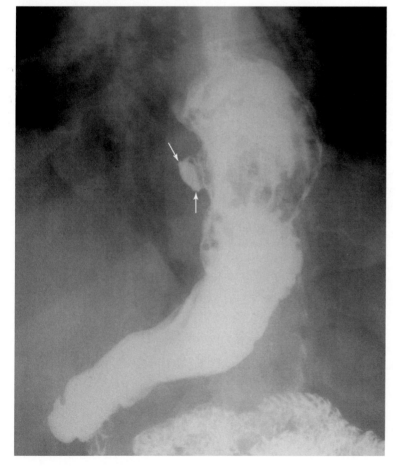

FIGURE 3-51. Gastric ulcer, upper GI series. The lesser curvature ulcer (*arrows*) protrudes from the stomach lumen.

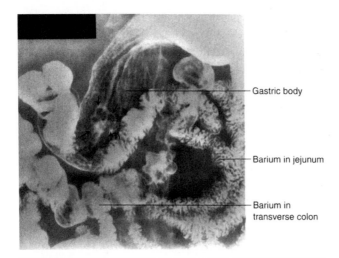

FIGURE 3-53. Double-contrast upper GI series. Gastric polyp. The stalk (*curved arrow*) of the benign polyp (*straight arrows*) is clearly visible.

(Fig. 3-55). The mucosal surface shows tiny ulcerations in a uniform nature throughout the affected area, often accompanied by loss of haustrations (the lead pipe colon). Crohn's disease affecting the colon (Fig. 3-56) often spares the rectum, skip lesions are common, and deeper ulcerations occur.

The barium enema, particularly with double-contrast technique, is valuable in detecting colon polyps as well as colon cancer. Intraluminal polyps (Fig. 3-57) are more easily detected than those that are sessile (along the colon wall). Evolution of polyps into colon cancer does occur; the larger the polyp, the greater the chance the histology will show a malignant change. There are approximately 150,000 new cases of carcinoma in the colon and rectum reported each year in the United States. Early detection of this disease improves survival dramatically. As colon cancer progresses in size, it often surrounds the bowel lumen in a fashion described as an apple core or napkin ring (Fig. 3-58). Large advanced cancers are evident on CT (Fig. 3-59).

There are a number of syndromes characterized by multiple colonic polyps, sometimes with additional polyps of the small bowel or stomach. Prominent among these is familial polyposis of the colon, which is characterized by multiple adenomas, all with malignant potential (Fig. 3-60).

Acute appendicitis is the most common surgical disease of the abdomen. If clinical history and physical examination are strongly suggestive of appendicitis, further imaging examinations are not needed, as the accuracy of clinical findings approaches 90%. Plain films of the abdomen are not particularly helpful in the diagnosis of appendicitis, unless a calcified appendicolith is noted. Imaging studies are most valuable in those individuals with

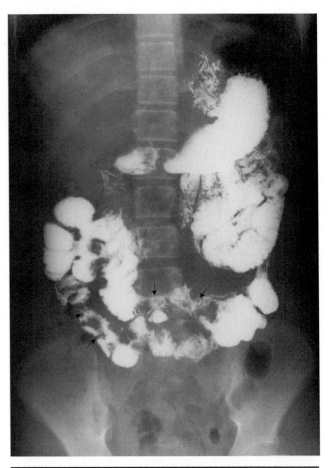

FIGURE 3-54. Crohn's disease of the ileum. Antegrade small bowel examination. The affected small bowel (*arrows*) is narrowed; the adjacent space between small bowel loops indicates bowel wall thickening.

low to moderate probability of a positive diagnosis (Fig. 3-61). In children, careful ultrasound examination is frequently the study of choice; CT is sometimes difficult because of the small amount of periappendiceal fat in this age group. In adults, multislice CT of the right lower quadrant, with or without the use of contrast material, is recommended. The abnormal appendix can be identified in most cases as a small tubular structure with distended lumen, thickening of the periappendiceal wall, and inflammation of adjacent fat (Fig. 3-62). One can usually diagnose perforation of the appendix by changes adjacent to the organ.

IMAGING FEATURES OF GENITOURINARY ABNORMALITIES

Certain anomalies obstruct the flow of urine, producing proximal obstruction. Congenital ureteropelvic junction (UPJ) obstructions can sometimes be diagnosed

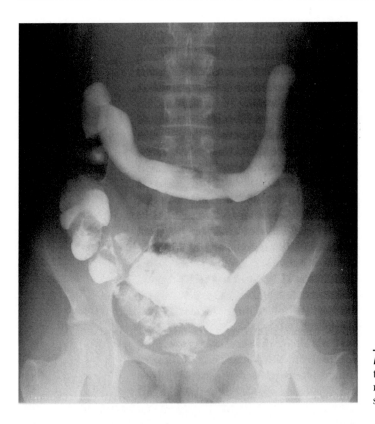

FIGURE 3-55. Ulcerative colitis. Barium enema. The entire colon, except the cecum, is uniformly narrowed, the mucosal surface is irregular, and the overall configuration suggests a lead pipe appearance.

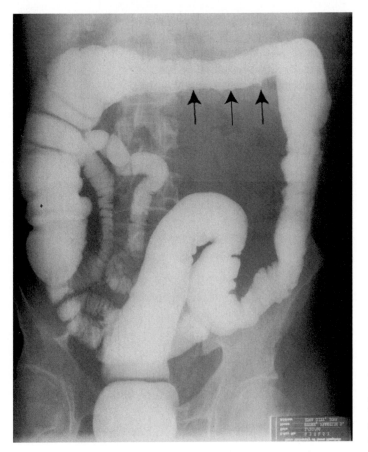

FIGURE 3-56. Crohn's disease of the colon. Barium enema. The rectum, sigmoid, and ascending colon are normal. The descending and transverse colon are slightly narrowed, and the mucosa is nodular with small ulcerations (*arrows*) extending from the colon lumen.

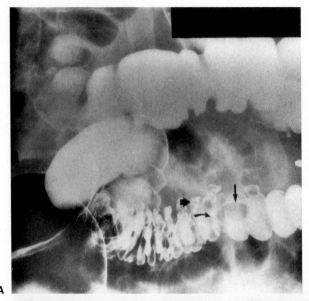

A

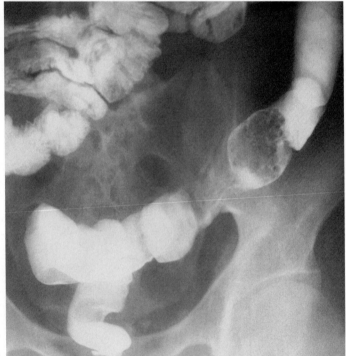

B

FIGURE 3-57. A: Double-contrast colon examination. Sigmoid colon benign polyp. The body of the polyp is indicated by the *long straight arrow,* and the polyp stalk (*curved arrow*) is clearly visible. Multiple diverticula (*short straight arrowhead*) are present in the sigmoid colon. **B:** Villous adenoma with focal carcinoma in the polyp mucosa. Barium enema. A large, lobulated mass fills the lumen of the sigmoid colon.

in utero; less severe cases do not present until later in life. Ultrasound is an excellent technique for demonstrating UPJ obstruction, showing the amount of pelvicalyceal dilatation and its effect on the renal parenchyma (Fig. 3-63). Congenital vesicoureteral junction obstruction is less frequent but usually bilateral.

Embryologically, the kidneys develop in the pelvis and migrate cephalad into the abdomen. The kidney that fails to migrate cephalad into the abdomen is called a pelvic kidney, sacral kidney, or simple ectopia (Fig. 3-64). Occasionally, a kidney will migrate to the side opposite

where it should normally reside, called crossed ectopia (Fig. 3-65). In a horseshoe kidney, the lower poles of the right and left kidneys are connected by a bridge, or isthmus, of renal tissue (Fig. 3-66).

Ureterocele (Fig. 3-67) refers to a dilated intramural ureteral segment that protrudes into the bladder, simulating a cobra's head. Ureteroceles result from either congenital or acquired stenosis at the ureteral orifice and can cause partial ureteral obstruction. Bladder diverticula generally are acquired but on occasion are congenital (Fig. 3-68).

(*text continues on page 122*)

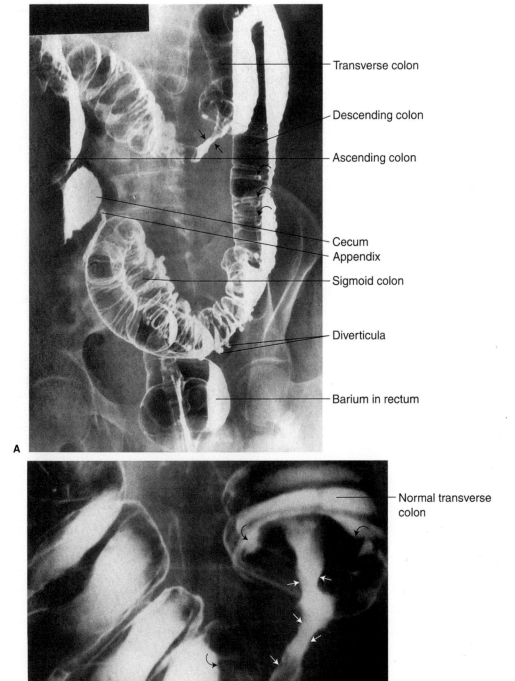

FIGURE 3-58. **A:** Adenocarcinoma of the transverse colon. Double-contrast colon examination. Note the classic apple core appearance of the colon cancer. The core represents the patent portion of the bowel lumen (*straight arrows*). Diverticula of the descending colon are seen *en face*. **B:** Close-up view of the tumor mass in A. Note the irregular mucosa of the narrowed lumen of the apple core lesion (*straight arrows*). The mass creates a shouldering (*curved arrows*) deformity in the neighboring transverse colon both proximally and distally.

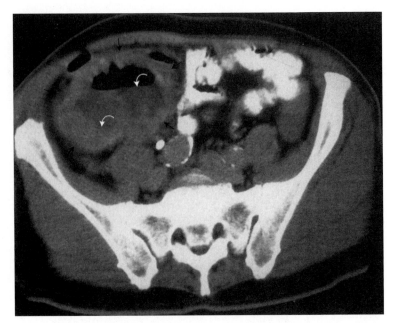

FIGURE 3-59. Lower abdomen axial CT image. The *white arrows* outline a large cecal neoplasm. The *curved arrows* show an air–fluid level within the tumor mass secondary to necrosis.

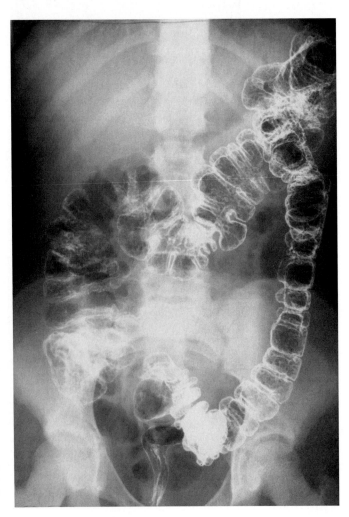

FIGURE 3-60. Familial polyposis of the colon. Double-contrast barium enema. There are innumerable tiny polyps throughout the colon.

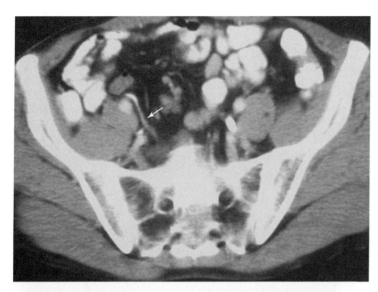

FIGURE 3-61. Normal appendix. Abdominal CT. The appendix is the wormlike, barium-filled density (*arrows*) in the right lower quadrant. (Courtesy of Bruce Brown, M.D.)

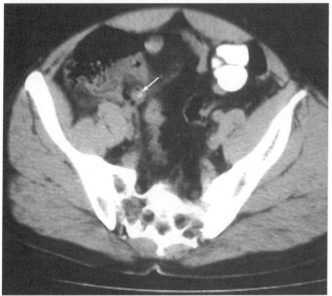

FIGURE 3-62. Abdominal CT transverse view of appendix. Appendicitis with perforation. A calcified appendicolith is in the lumen of the appendix (*arrow*). There is gas in the appendiceal wall and periappendiceal fluid. (Courtesy of Bruce Brown, M.D.)

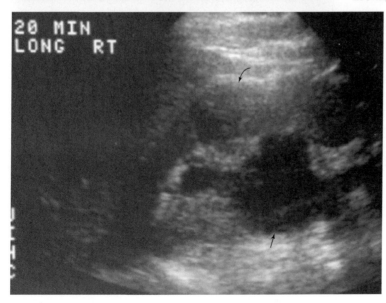

FIGURE 3-63. Abdominal sonogram. Ureteropelvic junction obstruction. The echo-free renal pelvis and associated calyces (*arrows*) are dilated. Renal–cortical borders are outlined by *curved arrows*. (Courtesy of Monzer Abu-Yousef, M.D.)

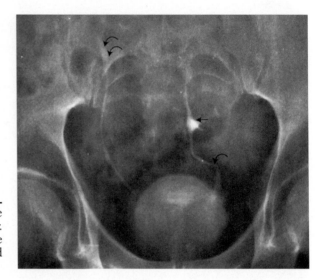

FIGURE 3-64. Abdomen AP EU. Pelvic kidney (simple ectopia). The left kidney is situated in the pelvis, just cephalad to the urinary bladder. The upper collecting system of the pelvic kidney is indicated by the *straight arrow*. Note the foreshortened left ureter (*curved arrow*) and the normal right ureter (*double curved arrows*).

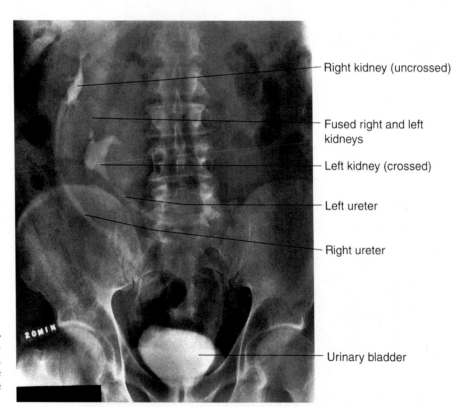

Right kidney (uncrossed)

Fused right and left kidneys

Left kidney (crossed)

Left ureter

Right ureter

Urinary bladder

FIGURE 3-65. Abdomen AP 20-minute EU. Crossed fused ectopia. In this anomaly, the upper pole of the crossed kidney is usually fused to the lower pole of the uncrossed kidney.

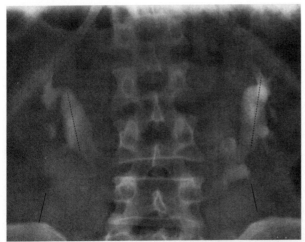

A

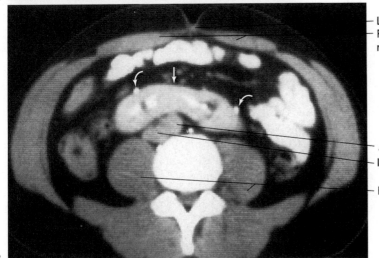

B

— Linea alba
— Rectus abdominis
   muscle

— Aorta
— Inferior vena cava

— Psoas muscle's

FIGURE 3-66. A: Abdomen AP EU. Horseshoe kidney. The lower poles of the kidneys are oriented medially. A helpful clue to the diagnosis is that the renal axes (*dotted lines*) are not parallel with the psoas muscle margins (*solid lines*). **B:** Lower abdomen axial CT with intravenous contrast media. A bridge of renal tissue or isthmus (*straight arrow*) connects the renal lower poles, which are anterior to the aorta and inferior vena cava. The ureters cross the isthmus anteriorly (*curved arrows*), and the upper collecting systems are indicated by the *double straight arrows*.

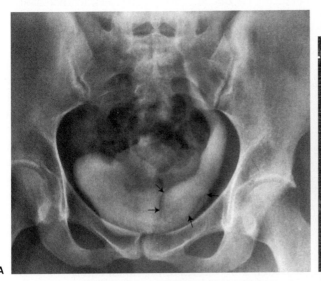

A

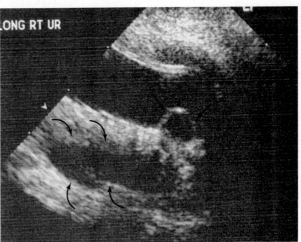

B

FIGURE 3-67. A: Pelvis AP EU. Ureterocele. Note the cobra head appearance (*straight arrows*) of the ureterocele. The left ureter is moderately dilated. **B:** Ureterocele, pelvic ultrasound. The wall of the ureterocele (*arrows*) is visualized by echo-free urine in the bladder and within the ureterocele. A dilated ureter (*curved arrows*) is noted posterior to the bladder.

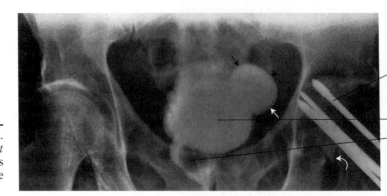

Metallic orthopedic pins

Urinary bladder

Foley catheter balloon

FIGURE 3-68. Cystogram. Bladder diverticulum (*straight arrow*). There are unilateral pins traversing a left hip fracture (*curved arrow*).

Urolithiasis is one of the most common urologic problems encountered in the everyday practice of medicine. Most ureteral stones are less than 1 cm in diameter, and approximately 75% of acutely symptomatic stones are located in the distal third of the ureter. Approximately 90% of all genitourinary (GU) calculi are radiopaque on plain film.

Some radiopaque renal calculi actually fill all or part of an upper collecting system and are called staghorn calculi (Fig. 3-69). When such calculi are bilateral, their appearance should not be mistaken for contrast media in the upper collecting systems. Obviously, calculi can occur at any location in the urinary tract (Fig. 3-70). The differential diagnosis for a renal pelvis filling (nonradiopaque) defect is listed in Table 3-6.

Multiple unilateral or bilateral interstitial renal calcifications are referred to as nephrocalcinosis. Nephrolithiasis, or calcification in the renal tubules, occurs with metabolic abnormalities (hypercalcemia) or with congenitally dilated collecting tubules (medullary sponge kidney). The plain film appearance (Fig. 3-71) is pathognomic—another Aunt Minnie.

Although EU is often used to diagnose urolithiasis (it is valuable in quantitating the degree of ureteral obstruction), it is considerably less sensitive than CT. Current protocol for patients with suspected ureteral stones calls for multislice CT through the regions of the kidneys and ureters without intravenous contrast material (Fig. 3-72).

Therapeutic ultrasound has become a useful tool for breaking up calculi. This is called extracorporeal sound wave lithotripsy, or ESWL (Fig. 3-73). The fragmented calculi usually pass spontaneously without surgical intervention.

GU infections are a common occurrence in medicine and usually do not require diagnostic imaging procedures. In children, especially males, with documented urinary infection, study for vesicoureteral reflux is recommended (Fig. 3-28), and ultrasound study of the kidneys is often of value. Severity of infection ranges from mild cystitis to perinephric abscess (Fig. 3-74). Acute pyelonephritis usually causes renal enlargement, which may be focal (Fig. 3-75); with atrophic pyelonephritis, the kidney may shrink.

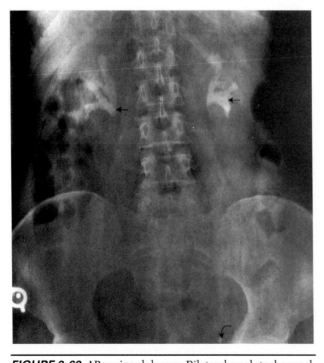

FIGURE 3-69. AP supine abdomen. Bilateral renal staghorn calculi. The calculi (*straight arrows*) closely resemble contrast media in upper collecting systems, demonstrating the importance of the preliminary radiograph. Incidentally noted is a left pelvic phlebolith (*curved arrow*).

▶ TABLE 3-6   Masses in the Renal Pelvis

- Stones
- Tumor
- Mycetoma (fungus ball)
- Blood clot
- Necrotic renal papillae

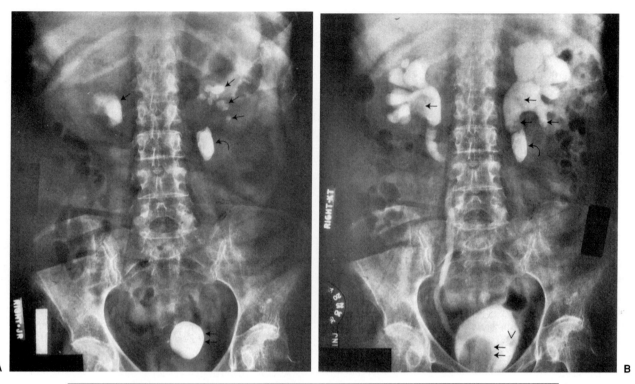

A   B

FIGURE 3-70. A: Abdomen preliminary radiograph. There are bilateral radiopaque renal calculi (*straight arrows*), a large radiopaque calculus in the proximal left ureter (*curved arrow*), and a large radiopaque calculus in the urinary bladder (*double straight arrows*). **B:** Abdomen AP 5-minute EU in the same patient as A. Bilateral dilated upper collecting systems contain multiple filling defects secondary to calculi (*straight arrows*). The proximal left ureter is obstructed by a large calculus (*curved arrows*), and the entire right ureter is dilated, suggesting an obstructing calculus at the ureterovesical junction. The opaque urinary bladder calculus (*double straight arrows*) now appears nonopaque relative to the more dense surrounding contrast media. Note bladder catheter (*arrowhead*).

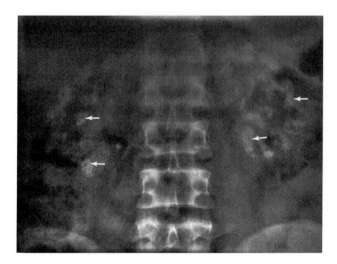

FIGURE 3-71. Nephrolithiasis. The abdominal radiograph shows extensive bilateral calculi (*arrows*) in a radial distribution.

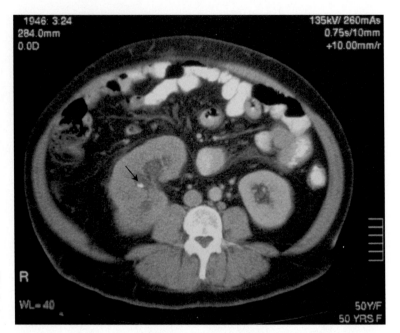

FIGURE 3-72. Abdominal axial CT at the level of the kidneys. A renal stone (*arrow*) is in a calyx of the right kidney (it was invisible on the abdominal radiograph). (Courtesy of Rommel Dhadha, M.D.)

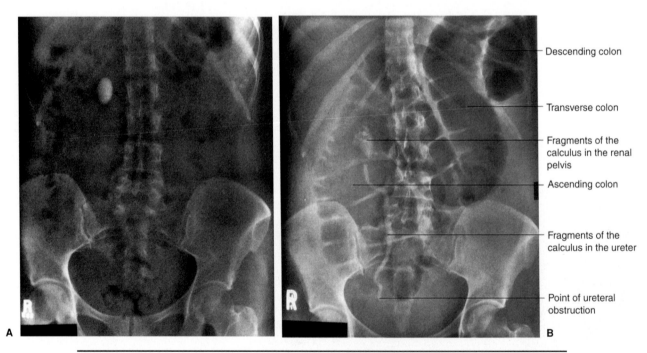

FIGURE 3-73. A: Abdomen AP radiograph. Solitary radiopaque calculus in the right renal pelvis (*straight arrow*). **B:** Abdomen AP radiograph 24 hours post–extracorporeal sound wave lithotripsy (ESWL). The obstructed ureter is filled with multiple small fragments of the calculus, referred to as "steinstrasse" (or "stone street"). The colon is air-filled and dilated (adynamic ileus), owing to pain of renal colic.

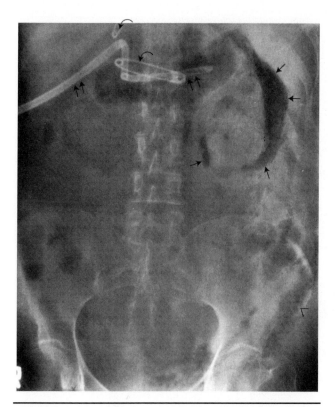

FIGURE 3-74. Abdomen AP supine radiograph. Left perinephric abscess. There is gas in the abscess surrounding the left kidney (*straight arrows*). An abscess drain (*double straight arrows*) is in place, and common safety pins (*curved arrows*) project over the abdomen. There is gas in the subcutaneous tissues of the left flank (*arrowhead*) secondary to extension of infection.

Renal cysts may be single, multiple, unilateral, or bilateral. These lesions are usually asymptomatic and often are an incidental finding on EU, US, or CT performed for other reasons. Although cysts are of no clinical significance, they must be evaluated closely to distinguish them from solid tumors. This is easily done with US (Fig. 3-76) or CT (Fig. 3-77) as the water density and sharp borders of cysts are apparent. Other benign renal tumors are uncommon.

Malignant renal tumors are solid masses. Approximately 90% are renal cell carcinomas. Patients with renal cell carcinomas may present with gross or microscopic hematuria, pain, or other symptoms. US (Fig. 3-78) determines the solid nature of the mass. CT and/or MRI is the proven method of diagnosis. EU is less sensitive and accurate. The radiologic features of primary renal malignancies are shown in Table 3-8, and some examples of these tumors are shown in Figs. 3-79 and 3-80.

Malignant tumors of the urothelium occur in the renal pelvis, ureter, or bladder. As they often cause urinary obstruction, ureteral opacification displays them best (Figs. 3-81 and 3-82).

Extrinsic malignancies, such as retroperitoneal tumors, can displace or obstruct the ureter (Fig. 3-83). Primary and secondary neoplasms can also involve the ureter and bladder (Figs. 3-84 and 3-85).

OBSTETRIC AND GYNECOLOGICAL IMAGING

There is seldom a need today for abdominal plain films in the diagnosis of pregnancy; however, when such a study is done (for necessity or by accident; Fig. 3-86), the risk of damage to the fetus from radiation is extremely low. Here is another Aunt Minnie—a radiograph showing an intrauterine contraceptive device (Fig. 3-87).

(*text continues on page 130*)

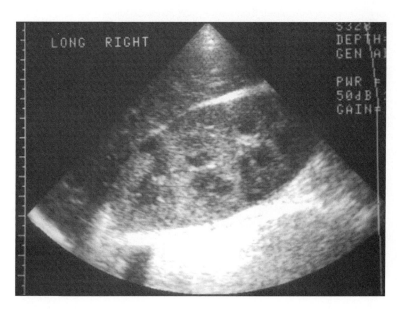

FIGURE 3-75. Sagittal sonogram of right kidney. Segmental pyelonephritis. Note the increased echogenicity of the upper pole. The foci of decreased lucency in both upper and lower poles are the renal pyramids. (Courtesy of Monzer Abu-Yousef, M.D.)

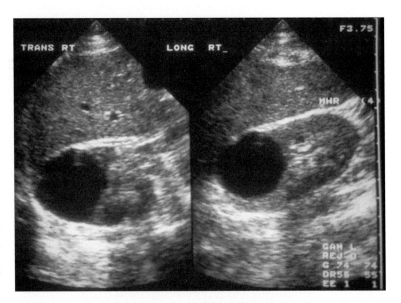

FIGURE 3-76. Transverse and longitudinal sonograms of the right kidney. Renal cyst of the upper pole. The cyst is echolucent, has sharp borders, and shows posterior enhancement. (Courtesy of Monzer Abu-Yousef, M.D.)

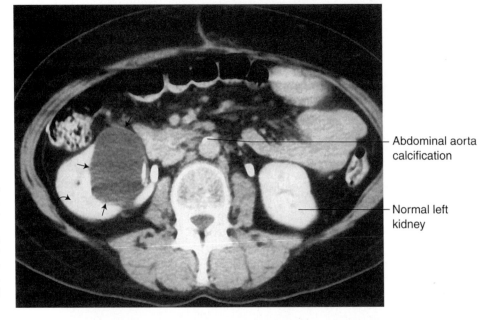

FIGURE 3-77. Abdomen axial CT image through the kidneys after intravenous contrast media. Right renal cyst. The cyst has sharp, smooth margins (*straight arrows*) and a low tissue density when compared with the remainder of the right kidney (*curved arrow*).

Abdominal aorta
calcification

Normal left
kidney

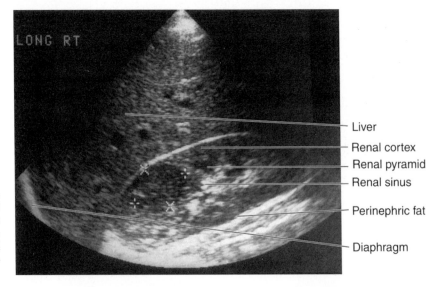

FIGURE 3-78. Renal cell carcinoma. Right renal longitudinal sonogram. The electronic caliper *X marks* and *crosses* delineate an upper pole renal mass. The numerous internal echoes (hyperechoic) within the mass indicate it is solid.

Liver

Renal cortex

Renal pyramid

Renal sinus

Perinephric fat

Diaphragm

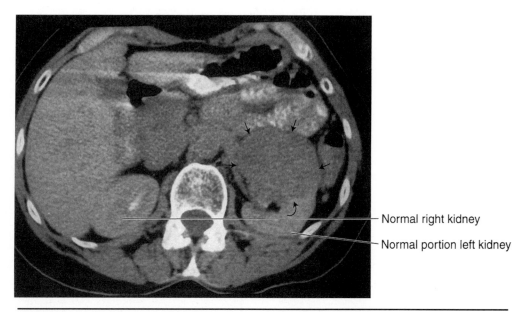

Normal right kidney

Normal portion left kidney

FIGURE 3-79. Abdomen axial CT. Left renal cell carcinoma (*straight arrows*). The mass lesion is solid, and its border with the normal kidney (*curved arrow*) is poorly defined.

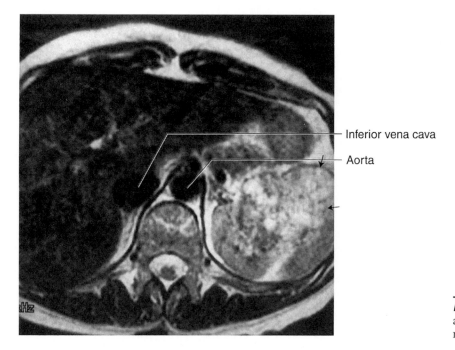

Inferior vena cava

Aorta

FIGURE 3-80. Abdomen axial T2 MR image. There is a large left renal cell carcinoma (*arrows*).

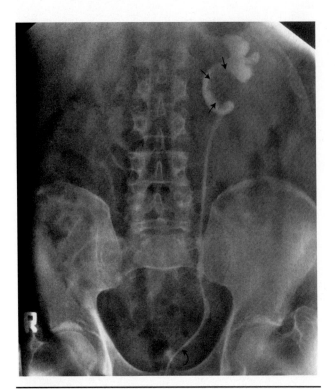

FIGURE 3-81. Left retrograde pyelogram. Transitional cell carcinoma of the left renal pelvis (*straight arrows*). A left ureter retrograde catheter (*curved arrow*) is in place.

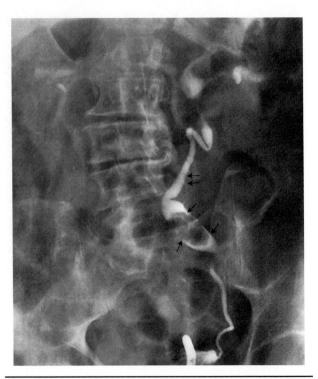

FIGURE 3-82. Left retrograde pyelogram. A partially obstructing ureteral carcinoma (*straight arrows*) has resulted in a dilated proximal ureter (*double straight arrows*). A cystoscope is in the bladder.

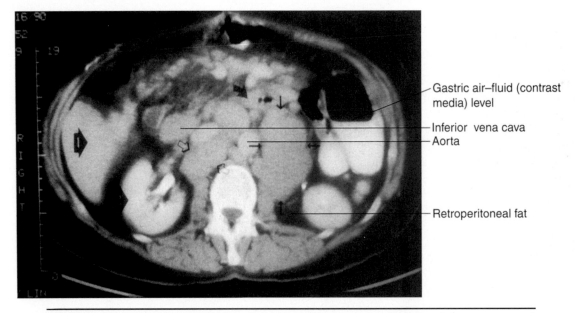

Gastric air–fluid (contrast media) level

Inferior vena cava

Aorta

Retroperitoneal fat

FIGURE 3-83. Abdomen axial CT image. Lymphoma. The tumor (*small black* and *short open arrows*) involves lymph nodes in the retroperitoneum and surrounds the enhanced aorta and inferior vena cava. The arrow labeled **1** indicates the inferior aspect of the liver.

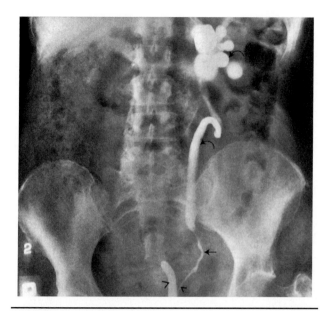

FIGURE 3-84. Left retrograde pyelogram. Encasement of the distal left ureter by cancer of the cervix has resulted in stricture and partial obstruction of the distal left ureter (*straight arrow*). The left ureter proximal to the stricture is dilated (*curved arrows*). The cystoscope and retrograde catheter (*arrowheads*) can be seen.

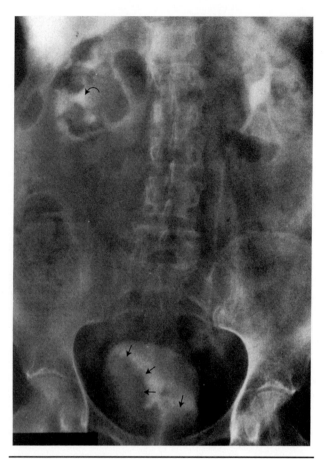

FIGURE 3-85. Abdomen AP EU. Transitional cell carcinoma of the bladder. The bladder mass (*straight arrows*) is partially obstructing the right ureteral orifice, resulting in a dilated right upper collecting system (*curved arrow*). The left kidney and ureter are normal.

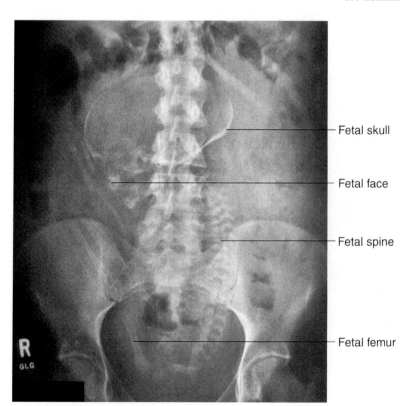

Fetal skull

Fetal face

Fetal spine

Fetal femur

FIGURE 3-86. Abdomen AP radiograph. Third-trimester intrauterine pregnancy in a breech presentation.

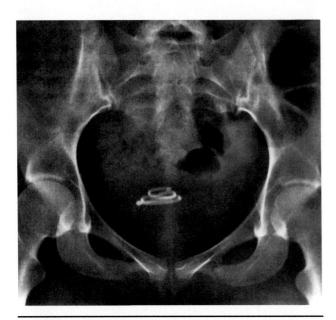

FIGURE 3-87. Pelvis AP radiograph. Intrauterine contraceptive device (IUD). The *straight arrow* indicates the normal position and appearance of the IUD.

Routine ultrasound evaluation of the pregnant woman and her fetus, a standard practice in the developed world, is of considerable value in obstetrics. Fetal maturation, major anomalies, placental assessment, and many associated maternal conditions can be evaluated (Figs. 3-88 and 3-89). Ectopic (tubal) pregnancy is readily diagnosed with ultrasound (Fig. 3-90).

Uterine anomalies and tubal diseases affecting fertility are often studied with hysterosalpingography. In this examination, contrast material is injected into the cervix, outlining the uterine cavity and fallopian tubes (Fig. 3-91). In the normal woman, contrast spills into the peritoneal cavity. Uterine anomalies can be detected with US, CT, and MRI (Fig. 3-92). Infected fallopian tubes typically fill with pus (pyosalpinx) and have characteristic ultrasound features (Fig. 3-93).

Benign uterine fibroids (leiomyomatosis), the most common gynecologic tumor, can (if calcified) be recognized by their classic appearance in the abdominal radiograph (Fig. 3-94). They are often seen on other imaging modalities (Fig. 3-95 and 3-96).

Imaging has, to date, played a minor role in evaluating carcinoma of the endometrium. MRI may be useful in staging cervical cancer (Fig. 3-97).

Detectability of ovarian tumors is much better with imaging studies than with physical examination. Tumors are seldom diagnosed on plain film unless they are huge or have typical features (Fig. 3-98). Both benign and malignant neoplasms have characteristic features on US, CT, and MRI. As in the kidney, ultrasound separates solid and cystic (usually benign) masses (Fig. 3-99).

(*text continues on page 136*)

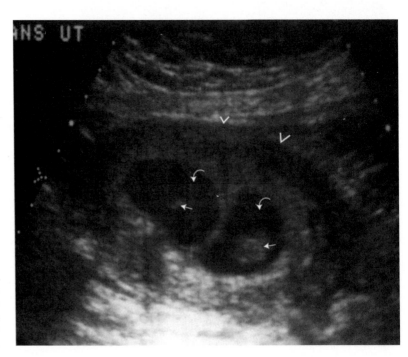

FIGURE 3-88. Transabdominal transverse obstetrical sonogram. Twin pregnancy. The twin fetuses (*straight arrows*) are located in separate sacs and are surrounded by amniotic fluid (*curved arrows*). The uterine wall is indicated by *arrowheads*.

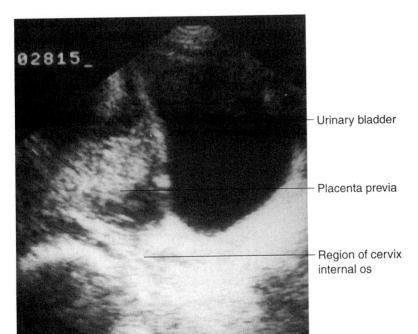

— Urinary bladder

— Placenta previa

— Region of cervix
internal os

FIGURE 3-89. Transabdominal longitudinal (sagittal) sonogram. Placenta previa. The sonogram shows the placenta covering the internal cervical os, thus precluding vaginal delivery.

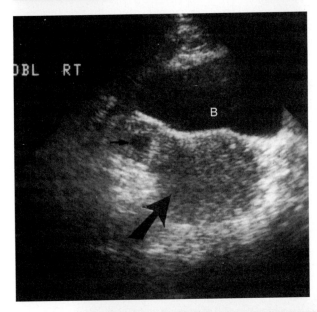

FIGURE 3-90. Transabdominal oblique sonogram. Ectopic pregnancy. The *large arrow* indicates a hyperechoic, blood-filled uterus. The *small arrow* indicates the gestational sac in the right fallopian tube (B, urinary bladder).

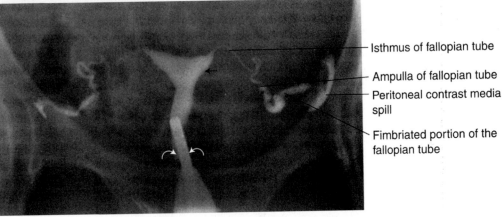

— Isthmus of fallopian tube

— Ampulla of fallopian tube

— Peritoneal contrast media spill

— Fimbriated portion of the fallopian tube

FIGURE 3-91. Hysterosalpingogram. Normal uterus (*straight arrow*) and fallopian tubes. Contrast media injected into the uterus via a cervical cannula (*curved arrows*) spills into the peritoneal space, indicating fallopian tube patency.

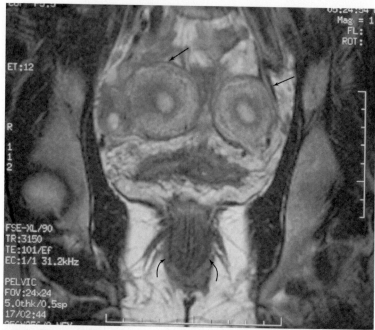

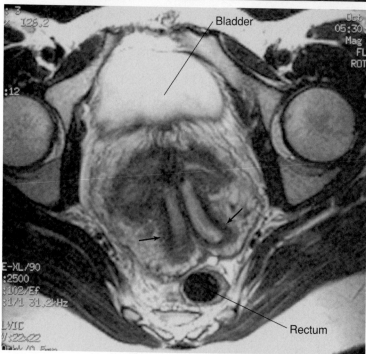

FIGURE 3-92. Coronal (**A**) and axial (**B**) pelvic MRI. Uterine didelphys, demonstrating two separate uteri (*arrows*) with their endometrial cavities two uterine cervices, and two vaginas (*curved arrows*). (Courtesy of Alan Stolpen, M.D.)

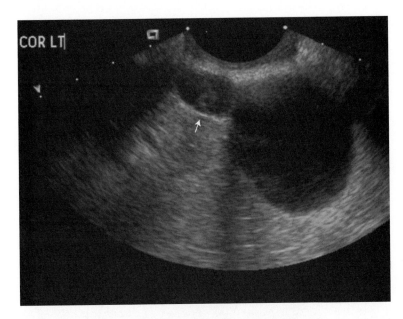

FIGURE 3-93. Coronal transvaginal sonogram. Hydro(pyo)salpinx. The fluid collection has some internal echoes; its configuration is oval with a smaller oval communication (*arrow*) at the apex; this establishes the fallopian tube as the locale of the abnormality. (Courtesy of Monzer Abu-Yousef, M.D.)

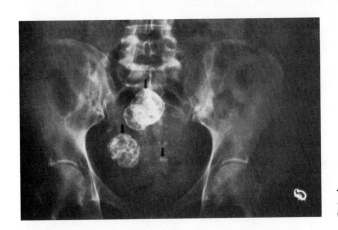

FIGURE 3-94. Pelvic radiograph. The calcified uterine fibroids (*arrows*) are an Aunt Minnie.

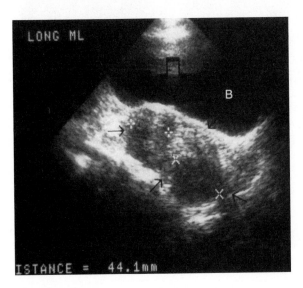

FIGURE 3-95. Transabdominal longitudinal (sagittal) sonogram. The uterus is outlined by the *black straight arrows*. The electronic caliper *X marks* and *crosses* outline two large fibroids. The many internal echoes within the masses indicate that they are solid.

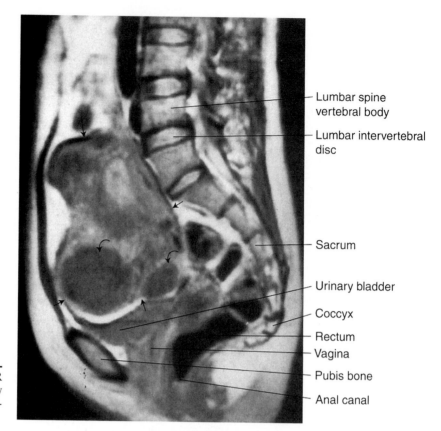

Lumbar spine
vertebral body

Lumbar intervertebral
disc

Sacrum

Urinary bladder

Coccyx

Rectum

Vagina

Pubis bone

Anal canal

FIGURE 3-96. Pelvis midline sagittal T1 MR image. The enlarged uterus is outlined by *straight arrows*. Two large fibroids are indicated by the *curved arrows*.

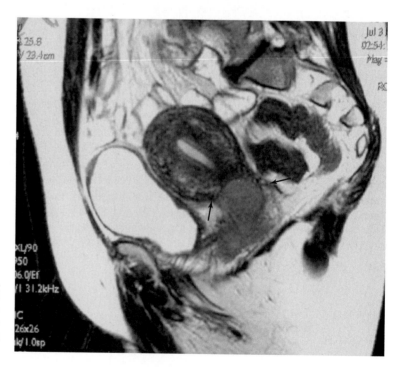

FIGURE 3-97. Sagittal pelvic MR image. Cervical carcinoma. There is abrupt transition of normal uterine mucosa at the tumor margin (*arrows*). Inferiorly, the tumor is more infiltrative. (Courtesy of Alan Stolpen, M.D.)

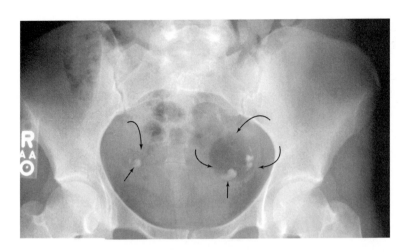

FIGURE 3-98. Pelvic radiograph. Bilateral ovarian teratoma. Each tumor contains teeth (*arrows*) and substantial intratumor fat (*curved arrows*) allowing the tumors to be better visualized. (Courtesy of Alan Stolpen, M.D.)

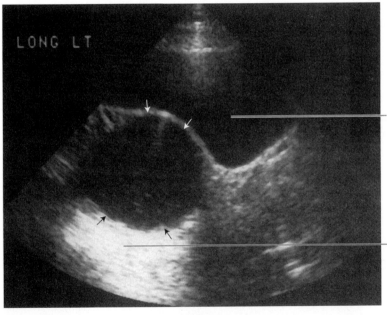

Urinary bladder

Posterior enhancement

FIGURE 3-99. Transabdominal sagittal sonogram. Mucinous cystadenoma of the left ovary. The ovarian mass has only a few internal echoes and demonstrates posterior enhancement typical of a cyst.

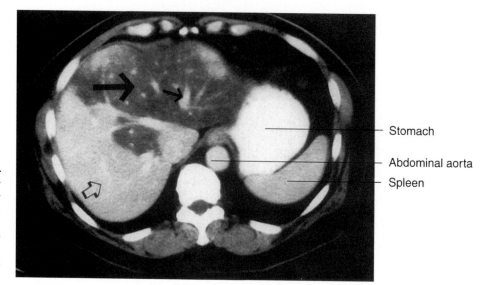

Stomach

Abdominal aorta

Spleen

FIGURE 3-100. Axial abdominal CT. Fatty liver (not in a cirrhotic patient). The *large black arrow* indicates the fatty changes. The *small black arrow* indicates vessels within the fat. The *open arrow* indicates a normal enhanced liver.

ACCESSORY DIGESTIVE ORGANS—IMAGING

Almost all imaging modalities can be used for the evaluation of liver disease. In general, the plain film is relatively insensitive, although it will show calcifications or gas in the liver. Evaluation for hepatomegaly is probably best by CT, although nuclear medicine scans or ultrasound examinations are also useful. MRI of liver disease is usually reserved for circumstances in which a definitive diagnosis is not possible with another modality.

Cirrhosis in North America is most often related to chronic alcoholism or as a complication of hepatitis. The severity of cirrhosis is primarily evaluated by physical examination and laboratory tests, but imaging is often useful.

Early changes include hepatomegaly with fatty infiltration of the liver, easily detected on CT (Fig. 3-100). As cirrhosis progresses, there is diminution in the size of the liver and development of heterogeneous density of the liver parenchyma with a knobby surface related to coexisting scarring and regeneration of liver nodules (Fig. 3-101). Changes of portal hypertension (splenomegaly, ascites, and dilated portal veins and tributaries) can be found in severe disease. Portal venous flow may be reduced or even reversed in severe cirrhosis, and secondary hepatic venous occlusion can occur. These can be delineated with Doppler ultrasound examination (Fig. 3-102).

The liver is the most common site for metastases from intraabdominal organs and often from tumors elsewhere in the body (lung and breast). Metastatic tumors in the

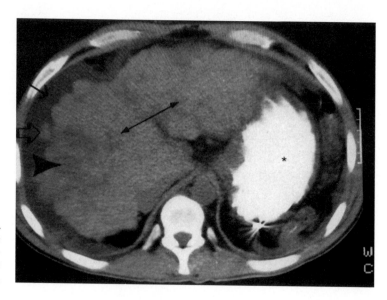

FIGURE 3-101. Axial abdominal CT. Cirrhosis. The liver margins (open area) are nodular. There are scattered fatty changes (*arrowhead*) and ascites (*short black arrow*). Both lobes (*long two-headed arrow*) are involved.

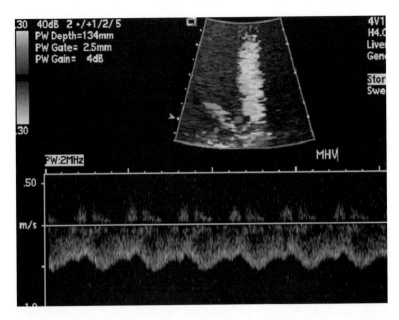

FIGURE 3-102. Hepatic versus Doppler ultrasound in a cirrhotic patient. The study shows patent hepatic veins (*arrows*) converging. The up-and-down Doppler signal indicates normal venous flow. (Courtesy of Monzer Abu-Yousef, M.D.)

liver are found 10 to 20 times more often than primary malignant tumors. Often, the hepatic metastatic disease is the first clinical indication of tumor. Imaging of metastatic liver disease is best done with CT using intravenous contrast material. Metastatic lesions are most often of reduced density when compared with the liver parenchyma (Fig. 3-103).

Benign primary tumors of the liver include hepatic cysts and cavernous hemangiomas; both are incidental findings and of no clinical significance. Larger hemangiomas or others with bizarre features may require MRI to be separated from malignant lesions (Fig. 3-104). Primary hepatoma occurs primarily in patients with preexisting liver disease. Hepatoma is less dense than normal liver parenchyma and has ill-defined margins. CT and MRI are useful for defining hepatic anatomy to determine resectability of tumors.

There are many methods to image biliary tract abnormalities. Ultrasound is the workhorse. Gallstones are the most common abnormalities of the gallbladder. About 10% of stones are calcified and visible on plain films (Fig. 3-9). Ultrasonography is effective in detecting gallstones, as the highly echogenic stones are surrounded by echo-free bile. Failure to propagate the sound wave distally causes shadowing (Fig. 3-105). The common duct is also studied during gallbladder examinations.

Acute cholecystitis can be confirmed, if ultrasound shows gallstones, with thickening of the gallbladder wall and localized tenderness. In ambiguous cases, radionuclide cholescintigraphy is performed. In acute cholecystitis, there is obstruction of the cystic duct so that radioactive material secreted from the liver fills the biliary tract, including the common duct but not the gallbladder (Fig. 9-12 in Chapter 9).

With distal obstruction, such as common duct stones or pancreatic tumors, the proximal biliary tract dilates. Recent technical developments in MRI allow the evaluation of the biliary tract and pancreatic duct noninvasively.

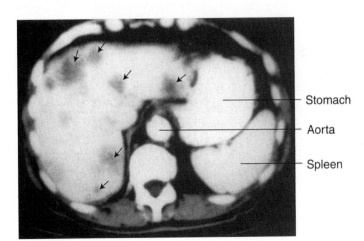

— Stomach

— Aorta

— Spleen

FIGURE 3-103. Abdomen axial CT. Right and left hepatic lobe metastases. The metastases (*straight arrows*) appear hypodense compared with the enhanced normal liver. Liver enhancement was accomplished by intravenous injection of contrast media.

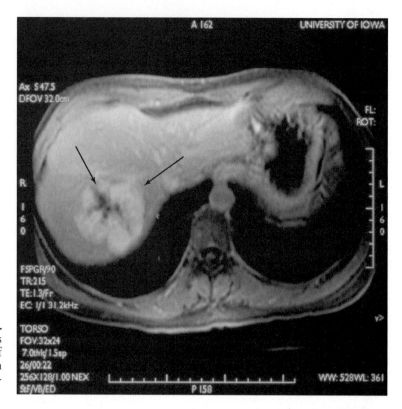

FIGURE 3-104. Axial MRI. Liver hemangioma. This study performed after intravenous administration of gadolinium shows a high signal mass (*arrows*) with bright walls characteristic of a hemangioma. (Courtesy of Alan Stolpen, M.D.)

MRI offers spectacular imaging of biliary obstruction (Fig. 3-106).

Splenomegaly is sometimes evident on the abdominal radiograph (Fig. 3-3), but is more reliably evaluated by US or CT. There are measurements available to separate the normal-sized from the enlarged spleen, although considerable overlap exists. Perhaps this is an appropriate time to again quote Ben Felson, "A radiologist with a ruler in his hand is a dangerous person."

Pancreatitis occurs as a complication of alcoholism, biliary tract disease, and sometimes trauma. Although the inflamed pancreas sometimes appears normal on US or CT examination (Fig. 3-107A), more often there is diffuse or localized swelling of the gland and inhomogenicity of US signal and CT as well as adjacent fluid (Fig. 3-107B). An important complication of acute pancreatitis is pseudocyst formation. The large, frequently multiloculated cysts are visible on either US or CT (Fig. 3-108).

In pancreatic carcinoma, clinical manifestations are infrequent before metastases have occurred. Both US and CT are useful for detecting pancreatic neoplasms as well as for staging the extent of metastatic disease. Tumor involvement of the celiac or superior mesenteric vessels makes resection impossible (Fig. 3-109).

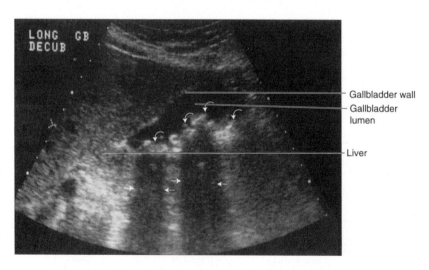

Gallbladder wall
Gallbladder lumen
Liver

FIGURE 3-105. Longitudinal decubitus sonogram. Cholelithiasis. Note how the dense gallstones (calculi, *curved arrows*) cast acoustic shadows (between the *straight arrows*) because the sound waves are unable to penetrate or traverse the dense calculi. This is similar to a shadow cast by a tree or building.

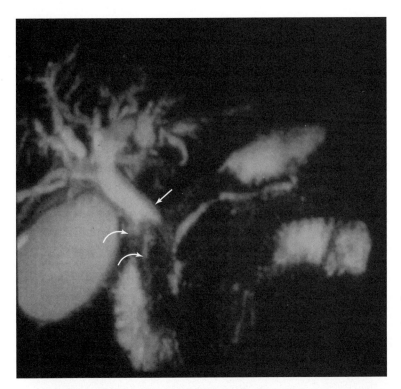

FIGURE 3-106. MRI cholangiopancreatogram. The common bile duct (*arrow*) and its proximal branches are dilated, owing to obstruction (*curved arrows*) from pancreatic carcinoma. The pancreatic duct (*open arrows*), gallbladder, and duodenal lumen are also visualized. (Courtesy of E. Scott Pretorius, M.D.)

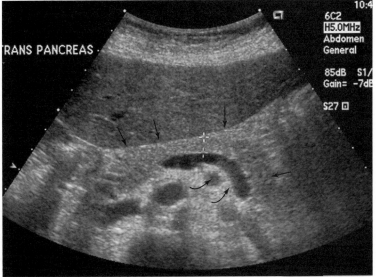

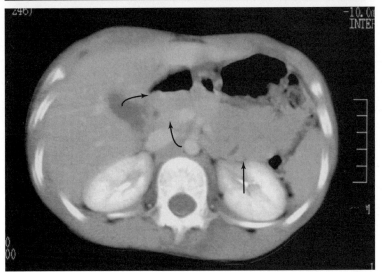

FIGURE 3-107. A: Transverse abdominal sonogram. Normal pancreas. The pancreas (*arrows*) is posterior to the liver (L) and anterior to the splenic vein (*curved arrows*). *Crosses* are in place to measure transverse pancreatic diameter. (Courtesy of Monzer Abu-Yousef, M.D.) **B:** Abdominal CT. Traumatic pancreatitis. The pancreatic body and tail (*arrows*) are enlarged and of uneven density. The mass (*curved arrows*) in the region of the pancreatic head is a hematoma.

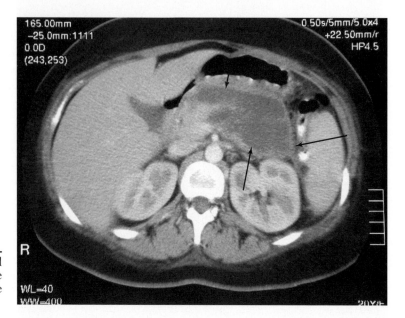

FIGURE 3-108. Pancreatic pseudocyst. Abdominal CT. The hypodense pseudocyst (*arrows*) replaces the body and tail of the pancreas. (Courtesy of Bruce Brown, M.D.)

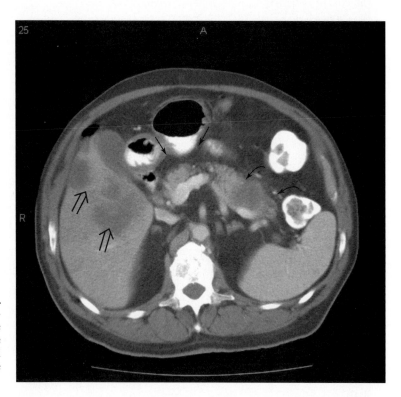

FIGURE 3-109. Abdominal CT. Pancreatic carcinoma. The pancreatic head and body (*arrows*) are normal. There is a poorly marginated hypodense mass (*curved arrows*) in the pancreatic tail. Several hypodense metastases (*open arrows*) are noted in the liver.

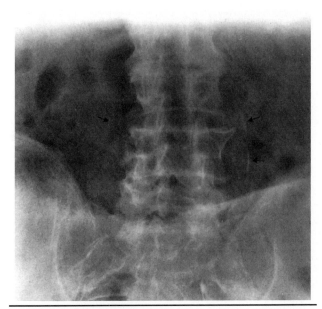

FIGURE 3-110. AP abdominal radiograph. Aortic aneurysm. The *straight arrow* indicate the calcified aneurysmal wall.

Abscess can occur anywhere in the abdomen—in a solid organ such as the liver or loculated anywhere in the peritoneal cavity (Fig. 3-19). CT is probably the best modality to detect and locate an intraabdominal abscess. Percutaneous drainage with CT guidance is often possible.

Abdominal aortic aneurysm is a common malady, particularly of the elderly. Calcification of the wall of the aneurysm is occasionally seen on plain films (Fig. 3-110). Abdominal ultrasound detects abdominal aneurysms, often when they are relatively small. In such circumstances, serial ultrasound examinations to evaluate the progression of disease may ultimately determine the need for repair. In larger aneurysms, extensive thrombosis occurs (Fig. 3-111). Dissection of an aneurysm occurs as a complication of atherosclerosis or other disease of the aortic wall. Here, blood dissects into the vessel media, producing a false channel and compromising the true lumen. As dissection progresses, there is hemorrhage into the retroperitoneum with shock and substantial mortality. CT is a valuable method of diagnosing and staging this disease.

SPECIAL PROBLEMS IN ABDOMINAL IMAGING

Trauma

In all age groups, trauma is the most common cause of preventable disease. Major types of abdominal trauma include motor vehicle accidents, falls, and assault. Imaging studies are important in the evaluation of abdominal trauma as clinical evaluation is unreliable.

The first decision in dealing with a trauma victim is, "Is there any clinical evidence of abdominal abnormality?" Unless there is at least some clinical suspicion (e.g., abdominal pain, contusion, or guarding), the likelihood of finding significant disease with special studies is very low.

If there is concern about abdominal injury, minimal imaging examination includes plain film with supplemental horizontal beam film (upright, decubitus, lateral). Although not a particularly sensitive examination, it is useful for orientation in subsequent studies and allows diagnosis of pneumoperitoneum, massive intraperitoneal fluid, or large soft tissue masses. Contrast studies of the gut, particularly with barium, are less sensitive than other imaging modalities, can cause significant imaging artifacts, and play no major role in acute trauma. Excretory urography is seldom performed because it is considerably less sensitive than other modalities. US, although useful in diagnosing large amounts of intraperitoneal fluid, is less sensitive than CT. Angiography plays a minor role, unless there is strong suspicion for vascular injury (e.g., a cold leg after pelvic trauma); it may have a therapeutic role in trauma patients, such as those with embolization of a bleeding spleen.

CT, particularly with multislice equipment, is the study of choice for evaluating abdominal trauma. With current equipment, the examination can be completed in less than one minute. Previously, most radiologists regarded patient hemodynamic stability necessary before CT could be performed. With the rapid procedure time available today, some compromise in the degree of stability is possible. Most examinations are done with administration of intravenous material. Oral contrast is customarily not given, because of the time involved for it to pass through the gut and its lesser value in diagnosis, unless bowel or pancreatic injury is suspected.

Hemoperitoneum from any source can be identified on CT, and the amount of blood can be quantified (Fig. 3-112). Multiple organ injuries are common; the liver, spleen, and kidney are affected more than other structures. Injuries to these organs are diagnosed with an accuracy of well over 95%. CT detects both the type and the severity of injury, an aid in determining which patients need immediate surgery versus nonoperative treatment (Figs. 3-112 to 3-114).

Gastrointestinal Bleeding

In acute gastrointestinal bleeding, a major concern is to decide if the source of blood loss is from the upper or lower gastrointestinal tract. Statistically, about two-thirds of patients have upper GI bleeding. Some common causes are listed in Table 3-7. Clinical clues are hematemesis, seen in bleeding from the upper GI tract, and hematochezia, from the colon. Melena can occur in either group but is more often associated with upper GI bleed.

(*text continues on page 144*)

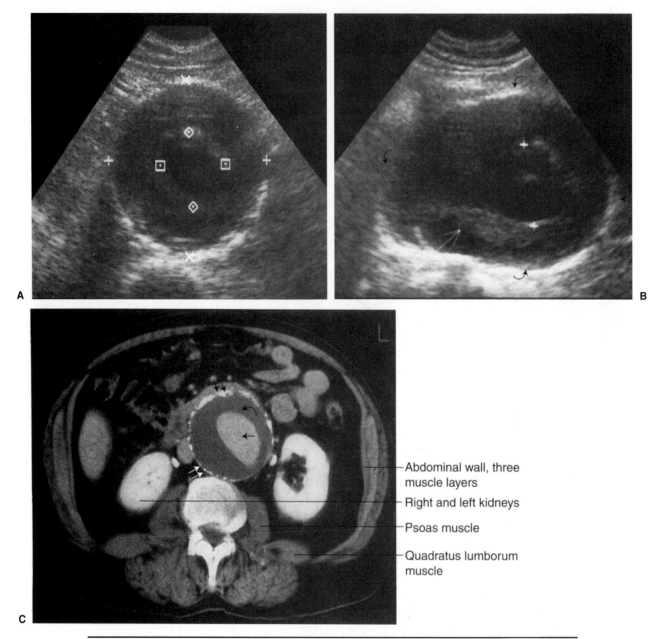

FIGURE 3-111. A: Transverse and **B:** longitudinal sonograms. Abdominal aortic aneurysm. Thrombus extends from the aortic wall, restricting blood flow to the midportion (outlined by *markers*) of the aorta. **C:** Axial abdominal CT. The *straight arrow* indicates the patent central lumen with thrombus (*curved arrow*) peripherally. The aortic wall (*double straight arrows*) is partially calcified.

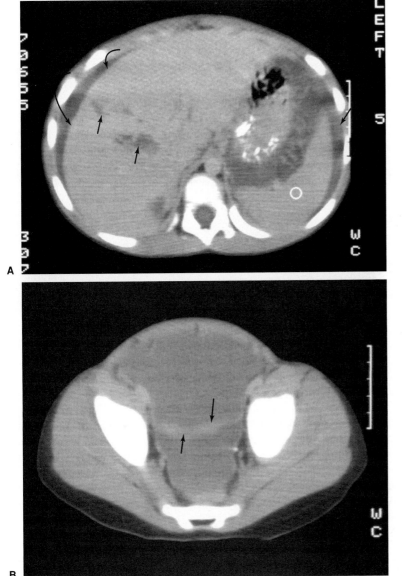

A

B

FIGURE 3-112. Abdominal CT. Hemoperitoneum, owing to liver laceration in a child. **A:** An irregular laceration (*arrows*) is seen in the hepatic parenchyma. Blood (*curved arrows*) surrounds the borders of the liver and spleen. **B:** In the pelvis, blood fills the peritoneal cavity, outlining the infantile uterus (*arrows*).

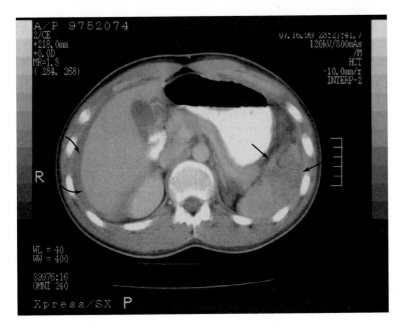

FIGURE 3-113. Abdominal CT after intravenous contrast material. Splenic laceration. The anterior portion of the spleen (*arrows*) has irregular density and does not opacify. Hemoperitoneum is evident by the hypodense fluid at the margins of the liver (*curved arrows*).

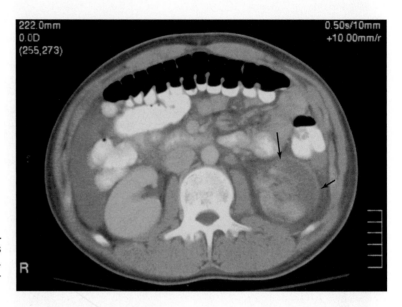

FIGURE 3-114. Abdominal CT after intravenous contrast material. Left kidney, traumatic laceration. Renal density is irregular anteriorly (*arrows*), indicating renal parenchyma admixed with blood.

Endoscopy is the procedure of choice for evaluating upper GI bleeding. It allows better localization than imaging examinations, and endoscopic treatment of the bleeding site is often possible. Imaging studies are used when bleeding is so massive that endoscopy is not practical. In these circumstances, angiography is often diagnostic and can be used therapeutically to occlude sites of bleeding (Fig. 3-115). CT is less valuable for acute bleeding, and barium is seldom indicated. For acute lower GI bleeding, proctosigmoidoscopy is the first procedure, followed by angiography, if needed.

In chronic gastrointestinal bleeding, nuclear medicine studies are more sensitive than other imaging studies. Either technetium-labeled sulfur colloid or red cells can be used. These examinations allow detection of active bleeding as low as 0.05 to 0.1 cc/min, and the examination can be done in less than an hour. Technical reasons favor one over the other in specific situations.

Acute Abdomen

A rough definition of *acute abdomen* is a situation involving a patient with acute abdominal pain and related signs wherein emergency surgery is being considered. Some common causes are listed in Table 3-8. In years past, exploratory surgery in the acute abdomen was often necessary, causing considerable morbidity and often unnecessary surgery. Imaging allows discrimination of nonsurgical disease (e.g., acute regional enteritis) versus diseases requiring surgery. It is of considerable value in delineation of the type of surgical disease—for instance, appendicitis versus ectopic pregnancy.

Traditionally, abdominal plain film and horizontal beam film are performed in all but those with the most urgent abdominal disease. Evaluation of the gas pattern and detection of pneumoperitoneum are its strong points. US is of value in certain situations, especially for gynecologic diagnosis; CT is generally more accurate in other areas.

▌ **TABLE 3-7 Etiology of Gastrointestinal Bleeding**

Esophagus, stomach, duodenum
- Varices with portal hypertension
- Peptic ulcer

Small bowel
- Duplication
- Mesenteric vascular disease
- Meckel's diverticulum

Colon
- Angiodysplasia
- Polyp or tumor
- Colitis

▌ **TABLE 3-8 Common Causes of Acute Abdomen**

Medical	*Surgical*
Chest disease—Pneumonia, infarct, pleurisy	Appendicitis
	Cholecystitis
Cardiac disease—Myocardial infarct, pericarditis	Bowel perforation
	Intestinal obstruction
Mesenteric adenitis	Pancreatitis
Ileitis, colitis	Mesenteric vascular ischemia
Renal colic	Salpingitis
Drugs	Ectopic pregnancy
Metabolic disease	Leaking abdominal aneurysm

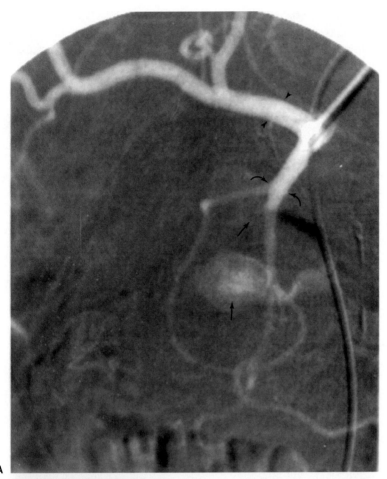

A

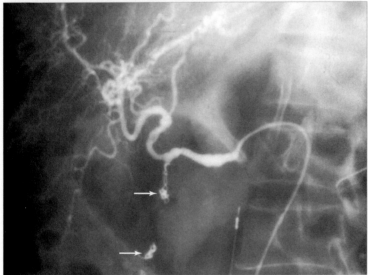

B

FIGURE 3-115. **A:** Selective angiogram opacities of hepatic (*arrowheads*) and gastroduodenal (*curved arrows*) arteries. Bleeding duodenal ulcer. Contrast material (*straight arrows*) extravasates into the duodenal lumen, indicating an actively bleeding ulcer. **B:** Coils were introduced into the gastroduodenal artery. The follow-up angiogram shows the coils (*arrows*) in place with occlusion of the gastroduodenal artery. There was immediate cessation of the gastrointestinal bleeding. (Courtesy of Shiliang Sun, M.D.)

Multislice CT is performed in most patients with acute abdomen, except those in whom clinical diagnosis is certain without imaging. These cases are done with the use of intravenous contrast (exception: suspected urolithiasis). Oral contrast and rectal contrast use have their proponents in the patient with acute abdomen, but others point out their disadvantages, particularly the increased time involved in the study.

The technique of CT examination is somewhat modified by the likely diagnosis suspected. Some common surgical causes of acute abdomen diagnosable on CT include appendicitis, bowel obstruction, urolithiasis, bowel perforation (most often peptic ulcer), gynecologic disease, pancreatitis, and aortic aneurysm. Less frequent causes include small bowel and colon disease, ischemic gut disease, and infections of solid organs.

KEY POINTS

- Imaging evaluation of the abdomen usually begins with an AP supine abdominal radiograph. This is particularly helpful in evaluating the gas pattern.
- Small bowel obstruction is characterized by dilated small bowel proximally with collapsed colon and minimal rectal gas.
- In adynamic ileus, there is proportional dilatation of both small and large bowel with gas throughout the gut.
- If bowel perforation is suspected, it is critical to perform horizontal beam films (upright, decubitus, or cross-table lateral) inasmuch as 2 cc of free intraperitoneal air can be identified.

- Contrast studies of the gut remain a valuable method to detect intraluminal and mural diseases such as tumors, mucosal disease, and ulcerations. They are particularly useful in the small bowel, where endoscopy is technically difficult.
- Ultrasound is the primary imaging modality for obstetrics and useful for detecting gallstones, renal and gynecologic disease, and abdominal aortic abnormalities.
- Abdominal CT is the method of choice for detection, localization, and characterization of tumors.
- CT diagnosis of appendicitis is very reliable, with direct visualization of the inflamed appendix in most cases.
- CT without intravenous contrast material initially is the preferred method for evaluating suspected renal and ureteral stones.
- CT is the study of choice in evaluating the trauma patient.
- MRI is useful in a variety of special situations in the abdomen.

REFERENCES

1. Brant WE, Helms CA. *Fundamentals of diagnostic radiology*, 2nd ed. Philadelphia: Lippincott Williams & Wilkins, 1999.
2. Gore RM, Levine MS. *Textbook of gastrointestinal radiology*, 2nd ed. Philadelphia: WB Saunders, 2000.
3. Kim SH. *Radiology illustrated: uroradiology*. Philadelphia: WB Saunders, 2003.

SUGGESTED READING

Haaga JR, Lanzieri CV, Gilkeson RC, eds. *CT and MR imaging of the whole body*, 4th ed. St. Louis, MO: Mosby, 2003.

Pediatric Imaging

Wilbur L. Smith

NORMAL

Children are not merely small adults. Sure, the body parts (hearts, eyes, noses) are the same, but the fact that children are growing and changing subjects them to different diseases as well as to different structural appearances. Chest radiographs of young children, for instance, feature that ubiquitous but often misdiagnosed anterior mediastinal mass, the thymus (Fig. 4-1). This organ, important in the immune response, usually becomes inconspicuous by age 5 or so; however, its involution is extremely variable, and it is not uncommon to find thymic remnants on chest CT scans up to age 20 years (Figs. 4-2 and 4-3). The thymus is a living piece of tissue that changes its configuration in a number of ways. In response to stress, it may shrink. When indented by the ribs, it may form a wavy border; in pathologic conditions, such as a pneumomediastinum, it may even be displaced superiorly and laterally over the lung fields (Figs. 4-4 to 4-6). The first rule in looking at children's radiographs is, expect change and variation and consider those factors before inventing a disorder that isn't real.

In general, congenital abnormalities are much more likely to present as clinical problems in neonates than they are in adults. Another way to look at it is if you got to adulthood without a congenital anomaly bothering you, it is likely that you will carry that anomaly to your grave. When you deal with an abnormal abdomen in a neonate, a congenital anomaly is extremely likely; in a 4-year-old it is somewhat likely; and in a 15-year-old it is less likely. If you play by the 99% rule in an 80-year-old, you probably shouldn't even think of congenital abnormalities as the cause of an acute abdomen. Having said this, I know that everyone will be able to find the unusual case of a congenital defect causing grief to an 80-year-old, but remember that's the zebra, not the horse!

Abdominal radiographs of neonates are very different from those of adults, whereas radiographs of older children and teenagers begin to have a lot of similarities with those of adults. Abdominal films of neonates are especially discrepant because of a number of physiologic factors. First and foremost, neonates swallow a tremendous amount of air during their relatively inefficient breathing and eating. It is, therefore, not at all unusual to find many

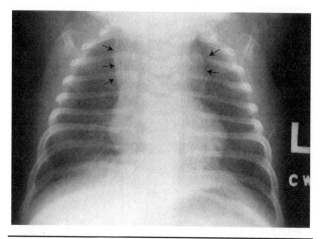

FIGURE 4-1. The large superior mediastinal mass that bulges both to the right and to the left is the thymus in this normal 3-month-old infant.

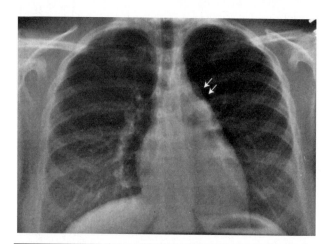

FIGURE 4-2. This teenager has a clearly visible thymic edge *(arrows)* on chest radiograph. Visualization of the thymus in normal teenagers is an unusual, but not rare, finding.

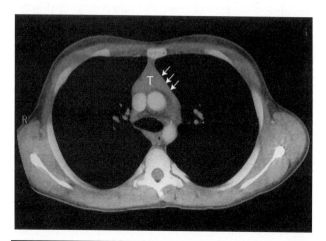

FIGURE 4-3. Chest CT of a 16-year-old patient shows a large thymus anterior to the opacified vessels. Note how the left lobe of the thymus (T) sticks out to abut the lung *(arrows)*.

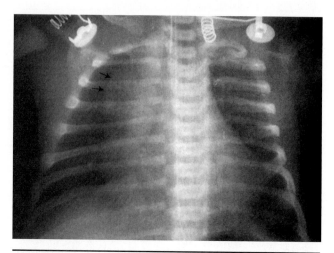

FIGURE 4-4. The large anterior mediastinal mass with the irregular margin *(arrows)* is the thymus. The thymic wave sign or undulating thymic border occurs because the costal cartilages are made of more firm tissue than the thymus; therefore, the thymus itself is indented. This is a normal finding.

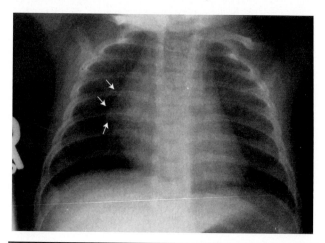

FIGURE 4-5. The so-called thymic sail sign shows the sharp edge of the thymus, somewhat like a boat sail, projected against the lung.

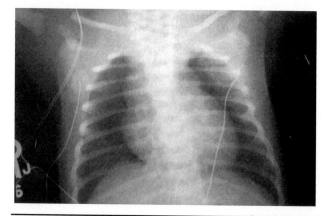

FIGURE 4-6. The large superior mediastinal mass in this otherwise well-term neonate is the thymus. If you call anything in the anterior superior mediastinum of a neonate normal thymus, you will be right 99% of the time.

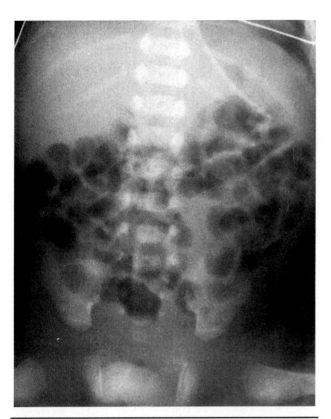

FIGURE 4-7. This abdominal film shows the bowel gas pattern of a normal newborn baby. Notice there are a number of nondistended bowel loops with considerable small bowel gas. The loops lie next to each other and are thin walled. This is a good visual picture to remember for the normal bowel gas appearance of a neonate. Older children do not have this much gas, and adults have very little small bowel gas, visible on plain films. Contrast this with Fig. 4-9, a baby with sepsis and some bowel wall edema.

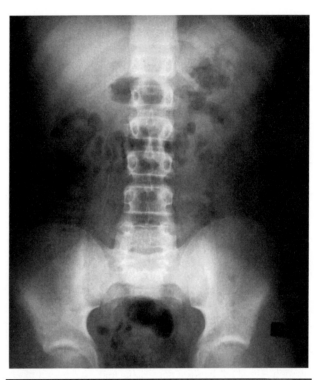

FIGURE 4-8. This plain film of the abdomen was obtained on a normal child with constipation. There is gas in the colon and stomach but very little gas in the small bowel. Contrast this to the appearance of Fig. 4-7, the neonate, where there is normally considerable small bowel gas.

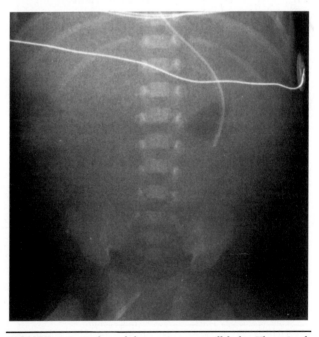

FIGURE 4-9. Gasless abdomen in a very ill baby. There is almost always some gas in the stomach but very little gas distal. This is abnormal and can occur as a result of the baby being too ill to swallow or a systemic illness. In this case, the baby was immobilized so that he would not fight the ventilator and this gasless abdomen resulted. Normally, babies should have gas in both large and small bowel.

loops of small bowel in the plain film of a normal neonate (Fig. 4-7), whereas in an adult or older child it is unusual to see so much small bowel gas (Fig. 4-8). In fact, it is abnormal to see a gasless abdomen in a neonate! Such a finding usually means that the infant is so obtunded that it cannot swallow air, that there is a discontinuity of the gastrointestinal (GI) tract preventing air from entering the bowel, or that the infant is septic or otherwise critically ill (Fig. 4-9). All of this air in the small bowel makes the interpretation of the films difficult as far as determining bowel distention. The best rule to remember is that the bowel loops of a normal neonate are thin walled and lie in close proximity to each other. The appearance of thick-walled bowel or marked separation of the bowel loops suggest an abnormal intraabdominal process (Fig. 4-10). Comparison of Figs. 4-7 and 4-10 illustrates this point.

The haustra of the colon are notoriously variable in their development and do not become prominent until about 6 months of age. For this reason trying to differentiate

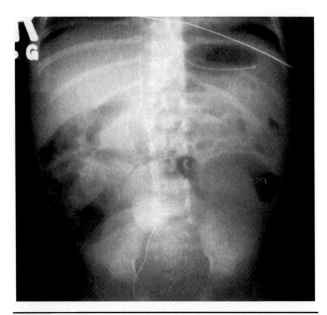

FIGURE 4-10. Contrast the abdominal plain film in this critically ill and septic neonate with the normal bubbly pattern of bowel gas shown in Fig. 4-7. The loops of bowel are separated, and some of the bowel shows evidence of a moderate degree of dilation. These findings are nonspecific and can be seen in any severely ill infant. In this case, sepsis caused abnormal bowel motility in this abnormal appearing radiograph.

TABLE 4-1 Causes of Bowel Obstruction in the Neonate

Atresia
Malrotation
Hernia
Meconium ileus
Hirschsprung's disease
Bowel duplications

large from small bowel on the plain radiographs of a neonate's abdomen is fraught with difficulty. Occasionally, you can get lucky and be reasonably certain in differentiation; however, most of the time it isn't even worth guessing. This makes the determination of whether there is rectal gas or not even more critical. The vast majority of newborns will have gas all the way through their GI tract by 24 hours after birth. If there is any doubt as to whether a child has

rectal gas or has obstruction, the prone cross-table lateral film is invaluable in making this distinction (Fig. 4-11). Remember: if you are looking for distal gas in an infant in whom you are considering bowel obstruction, go right for the rectum! (Table 4-1).

Another big difference between neonates and older children or adults is the presence of the belly button. This necessary structure and the appurtenances appended to it make for some weird shadows on abdominal films of babies. Many an unsuspecting physician has called an umbilical clamp a bone or a foreign body (Fig. 4-12). The umbilicus itself protrudes much farther in a neonate than in an adult. Any coin-shaped lesion in the lower midabdomen of a neonate should be considered the umbilical remnant until proven otherwise. A good clue is that, owing to the air surrounding the protruding umbilical stump, the edges of the umbilicus are very sharply defined, particularly the inferior edge (Fig. 4-13).

In this chapter I will discuss some of the common radiographic diagnoses of children, first neonates, then the older child. The intent is not to be comprehensive, as there are 1,000-page tomes for that; rather, this is intended to show practical imaging approaches to common diagnoses.

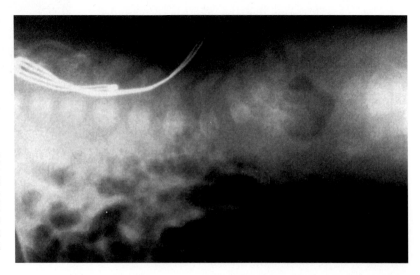

FIGURE 4-11. A prone cross-lateral view of the abdomen can often be helpful in showing whether or not gas is present in the rectum. Remember that because you cannot tell large bowel from small bowel in neonates, it is important to identify the rectum when you are trying to look for distal gas. Rectal gas usually is identified in the hollow of the sacrum, as in this infant.

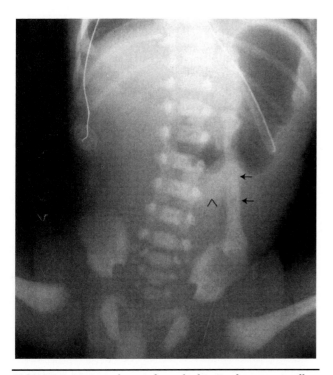

FIGURE 4-12. A newborn infant who has just begun to swallow air. Notice the nasogastric tube marking the stomach. The oblong structure to the left of the spine *(arrows)* almost looks like a bone of some sort; however, it is clearly attached to the umbilical stump *(arrowhead)* and in fact represents an umbilical cord clamp superimposed on the abdominal film.

FIGURE 4-13. This baby undergoing an upper GI has a circular, bowel-filled mass in the lower midabdomen. The mass projects slightly to the left because the baby is in an oblique position *(arrows)*. Note the very sharp margin, indicating that the mass protrudes off the abdominal wall. Anytime you see an extremely sharp border on a plain film of the abdomen, there has to be either air or fat surrounding that structure. In this case, air surrounds the structure because the umbilicus protrudes out from the abdominal wall. This is a typical umbilical hernia.

NEONATAL CHEST

The newborn's chest radiograph is a complex study with a substantial number of differences from that of an adult (Fig. 4-14). All babies have to change from an intrauterine environment where their lungs are fluid filled to one where they are breathing air. This transformation, which must occur within moments of birth, involves interaction of the pulmonary lymphatics, capillary vessels, and chest compression. This normal biologic process is not always smooth. In fact, many babies, if not all, have some very short-lived tachypnea in the first minute or two after being born, owing to the vagaries of clearing their normal *in utero* lung fluid. The physiologic phenomenon is reflected as the pleural effusions and streaky densities seen in the lungs on radiographs taken shortly after birth.

In an insignificant number of babies, it takes longer than a few moments to clear all of the *in utero* lung fluid. This condition has been aptly termed *transient tachypnea of the newborn* (TTN; Fig. 4-15). TTN should resolve clinically and radiographically within 24 hours, leaving behind a normal chest. In the first hours of life, however, this picture leads to a great clinical quandary because the radiograph of the neonate with TTN is indistinguishable from the radiograph of early neonatal pneumonia.

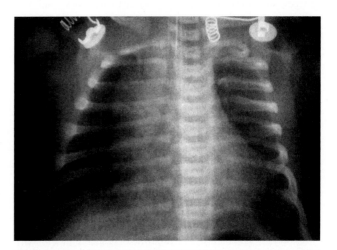

FIGURE 4-14. A normal newborn infant's chest. Notice the very different appearance from an adult chest. First, the heart and thymus are much larger than the cardiomediastinal silhouette of an adult. If you measure the heart and thymus (cardiothymic structures) and compare them to the diameter of the chest, often a baby's cardiothymic ratio will exceed 60% of the chest diameter. This is still normal. Notice also that the bones are very different, with a number of growth plates and other variants owing to infant development.

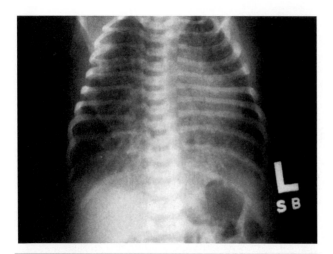

FIGURE 4-15. A: Chest film of a 4-hour-old baby shows bilateral streaky densities whose distribution is asymmetric. Note that the lungs are also very hyperinflated. All this cleared within 24 hours, and the findings were due to transient tachypnea of the newborn. On this film alone, however, you cannot exclude pneumonia. It is necessary to have the follow-up film to confirm the diagnosis of transient tachypnea.

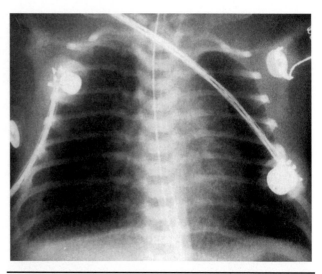

FIGURE 4-16. A very ill newborn with the streaky density pattern in both lungs and a large pleural effusion *(arrow)* on the right. Pneumonia plus a pleural effusion usually means group B strep infection in neonates.

There are a few clues, such as the presence of a large pleural effusion, which favors pneumonia; however, a definitive distinction can never be made. Here is a classic health care conundrum. TTN is much more common than neonatal pneumonia; however, conventional diagnostic tests cannot separate the two. The outcome of an untreated neonatal pneumonia is dire, so what do you do? Most prudent physicians bite the bullet and treat, knowing that in many instances the antibiotics are unnecessary. This situation demonstrates the principle that if the perceived severity of possible outcome is great, it alters the treatment choice when diagnosis is ambiguous. In other words, if you cannot tell, but the patient might die if you don't treat, overtreating is often acceptable.

There are other neonatal lung diseases that exhibit radiographs showing bilateral streaky densities. Transient tachypnea of the newborn is the prototype for this appearance; however, neonatal pneumonia, neonatal venous stasis, and neonatal congestive heart failure can be mimicked. A few points of differentiation are possible. A large pleural effusion usually favors pneumonia and specifically *reactive* pneumonia, owing to group B streptococcal infection (Fig. 4-16). Most neonatal pneumonias are acquired during the birth process, so that these pneumonias start small and tend to get dramatically worse over the first few days of life. If the streaky densities are associated with marked overaeration of the lungs, one might think of meconium aspiration. This disorder occurs when the newborns release their sphincters, spilling meconium into the amniotic fluid. This sphincter release, a response to stress, usually occurs *in utero* and the meconium is aspirated as the child begins

to try to breathe. This is a particularly nasty pneumonia because the meconium is both irritating and viscous so that it obstructs the airways as well as causing the reactive pneumonia. One of the tips for diagnosing meconium aspiration is the massive hyperinflation of the lungs usually seen on the chest film (Fig. 4-17).

Babies can get congestive heart failure for a number of reasons, some of which involve intrinsic heart disease and many of which do not (Fig. 4-18). Arrhythmias, anemia, and arteriovenous shunts can cause high-output failure that is indistinguishable by chest film from the failure caused by intrinsic heart lesions such as hypoplastic left heart. The best clue that the streaky density pattern you are looking at on the chest film is owing to heart disease is cardiomegaly. Beyond that, it is difficult to be more precise. The most important thing is to remember heart failure in your differential diagnosis.

HYALINE MEMBRANE DISEASE

A common disorder of neonates is hyaline membrane disease (HMD). Here the clinical information helps a lot, as most of these infants are premature and most do not have respiratory distress immediately after birth. The other good news is that the radiographs are virtually diagnostic in the vast majority of cases (Fig. 4-19). The HMD radiograph shows four characteristic features: (a) diffuse granularity, (b) uniform disease, (c) air bronchograms, and (d) a relatively small lung volume. Not all radiographs will show all of these features, but most will have at least three.

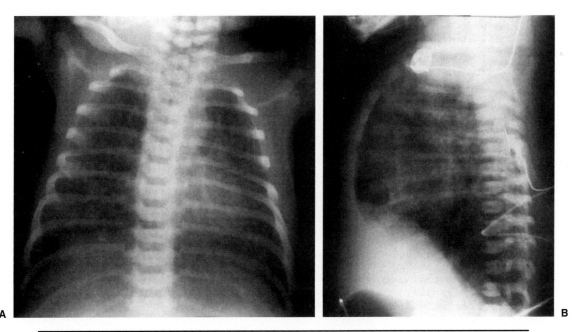

FIGURE 4-17. The anterior posterior radiograph **(A)** and lateral radiograph **(B)** of a 1-day-old infant with severe meconium aspiration, showing marked hyperinflation of the lungs and bilateral streaky densities in both lung fields consistent with meconium aspiration. Notice on the lateral view (B) how flat the diaphragms are and how prominent the anterior posterior diameter of the chest is. Meconium aspiration is highly associated with air-block phenomenon.

HMD occurs owing to a lack of the lipid chemical surfactant that is synthesized by the alveolar lining cells of term infants. These type 2 alveolar lining cells develop and mature during the third trimester of pregnancy; therefore, they are deficient among premature infants. Surfactant works by lowering the surface tension of the alveoli, allowing them to remain expanded. A simple analogy is that of a child's bubble pipe. You have to add soap to the water in the pipe to change the surface tension or you cannot blow many bubbles! If the surfactant is not present in the neonate's lung, the bubbles (alveoli) collapse. There you have it: The radiology of HMD is predominantly the radiology of profound atelectasis on an alveolar rather than a segmental level. In fact, some of the more forward-thinking clinicians propose changing the name of this disease to surfactant deficiency disorder.

SURGICAL CONDITIONS

Pediatric surgical disease of the chest of a neonate can be roughly defined as anything that needs prompt intervention (Table 4-2). By this definition, for example, a tension pneumothorax needing treatment with a chest tube is surgical disease. In assessing the newborn child's chest radiograph when surgical disease is suspected, you must take two steps. First, identify which side is the more abnormal (most surgical conditions are unilateral). Second,

determine the direction of shift of the mediastinum. This is best done by looking at the trachea, but the position of the heart and thymus can also be secondary clues (Fig. 4-20). As a general (99%) rule, surgical conditions will displace the mediastinum *away* from the more abnormal side. For example, in the instance of a diaphragmatic hernia (a condition owing to an *in utero* defect that allows the abdominal contents to protrude into the chest), the heart and mediastinum are clearly shifted away from the side of the hernia by the mass of the protruding guts (Fig. 4-21). Therefore, if you look at the radiograph and decide that the side with the bowel in the chest is the abnormal side, and then look at the mediastinal position, you can readily deduce that this is a surgical condition and an emergency.

When you are deciding on the more abnormal lung in neonates, remember that birth is a time of transition. In our example of a diaphragmatic hernia, *in utero* the bowel is filled with fluid. It isn't until the infant begins to breathe and swallow air that the gut assumes its normal

▶ **TABLE 4-2 Common Surgical Chest Conditions in Neonates**

Pneumothorax
Diaphragmatic hernia
Lobar emphysema
Cystic adenomatoid malformation
Pleural effusions (large)

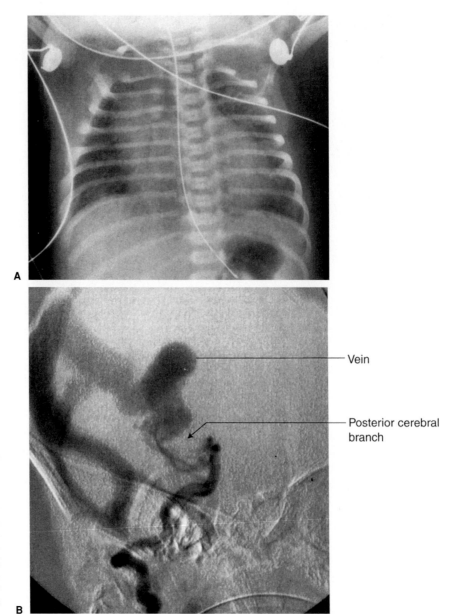

Vein

Posterior cerebral branch

FIGURE 4-18. **A:** Cardiomegaly with pulmonary congestion in a child with congestive heart failure. The findings are nonspecific, and failure can occur due to multiple causes. **B:** A lateral arteriogram of the head of the baby shown in A shows the carotid artery branches *(arrows)* connecting to a large venous sinus, creating an arterial venous fistula. This condition is called a vein of Galen aneurysm. The baby is in high-output congestive heart failure.

postnatal air-filled condition. Therefore the first film in a neonate may show a fluid density filling the chest, but within a few moments the normal swallowing of air results in replacement of this fluid density by the bubbly appearance of air-filled bowel.

In some conditions this transition to an air-filled mass can be even further delayed until 2 or 3 days after birth. This usually occurs in situations where the connection between the lung and the tracheobronchial tree is abnormal, and it can take a considerable period of time, up to several days, for the normal *in utero* lung fluid to empty out and the air to fill the lung anomaly. A good example of this is lobar emphysema, a condition whereby the tracheobronchial airway connects abnormally to a lobe of the lung,

allowing air to flow in but not out. The lobe, therefore, hyperinflates, becoming a tumor in the chest. Babies don't breathe air *in utero*; their lungs are fluid filled. Right after birth, this abnormally connected lobe is full of lung fluid as is the rest of the lung. The same mechanics that do not allow air to escape freely also do not allow the fluid to escape freely; therefore, it takes a long time for turnover of the fluid to take place, and the initial chest film looks like a solid (water) density mass with mediastinal displacement (Fig. 4-22). In a sense, it doesn't make any difference because criteria one and two for diagnosing a surgical condition are met no matter what the status of the mass; however, it's always nice to make a precise diagnosis.

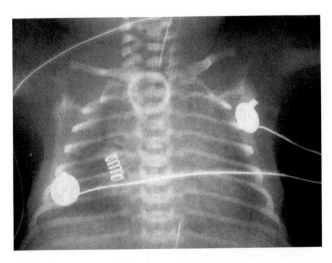

FIGURE 4-19. Classic radiograph of a patient with hyaline membrane disease. Note that the lungs are relatively small in volume.

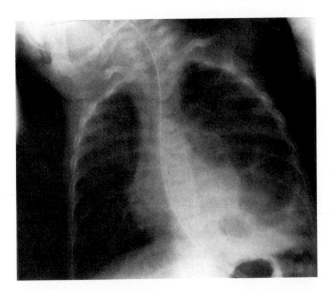

FIGURE 4-20. A very ill neonate. Note that the bubbly mass in the left lung base causes the heart and mediastinum to be shifted from left to right. First you decide which lung is abnormal (in this case, clearly the left). If the heart and mediastinum are shifted away from the abnormal lung, it is almost always surgical disease of the chest. Incidentally, the mass in this case is a cystic adenomatoid malformation, a benign tumor of the lung caused by abnormal budding of the foregut.

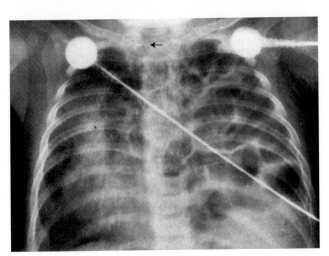

FIGURE 4-21. Bubbly material fills the left chest, displacing the heart and mediastinum far to the right. These bubbles actually are air-filled bowel. Notice the trachea area. Position of the trachea is the single best indicator of mediastinal displacement.

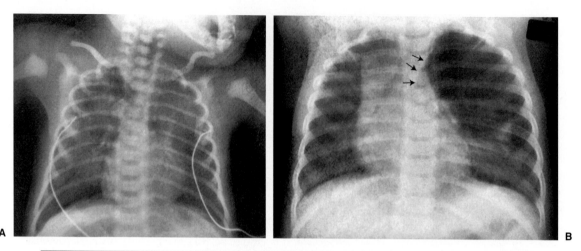

FIGURE 4-22. A: A neonatal chest film shows mediastinal shift from left to right and a partially opaque fluid density in the left upper lobe. This is a patient with congenital lobar emphysema and only partial emptying of the fluid from the emphysematous lobe. **B:** The same patient at age 11 months demonstrates findings more typical of lobar emphysema with the markedly hyperinflated upper lobe herniated across the midline *(arrows)*. The principle for surgical disease remains valid; mediastinal shift away from the abnormal side needs rapid intervention.

ESOPHAGEAL ATRESIA

Our discussion so far has focused on lung disease, but of course there are other significant organs in the pediatric chest, including the heart and the esophagus. Esophageal abnormalities that are of importance in children are usually related to esophageal atresia. The most common form of esophageal atresia is a blind-ending proximal esophagus with a fistula extending from the trachea or left main stem bronchus to a blind distal esophagus. Inhaled air travels through the fistula and into the rest of the GI tract; therefore, the initial films can look superficially normal. The clues are that the GI tract is more distended by air than usual and the proximal esophageal pouch is very dilated. Clinicians become alerted to this condition when the child chokes on feedings and the pediatrician cannot pass a nasogastric tube into the stomach (Fig. 4-23).

There are two less prevalent but still frequent variants of esophageal abnormalities. The first is esophageal atresia without fistula, in which case the abdomen is gasless because the infant cannot swallow any air to displace the fluid that is in the abdomen *in utero* (Fig. 4-24). Such infants are usually quite ill and need emergent surgery. The second variant is tracheoesophageal fistula without esophageal atresia. This so-called H-type fistula can be a difficult diagnosis. The nasogastric tube test is normal, so that the diagnosis is not readily apparent to the clinician. The child usually presents frequent pneumonias because each time the infant eats, some of the material goes into the lung. Whenever you have an infant with frequent and recurrent pneumonia, this entity, along with cystic fibrosis,

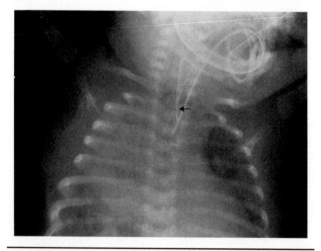

FIGURE 4-23. This very ill infant choked on being fed his first bottle. The chest radiograph shows a very dense right upper lobe infiltrate because of aspiration pneumonia. Note that the nasogastric tube won't go any farther than the upper esophagus *(arrows)*. A surgical clip was placed to identify the site of the tracheoesophageal fistula as this infant was too ill to undergo primary repair of the esophageal atresia; a first-step procedure, ligating and dividing the fistula, was undertaken to protect his lungs. Survival of children with tracheoesophageal fistula correlates directly with the amount of lung disease owing to aspiration.

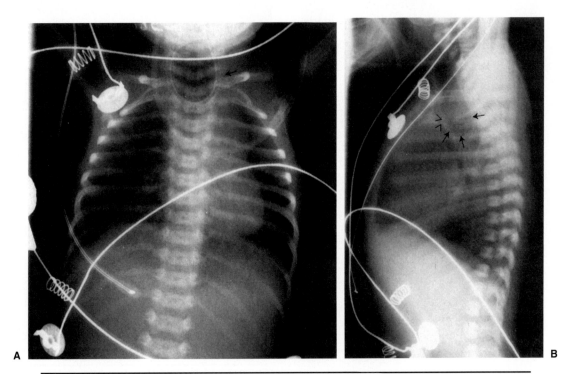

FIGURE 4-24. A: A typical radiograph of a child with esophageal atresia. Note the nasogastric tube *(arrow)* coiled in the upper esophagus. There are two major differences between this film and that of the child shown in Fig. 4-23. First, this child has not gotten aspiration pneumonia because this abnormality was recognized earlier and the child was not fed. Second, note that there is no gas in the abdomen. Patients with tracheoesophageal fistula always have the very distended stomach as each breath pumps air into that organ. The absence of gas in the abdomen makes the diagnosis of esophageal atresia without fistula. **B:** This lateral view of the same patient shows the very dilated proximal esophagus *(arrows)*. Note that the dilated esophageal pouch displaces the airway anteriorly *(arrowheads)*. These infants will often have abnormalities of the airway that accompany the abnormalities of the esophagus.

needs to be considered (Fig. 4-25). A barium esophagram is necessary to confirm the diagnosis.

CONGENITAL BOWEL ABNORMALITIES

Bowel Atresia

In babies, the commonest cause of bowel obstruction is atresia of the bowel. Atresia occurs owing to a number of complex intrauterine processes, most of which involve vascular supply to the wall of the bowel. Radiographs of the atresia vary tremendously according to the level at which the atresia occurs; however, they have common features. First, there is no gas distal to the level of the atresia, and second, the bowel proximal to the atresia is disproportionately dilated. Beyond that, it is just a matter of looking at the radiograph to try to guess how far down the bowel you can go before you encounter the atresia (Figs. 4-26 to 4-28). As a general rule to help you establish the level, remember that the duodenal bulb is located in the right upper quadrant of the abdomen; therefore, if you have a dilated stomach and loop only in the right upper quadrant, duodenal atresia is likely. The jejunum is predominantly in the upper abdomen and predominantly on the left side, whereas the ileum is in the right lower quadrant. If you see many dilated bowel loops and particularly large loops preponderantly to the right of the spine, it is probably an ileal atresia, whereas if the loops are confined to the upper abdomen and predominantly to the left, it is probably jejunal atresia. These are 70:30 rules, so don't get too preoccupied with them; on the other hand, they can be very helpful.

Meconium Ileus

Meconium ileus is a condition that mimics a distal bowel atresia and that deserves special note because of its prevalence in the white population. In meconium ileus, the contents of the bowel (meconium) are abnormal, becoming thick and viscous due to the lack of digestive enzymes. This material compacts in the ileum to cause a complete obstruction. One could think of it as analogous to filling a pipe with tar. Technically, this is not an atresia; however, it mimics an atresia because the bowel is completely

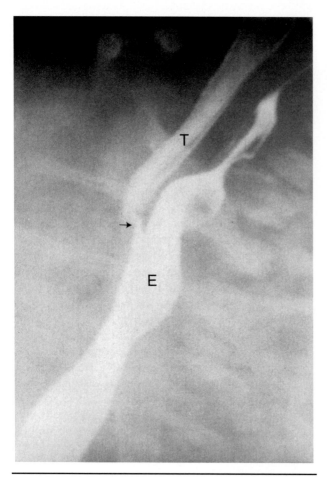

FIGURE 4-25. A barium esophagram on a baby with recurrent pneumonia shows a connection between the esophagus (E) and the trachea (T), a so-called H-type tracheal–esophageal fistula. This abnormality can sometimes be extremely difficult to detect.

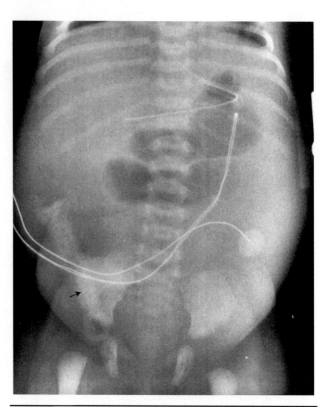

FIGURE 4-27. This infant had a moderate degree of abdominal distention at birth, which progressed to a worrisome abdominal distention within 6 hours. Note that there is no gas in the rectum and that only two dilated loops of bowel are identified, predominantly in the upper abdomen and to the left of the spine. These films are most consistent with abdominal obstruction very high in the bowel but distal to the duodenum. This is an example of surgically proven jejunal atresia.

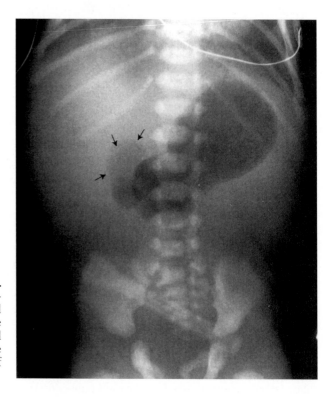

FIGURE 4-26. A newborn infant with marked abdominal distention. Note that the gas goes no farther than the very dilated duodenal bulb *(arrows)*. This is characteristic of the so-called double-bubble sign of duodenal atresia. Whenever you see a patient with duodenal atresia, think of the very frequent associations of Down syndrome and congenital heart disease and the less frequent association of esophageal atresia.

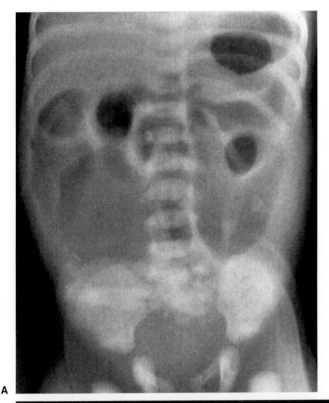

A

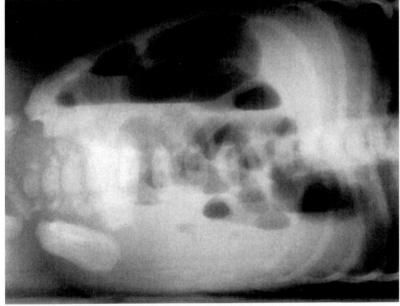

B

FIGURE 4-28. **A:** Abdominal radiograph of a 1-day-old baby with abdominal distention shows evidence of multiple dilated bowel loops and no gas in the rectum. The findings are consistent with an ileal atresia. **B:** A decubitus view of the same infant illustrated in A shows multiple air–fluid levels. The presence of air–fluid levels is sometimes valuable in distinguishing ileal atresia from meconium ileus. Air–fluid levels favor ileal atresia. Incidentally, note our old friend, the cord clamp.

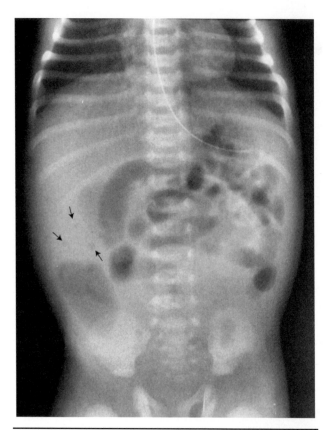

FIGURE 4-29. A newborn infant with a very distended abdomen. Note the bubbly appearance *(arrows)* in the right lower quadrant of the abdomen. These bubbles coupled with a paucity of gas in the rectum are characteristic of meconium ileus. The vast majority of babies with meconium ileus will also have cystic fibrosis.

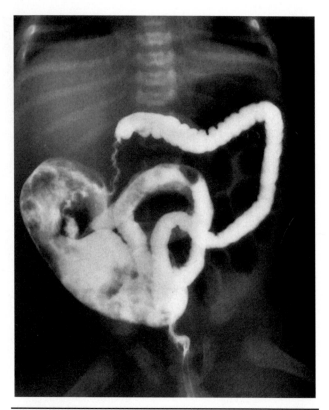

FIGURE 4-30. A contrast enema performed on the patient shown in Fig. 4-29 shows a very small (micro-) colon leading to a very dilated ileum distended with multiple filling defects. The filling defects are the impacted meconium, which gives meconium ileus its name. Remember that a microcolon means a distal obstruction.

obstructed by intraluminal content. There are a few signs that can be used to distinguish meconium ileus from ileal atresia. The meconium ileus usually entraps some air, so that one sees a bubbly appearance at the level of the meconium-filled bowel (Fig. 4-29). Also, the meconium is so thick and tarlike that it does not form air–fluid levels with the swallowed intestinal gas. This is in contradistinction to an ileal atresia, whereby the fluid intraluminal contents of the bowel interact with the swallowed gas to form multiple air–fluid levels.

No discussion of intestinal obstruction in neonates would be complete without mention of microcolon. *Microcolon* is another term for the small lumen colon that is encountered in babies with distal intestinal obstruction, usually either meconium ileus or ileal atresia. Babies' colons dilate because of the presence of intraluminal content, that is, meconium. This meconium is formed *in utero* by sloughing of the cells and mucus from the GI tract. If there is enough downstream bowel from an obstruction (e.g., in the instance of duodenal atresia), there will be enough cells and mucus sloughed to form meconium and the colon

will have this meconium content. If, however, the obstruction is low so that there is not enough bowel distal to the obstruction to form meconium, then one gets an unused or microcolon. Microcolon is therefore a common sign of distal bowel obstruction (Fig. 4-30). You can obviously be fooled, because diseases like Hirschsprung's disease, where the lumen is intact but the colon does not transport meconium normally, occasionally give you a microcolon. Again, the 99% rule prevails that microcolon means distal obstruction.

Hernias

Two other congenital anomalies merit discussion as the cause of abdominal catastrophes in neonates or in slightly older children. The first is the most common cause of bowel obstruction in children, the hernia. Hernias in children are usually congenital defects that allow the bowel to protrude into a space where it doesn't belong. The bowel then gets caught, swells, and complications ensue. The most common site of hernia is the inguinal area (Fig. 4-31), however, internal hernias, particularly in areas where the

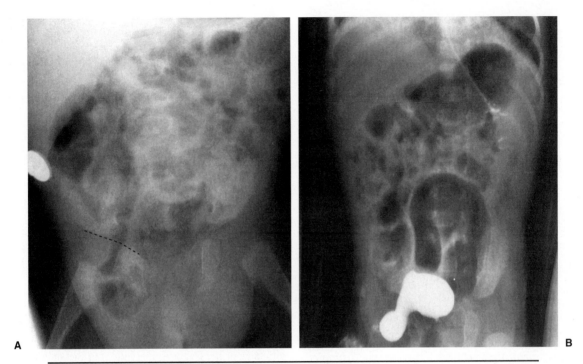

FIGURE 4-31. A: Plain radiograph of the abdomen shows bowel lying below the inguinal ligament *(dotted line)*. On a plain radiograph, the inguinal ligament is defined as the space between the symphysis pubis and the anterior superior iliac spine—in this case, the child had a large inguinal hernia filled with bowel. **B:** This baby, having a contrast study of the kidneys, had a protrusion of the lateral margin of his bladder into the right inguinal canal. A small protrusion can be normal; however, this large protrusion of bladder is associated with an inguinal hernia.

bowel goes from retroperitoneum to an intraperitoneal location, are also possible (Fig. 4-32). Hernias can go on for a long time if the bowel does not become compromised, but they can become very symptomatic very fast in instances where the bowel is compromised (Fig. 4-33). Some conditions of the neonate may enhance the possibility of a hernia, particularly conditions that involve chronic ascites, prematurity, or the presence of a ventricular peritoneal shunt for hydrocephalus (Fig. 4-34).

Malrotation

The other congenital abnormality worthy of special attention is that of malrotation. This condition occurs because of a congenital abnormality of fixation of the bowel. Remember that the bowel forms about the axis of the superior mesenteric artery (I bet you never thought you'd ever need that bit of embryology) and that the bowel herniates out of the body through the omphalus, then returns to the abdominal cavity. If, on return, the bowel does not rotate appropriately, it fixes in abnormal positions. This error in fixation of the bowel sets the scene for the bowel to twist and obstruct, causing the so-called midgut volvulus (Figs. 4-35 and 4-36). This is truly a surgical emergency and should be considered whenever you have an abnormal film suggesting obstruction, as well as the presence of bil-

ious vomiting in a child. Because the bowel twists about the superior mesenteric artery and vein, the major complication is vascular compromise of the bowel. If the bowel is not untwisted, the gut will die, leaving the child a nutritional cripple. Although malrotation is discussed with the neonatal diseases, be aware that it can present at any time in life. The majority of malrotation patients who get in trouble do so before 2 years of age; however, older children and adults can occasionally have malrotation-related problems.

CONGENITAL HEART DISEASE

Serious congenital heart disease has a prevalence of approximately 1 per 1000 live-born infants and therefore is a disease that you will likely encounter if you care for children. You could argue that this belongs in the neonatal section, but many children with serious heart disease present later, so I left it here—life is imperfect!

Although plain film is valuable for screening for congenital heart disease, it takes a tremendous amount of experience (and luck) before you can be specific as to the type of congenital heart disease. Several principles are very important. The first is that heart size in infants and children is more difficult to estimate than that in adults. The

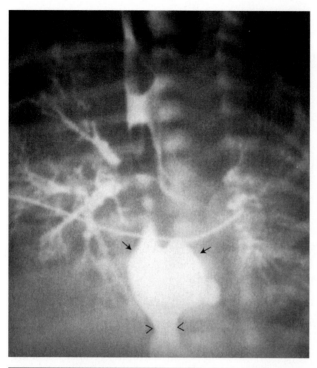

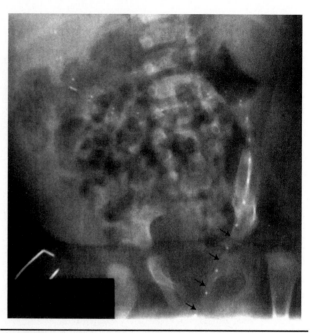

FIGURE 4-34. This baby with hydrocephalus had a ventricular peritoneal shunt. The radiopaque markers *(arrows)* show the course of the shunt. Notice that the shunt extends into an inguinal hernia. Because these babies have chronic ascites from the drainage of the cerebrospinal fluid into the abdomen, they are more prone to have inguinal hernias. Approximately one-third of babies with ventricular peritoneal shunts develop inguinal hernias.

FIGURE 4-32. This neonate has a large hiatus hernia or protrusion of stomach above the diaphragm. The hernia pouch *(arrows)* is shown in the chest, whereas the narrowing of the esophageal hiatus *(arrowheads)* shows the area where the stomach herniates through the periesophageal hiatus. Note that there is contrast in the lungs. This hernia was so large that it caused the baby to reflux contrast from his stomach to his esophagus and then aspirate. Unlike this one, most hiatus hernias are relatively benign.

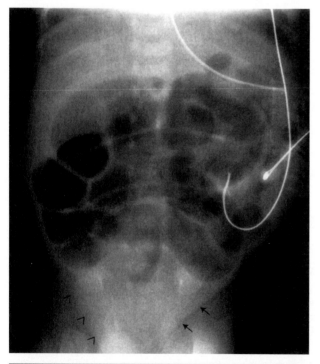

FIGURE 4-33. This premature infant developed signs of a bowel obstruction. Note the very dilated loops of small bowel on the film. The most important finding is the asymmetry of the inguinal folds, the right bulging in a concave fashion *(arrowheads)*, whereas the left is straight *(arrows)*. The bulge in the right groin is owing to an incarcerated inguinal hernia, a finding the clinician missed until they took off the patient's diaper.

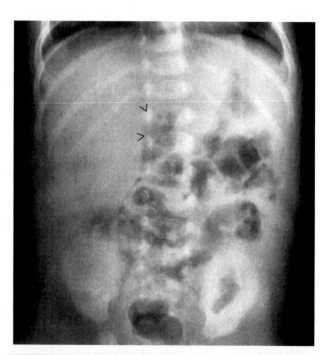

FIGURE 4-35. This 36-day-old infant began vomiting bilious material and became acutely ill. The plain abdominal radiograph is not diagnostic; however, note the gas-filled duodenal bulb *(arrowheads)*. It is very unusual to see gas in a normal duodenal bulb. The subsequent upper GI proved that this patient had a midgut volvulus. The plain film findings in midgut volvulus range from normal to complete bowel obstruction. When in doubt with an infant with bilious vomiting, note that an upper GI is always indicated.

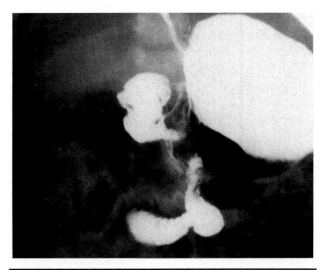

FIGURE 4-36. Upper GI in a 27-day-old baby who suddenly developed bilious vomiting. Note that the duodenum descends in the midline, then passes off to the right at the duodenal–jejunal junction *(arrows)*, never coming to the left of the spine and behind the stomach as is normal. This is characteristic of malrotation, an anomaly that occurs due to malfixation of the gut *in utero*. The greatest danger with these infants is midgut volvulus and infarction of the small bowel because of twisting about the vascular pedicle at the root of the mesentery.

rule of thumb of 50% cardiothoracic ratio is not valid in children. When you're looking for cardiomegaly in a child, you need to be sure *that you are not looking at thymus, that the film has been taken on a good breath, and that lateral views are used extensively*. If the heart protrudes signifi-

cantly beyond the visible airway on lateral view, the heart is usually enlarged. If on an anteroposterior (AP) view the heart appears large whereas on the lateral view it is normal, then you are usually dealing with a deceiving thymus (Fig. 4-37).

The second rule is that children can have very serious heart disease and a normal-sized heart. This is particularly true in conditions where blood flow to the lungs is insufficient because of right-to-left shunting. As a good general rule, children's hearts, being resilient, tend to dilate owing to a volume rather than a pressure overload. Conditions that cause right-to-left shunting, like tetralogy of Fallot, do not give you an enlarged heart because the volume of blood traversing the heart is actually diminished (Fig. 4-38). A truly cyanotic neonate with a normal chest film (including heart size) usually has some variant of tetralogy of Fallot.

Rule number three is that if you think the pulmonary vascularity is increased in a patient suspect for congenital heart disease, you are probably right; however, if you think it is decreased, you are probably wrong. For some reason, it is much easier for humans to perceive an increase in vascularity than a decrease in vascularity in a chest film, probably because of the way our brains are wired. An enlarged heart and increased vascularity in an older child who is not cyanotic usually means some form of left-to-right shunt such as a ventricular septal defect (Fig. 4-39).

Rule number four is applicable to neonates. We have already talked about the fact that being born is the ultimate time of transition. When you are *in utero*, very little

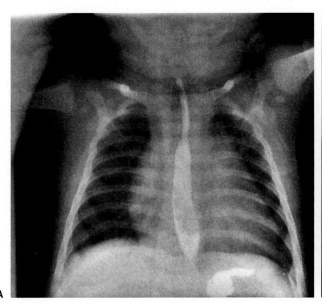

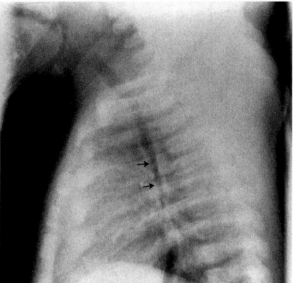

A

B

FIGURE 4-37. A: This child's heart measures over 60% of the transverse diameter of the chest on the radiograph. In an adult, this would be a large heart; however, this is a normal child with a large thymus simulating cardiomegaly. **B:** Note that on lateral view, the heart does not protrude posterior to the airway *(arrows)*.

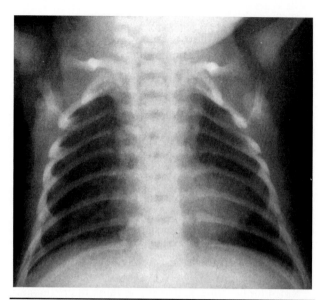

FIGURE 4-38. This cyanotic, extremely ill child has a relatively small but boot-shaped heart. The pulmonary vascularity is normal because of the presence of a patent ductus arteriosis. The findings are characteristic of a variant of tetralogy of Fallot.

flow to reach adult levels of blood flow through the lungs. All neonates, therefore, have a relative state of pulmonary hypertension. Early on, lesions that should have increased vascularity, such as transposition of the great vessels, are not revealed by radiograph (Fig. 4-40). The same logic explains why most left-to-right shunt lesions are not manifest until about 6 weeks of age (see rule three) when the pulmonary artery pressure has fallen significantly.

With those rules to consider, it is possible to set out a systematic approach to looking at the chest film of a newborn with congenital heart disease. First, see if the heart is enlarged and if you can determine which chamber is enlarged. Next, determine if the vascularity is normal or increased, keeping in mind that the younger the baby, the less confident you can be to find increased vascularity. Finally, you need to talk to your clinical colleagues and find out if the baby is truly cyanotic, as defined by arterial oxygen saturation of under 80% with a normal arterial CO_2 saturation. With those pieces of information you can look at Figures 4-41 and 4-42 and make a rough estimate as to what type of congenital heart disease the baby may have (Figs. 4-43 to 4-45).

blood goes through the pulmonary artery circuit. To understand this, think about physiology. *In utero*, the baby is not breathing air; therefore, there is no need for blood to bring oxygen to the baby from the lungs. Immediately following birth, the baby breathes air and the situation changes dramatically. It takes some time for the pulmonary arterial

MEDIASTINAL MASSES

Other than the thymus and bronchii, the remainder of the structures in the pediatric mediastinum are relatively inconspicuous unless abnormal. Pediatric mediastinal abnormalities (masses) conform to a compartmental scheme.

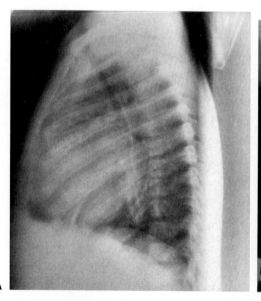
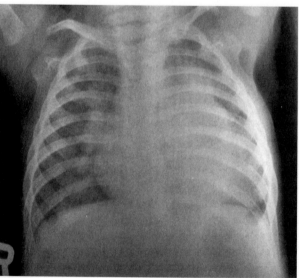

A   **B**

FIGURE 4-39. The AP **(A)** and lateral **(B)** radiographs of a 2-month-old infant with respiratory distress when feeding, but no evidence of cyanosis, shows a markedly increased pulmonary vascularity and a large heart. This combination in a child is characteristic of a congenital left-to-right shunt. The most common left-to-right shunt is a ventricular septal defect or a communication between the right and left ventricles.

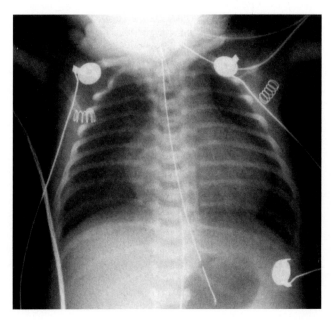

FIGURE 4-40. This very cyanotic patient has a chest radiograph showing a large heart, narrow superior mediastinum, and pulmonary vascularity that is slightly, but not dramatically, increased. The patient is a 3-day-old infant with transposition of the great vessels; the vascularity is going through the transition between the very high vascular resistance *in utero* and the lower vascular resistance of an air-breathing baby. Over the course of subsequent days, the vascular resistance will drop further and the lungs will become flooded.

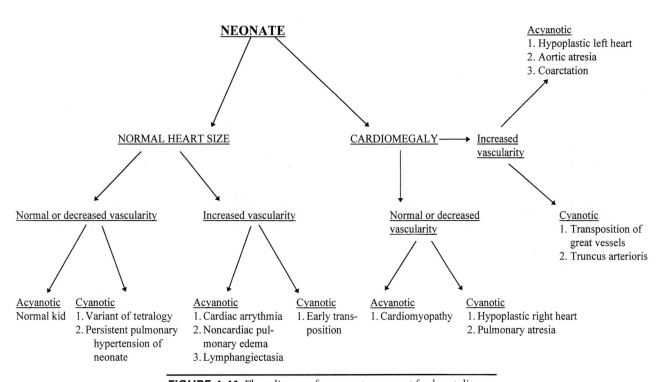

FIGURE 4-41. Flow diagram for neonates suspect for heart disease.

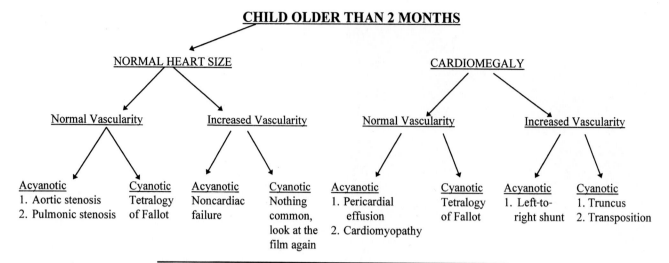

CHILD OLDER THAN 2 MONTHS

NORMAL HEART SIZE

CARDIOMEGALY

Normal Vascularity

Increased Vascularity

Normal Vascularity

Increased Vascularity

Acyanotic
1. Aortic stenosis
2. Pulmonic stenosis

Cyanotic
Tetralogy
of Fallot

Acyanotic
Noncardiac
failure

Cyanotic
Nothing
common,
look at the
film again

Acyanotic
1. Pericardial
    effusion
2. Cardiomyopathy

Cyanotic
Tetralogy
of Fallot

Acyanotic
1. Left-to-
    right shunt

Cyanotic
1. Truncus
2. Transposition

FIGURE 4-42. Flow diagram for older children suspect for heart disease.

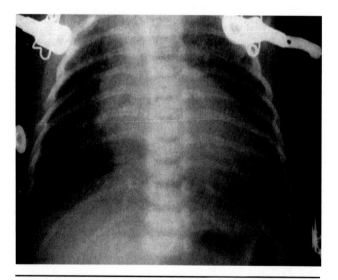

FIGURE 4-43. This child has a huge heart. Note that the superior mediastinum has a large shadow to the right of the trachea, a right aortic arch. The vessels are large, flooding the lung. If we add the information that the child was cyanotic, then this becomes a characteristic truncus arteriosis. Approximately 40% of truncus patients have a right arch.

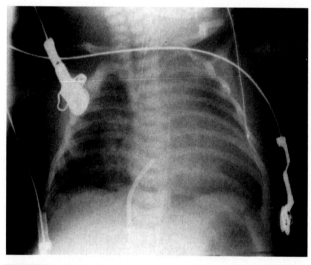

FIGURE 4-44. A large heart and increased vascularity; however, this time the child is not cyanotic. This usually means either a left heart obstructive lesion or failure for some other reason. The child has a hypoplastic left heart.

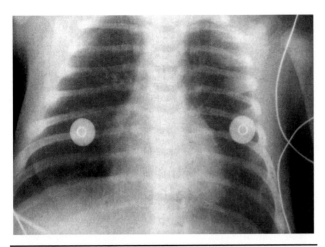

FIGURE 4-45. A large heart and increased vascularity in a 2-week-old baby—findings typical for transposition of the great vessels. Note the very thin mediastinum because the pulmonary artery is directly in front of the aorta as opposed to being slightly to the left of it. This is characteristic of the transposition of the great vessels.

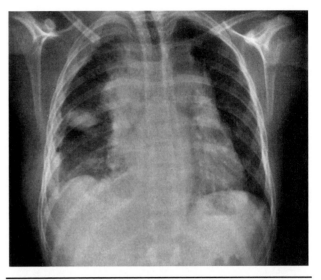

FIGURE 4-47. This anterior mediastinal lymphoma stops right at the undersurface of the clavicles. Remember that the anterior portion of the chest is physically lower than the posterior portion of the chest; therefore, any mass that has the clavicle as its superior margin must be an anterior mediastinal mass.

If you can accurately identify the compartment where a mass is located, you can provide an intelligent differential diagnosis. The anterior mediastinum is defined as part of the mediastinum visible in front of the airway on lateral view, and the posterior mediastinum is defined as that portion of the mediastinum just posterior to the anterior edge of the vertebral bodies on lateral view. Everything else is the middle mediastinal compartment (Fig. 4-46). The whole trick is telling these compartments apart, and there are a few rules:

1. *Clavicle cutoff sign:* The anterior chest is anatomically lower than the posterior chest, so if a mass stops at the inferior margin of the clavicle on the PA chest radiograph, it has to be in the anterior mediastinum (Fig. 4-47).
2. *Hilum overlay sign:* Structures in the far anterior mediastinum overlie the vessels at the lung hilum; therefore, the vessels are usually seen through these structures (Fig. 4-48).
3. *Posterior rib effacement:* Posterior mediastinal masses frequently spread the posterior ribs; therefore, distortion or asymmetry of the posterior ribs is a good sign that the mass is posterior (Fig. 4-49).
4. *Airway distortion sign:* Masses that distort the esophagus or compress the airways are almost surely middle mediastinum (Fig. 4-50).

Once you have applied these rules and decided in which compartment to look, the pathologic processes tend to categorize themselves fairly easily. Anterior mediastinal masses are almost always lymphoma or thymus related with the occasional thyroid mass or teratoma. An Aunt Minnie applies here: If the anterior mediastinal mass contains calcium, always go for teratoma (Fig. 4-51). Middle mediastinal masses are generally either lymph nodes or anomalous vessels related to the aortic arch. Esophageal and bronchial duplications are less frequent,

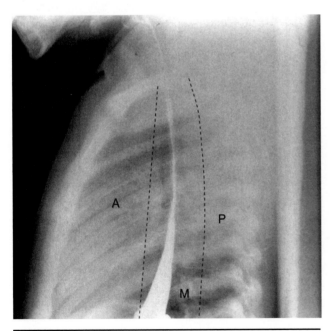

FIGURE 4-46. A normal lateral view of the chest, with barium in the esophagus, delineates the boundaries of the anterior (A), middle (M), and posterior (P) mediastinum. When you consider mediastinal masses, it is important mentally to divide the mediastinum into these components as it helps you to localize the likely diagnosis for the cause of the mass.

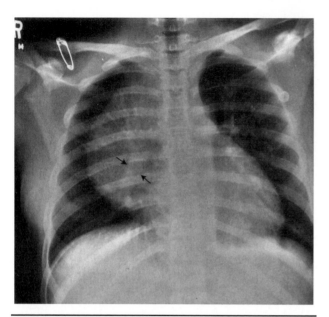

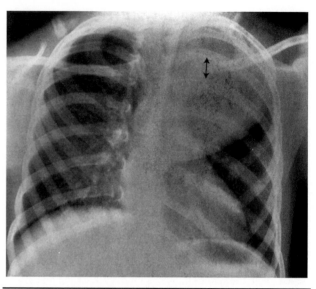

FIGURE 4-48. This teenager has an anterior mediastinal mass. Note that the descending branch of the right pulmonary artery *(arrows)* is visible through the mass, documenting that the tumor is not in the same plane as the vessel; otherwise, the silhouette sign would prevent the vessel from being visible. This is called the hilum overlay sign where masses out of plane of the hilum (usually anterior mediastinal masses) allow hilar structures to be visualized.

FIGURE 4-49. This child has a huge posterior mediastinal mass on the left. Note how the mass has spread the ribs posteriorly. Masses that distort the posterior ribs are almost always neural crest in origin, in this case a ganglioneuroblastoma.

but also occur in the middle mediastinum. Posterior mediastinum masses are neurogenic in origin, usually a neuroblastoma or ganglioneuroblastoma. When confronted with a suspected pediatric mediastinal mass, the first rule is to place it in the proper compartment; thereafter, it is a matter of pursuing the differential diagnosis.

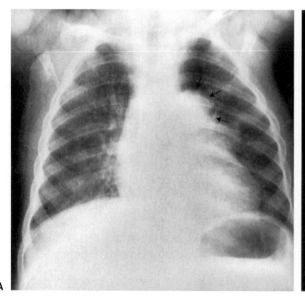

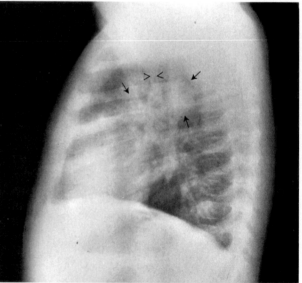

A

B

FIGURE 4-50. A: The large mass *(arrows)* near the mediastinum is displacing the upper lobe bronchus on the left. Note that the left lung is blacker than the right because the mass is causing partial obstruction of the left main stem bronchus, allowing air to get in but not to escape easily. The effect on the bronchus or blood vessels is characteristic of a middle mediastinum mass, in this case, a bronchogenic cyst. **B:** Lateral view shows the rounded mass *(arrows)* of the bronchogenic cyst in the same plane as the airway *(arrows)*.

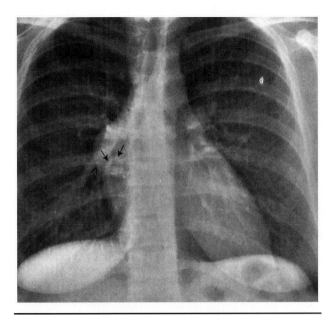

FIGURE 4-51. The mass lying anterior to the right hilum *(arrowheads)* contains a large glob of high-density calcium. Remember that anterior mediastinal mass plus calcium equals teratoma.

PYLORIC STENOSIS

A common intraabdominal condition worth discussion in babies (not brand new but 4 to 6 weeks old) is pyloric stenosis, which isn't a congenital anomaly. Pyloric stenosis is due to hypertrophy of the pyloric muscle induced by a heritable error in metabolism. Because of the heritable nature of the disease, it is somewhat a congenital defect, but it does not usually present right after birth because it takes some time for the abnormal chemistry to cause the pyloric muscle to hypertrophy to a sufficient degree to obstruct gastric outflow. The disease is male preponderant and classically presents with nonbilious vomiting and weight loss in a 6-week-old infant. The plain abdominal radiograph suggests a partial obstruction with a very dilated stomach. Upper GI will show elongation of the pyloric channel and the narrowing of that channel. Ultrasound is the current favored method for the definitive diagnosis, showing the very large pyloric muscle tumor in exquisite detail (Figs. 4-52 to 4-54).

CONDITIONS IN OLDER CHILDREN

CYSTIC FIBROSIS

When you are studying pediatric patients, it is always important to remember that the prevalence of congenital or heritable abnormalities is higher among the pediatric population than the adult population. Therefore, in looking at the radiographs of a child with recurrent pneumonias, you

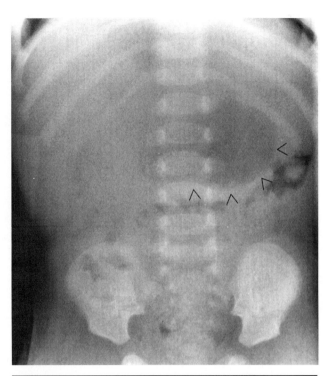

FIGURE 4-52. This 6-week-old infant had severe and pernicious vomiting that had become progressively worse over the course of a week. The impact on his nutrition was so severe that he had actually lost weight. Note the distended stomach *(arrowheads).* The presence of distal gas in his rectum shows that he was not completely obstructed, but the film is suggestive of a high-grade partial gastric outlet obstruction. About 90% of pyloric stenosis patients will have a plain film that looks like this.

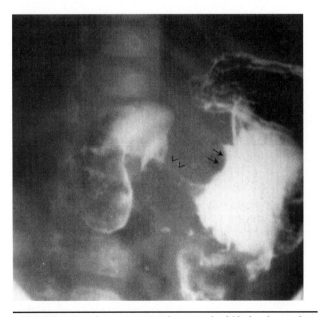

FIGURE 4-53. The upper GI in this 6-week-old baby shows elongation and narrowing of the pyloric channel *(arrowheads).* On the stomach side, notice the rounded indentation *(arrows)* caused by the very hypertrophied pyloric muscle. This is called the shoulder sign. Together this combination of signs is diagnostic for pyloric stenosis.

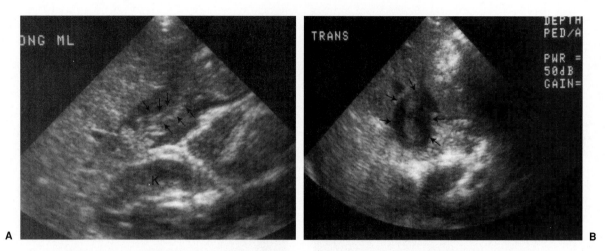

FIGURE 4-54. **A:** A longitudinal ultrasound view of the pylorus in a 6-week-old boy with vomiting. The pyloric muscle appears black, whereas the mucosa of the central lumen appears white *(arrows)*. During the entire period of observation, the configuration of the pyloric muscle did not change and measurement of the pyloric muscle revealed a thickness of 6 mm (normal is greater than 4 mm). This is diagnostic of pyloric stenosis. Note the intimate relationship of the pylorus to the right kidney (K). **B:** Transverse ultrasound view of the pylorus in the same infant as shown in A. Again the black or hypoechoic muscle surrounds the very echogenic mucosa. Arrows outline the transverse view of the pylorus. In pyloric stenosis, the muscle is thick and unchanging throughout the examination.

should think about heritable conditions that predispose the child to pneumonia, an example being cystic fibrosis. Cystic fibrosis, the most prevalent lethal genetic disease among the white population, begins with recurrent pneumonias but also has a number of features that allow a specific diagnosis from the films (Fig. 4-55). The lungs are usu-

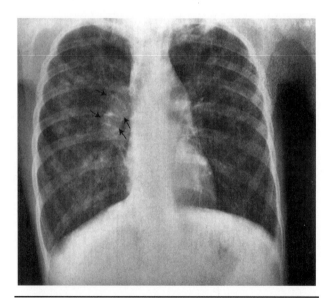

FIGURE 4-55. Typical chest film of a child with cystic fibrosis. Patchy infiltrates are present in both lung fields. The right hilus is very large and irregular owing to a combination of enlarged pulmonary artery and lymph nodes *(arrows)*. Note also that the heart is very small because of markedly overly expanded lungs. The pulmonary arteries are large because of a pulmonary hypertension. This is a very typical appearance for cystic fibrosis.

ally hyperexpanded because of the blockage of many of the smaller bronchi by mucous plugs. The presence of mucoid impactions, branch-shaped collections of intrabronchial mucus, is very suggestive of cystic fibrosis. Generally, the children have very prominent hili, due to the combination of the inflamed lymph nodes and pulmonary artery enlargement resulting from pulmonary hypertension caused by lung destruction. The last common finding of cystic fibrosis is that of peribronchial cuffing, or thickening of the walls of the bronchus, due to the intense inflammatory change induced by the disease (Fig. 4-56). None of these signs are pathognomonic for cystic fibrosis; however, all of these signs taken in combination make the likelihood of this disease very high.

INTUSSUSCEPTION

Intussusception, a disease in which one segment of bowel telescopes into another, has its maximum prevalence between the ages of 6 months and 2 years. The bowel is constantly in motion because of normal peristaltic activity. Theoretically, an inflamed intramural lymph node or some other structure alters this peristaltic activity, such that one segment of bowel begins to be propelled at a differential rate, leading to prolapse of one segment (intussusceptum) into the next contiguous portion of bowel (intussuscipiens). The intussusceptum becomes edematous because the blood supply of the prolapsed bowel is compromised and the intussusceptum begins to swell. This compounds the problem and leads to further extension

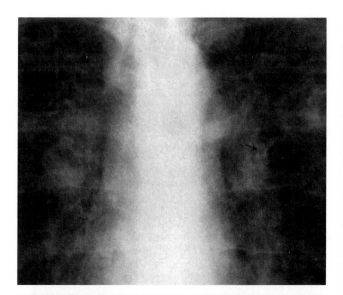

FIGURE 4-56. A close-up of the lung showing peribronchiolar thickening. Note that the bronchus appears as a black dot amidst a white cuff. This cuff is edema and inflammatory cage in the bronchial wall.

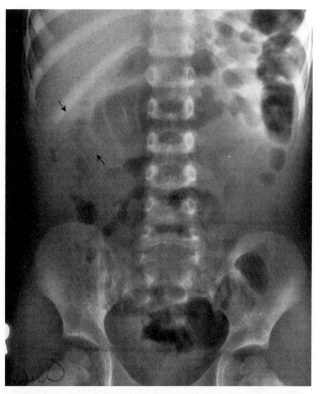

FIGURE 4-57. Notice the rounded density and a spiral gas pattern located in the right upper quadrant in this 2-year-old child with recurrent cramping, abdominal pain, and hematochazia *(arrows)*. This plain film alone, if not diagnostic, is certainly very suspicious of intussusception. About 80% of the time you can make the diagnosis of intussusception on plain film by looking for a rounded mass and the spiral air pattern that is so characteristic.

of the intussusception. The ultimate extension is protrusion of the intussusceptum from the rectum! In fact, in nineteenth century textbooks, the differential diagnosis of intussusception was rectal prolapse. The most common anatomic area involved in intussusception is the terminal ileum, and most intussusceptions are ileocecal.

Radiology plays a key role in the diagnosis as the child often presents with acute abdomen. Plain film shows evidence of partial bowel obstruction, and the intussusceptum is frequently visible on the plain film as a rounded density near the point of obstruction (Fig. 4-57). Diagnosis is confirmed either by ultrasound or by barium enema (Figs. 4-58 and 4-59). Radiology often plays both a diagnostic and a therapeutic role in intussusception. Between 50% and 80% of intussusceptions can be nonoperatively reduced using either an air enema or a contrast enema. These techniques are very specialized and should be performed only by trained personnel. They are, however, part of the standard armamentarium of any Board-certified radiologist.

APPENDICITIS

Appendicitis is the most common abdominal surgical emergency of later childhood. Appendicitis is one of the great mimics in that the symptoms can be fairly protean and the diagnosis in many instances is obscure (Table 4-3). There is an old adage that the clinical certainty of appendicitis should be about 85%, meaning that 15% of the appendices that a surgeon removes should be normal or the

surgeon is going to begin to miss some true-positive cases of appendicitis. Various radiology imaging techniques can narrow this false-positive rate somewhat, but really the value of imaging is in those cases where the diagnosis is in serious doubt. Look at it in another way. If imaging tests can give you 95% sensitivity, whereas clinical tests are 85% sensitive, the imaging doesn't add much in a situation where you are quite sure that appendicitis exists. On the other hand, in that case when you aren't sure or, let's say, you are only 30% sure, a 95% sensitivity test is crucial in deciding appropriate patient management. At current hospital prices, it is cheaper to do the test than to put the patient in the hospital overnight for observation.

▌ **TABLE 4-3 Classic Signs of Appendicitis**

1. Right lower quadrant pain
2. Leukocytosis
3. Anorexia/vomiting

Note: Only half of appendicitis patients under age 5 or over age 50 exhibit these signs!

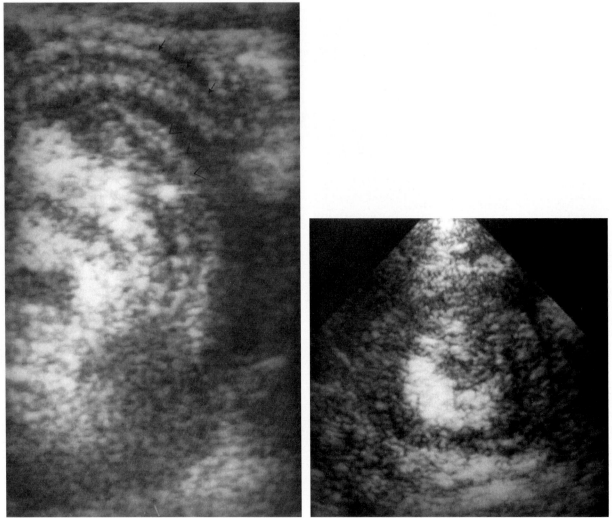

FIGURE 4-58. A: A longitudinal ultrasound view of an intussusception. Notice the intussusceptum *(arrowheads)* telescoping into the intussuscipiens. With a little imagination, you can almost see a coiled spring signal as the bowel wrinkles, with one loop of the bowel prolapsing into the other. **B:** A transverse view of an intussusception showing the target sign. The brightly echogenic material is the edematous mucosa, whereas the less echoic material is the wall of the intussusceptum.

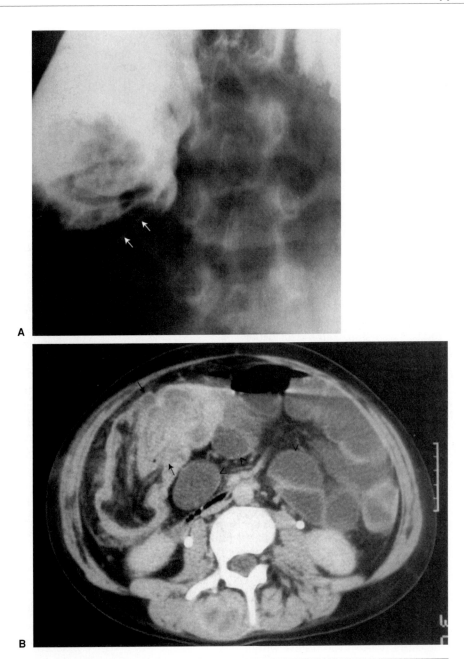

FIGURE 4-59. A: The barium enema in this 2-year-old child shows a round defect in the area of the cecum. Notice how the barium infiltrates in a spiral pattern as it pushes its way between the intussusceptum and the intussuscipiens. This so-called coiled spring *(arrows)* is characteristic of intussusception. **B:** This is a CT scan of a child with known tumor affecting the bowel wall. The child presented with abdominal pain owing to an intussusception *(arrows)* caused by a metastasis to a lymph node near his ileocecal valve. Note on this CT how you can see the same signs: the blunt-headed intussusceptum and the stretched fat of the mesentery, as the intussusceptum is propelled forward into the intussuscipiens. Note also the multiple fluid-filled bowel loops *(arrowheads)* from dilated small bowel secondary to the partial small bowel obstruction from the intussusception.

Appendicitis is discussed in detail in Chapter 3, so it will only be mentioned here.

SUMMARY

In this chapter, we have discussed the radiographs of children with particular emphasis on those conditions that are common and unique to pediatrics. As in any imaging, there will always be exceptions, but a few rules are key. Always remember the thymus as a deceiver in evaluating chest films in children, particularly younger children. Any anterior mediastinal mass is thymus, thymus, and thymus! Neonatal medical and surgical chest disease can be easily differentiated by remembering the rules of mediastinal shift and unilateral abnormality. If you apply carefully the rules of looking at congenital heart disease and mediastinal masses, you should be able to get into the ballpark about 80% of the time for making an accurate diagnosis of the correct lesion. That's a lot better than Babe Ruth did at batting, and look at how famous he is.

In summary, remember that it is normal for neonates to have considerable gas in their small bowel. As long as the walls are thin and the bowel loops are approximating each other, don't worry. Remember also that up to 6 months of age it is extremely difficult to tell large bowel from small bowel, and guesses as to whether a loop represents large or small bowel on plain film are exactly that—educated estimates. In babies with distended tummies, always look to the rectum to determine the presence of distal gas and thereby obstruction.

KEY POINTS—CHEST

- In some babies, *in utero* lung fluid takes more than a few minutes to clear, resulting in transient tachypnea of the newborn. This appears on radiographs as pleural effusions and streaky densities. TTN should resolve within the first 24 hours after birth.
- TTN is indistinguishable on radiographs from early neonatal pneumonia.
- The best clue to diagnosing congestive heart failure in babies is a radiograph displaying a streaky density pattern in the lungs and cardiomegaly. If the heart protrudes significantly beyond the visible airway on a lateral radiograph, the heart is generally enlarged.

- Hyaline membrane disease displays four characteristic radiographic features: diffuse granularity, uniform disease, air bronchograms, and a relatively small lung volume.
- Generally, surgical conditions are unilateral amd will displace the mediastinum away from the more abnormal side.
- Radiographic features of cystic fibrosis include hyperexpanded lungs, mucoid impactions, very prominent hili, and peribronchial cuffing.

KEY POINTS—ABDOMEN

- In summary, the rules for evaluating an infant's abdomen are different from those used for adults.
- The younger the child, the more discrepant the rules.
- Babies have a lot of air, and it is difficult to differentiate large from small bowel by plain film.
- Young children usually have congenital anomalies or atresias; slightly older children have manifestations of either congenital anomalies or heritable anomalies such as pyloric stenosis and malrotation.
- In children beyond 6 months, intussusception and appendicitis are the major clinical entities.
- In looking at abdominal films of children, remember that your odds are much better in diagnosing an unusual manifestation of a common disease (such as appendicitis) than in diagnosing a common manifestation of a rare disease.
- If you stick with the diagnosis and rules from this chapter, you will be right more often than you will be wrong.

REFERENCES

1. Silverman FN, Kuhn JP. *Caffey's pediatric x-ray diagnosis: an integrated imaging approach,* 9th ed., vols. 1 and 2. St. Louis, MO: Mosby, 1993.
2. Franken EA Jr, Smith WL. *Gastrointestinal imaging in pediatrics,* 2nd ed. New York: Harper & Row, 1982.

SUGGESTED READINGS

Strife JL, Bissett GS, Burrows PE. Cardiovascular system. In: Kirks DR, Griscom NT, eds. *Practical pediatric imaging: diagnostic radiology of infants and children.* Philadelphia: Lippincott-Raven Publishers, 1998.
Hedlund GL, Griscom NT, Cleveland RH, Kirks DR. Respiratory system. In: Kirks DR, Griscom NT, eds. *Practical pediatric imaging: diagnostic radiology of infants and children.* Philadelphia: Lippincott-Raven Publishers, 1998.

Chapter 5

Musculoskeletal System

William E. Erkonen and Carol A. Boles

NORMAL EXTREMITY IMAGES

When you think about it, bones are visible on nearly all radiographs. Therefore, radiologic anatomy of the musculoskeletal system is extremely important, but it is time-consuming to learn. Entire textbooks are dedicated to isolated joints, and there are just no shortcuts to mastering this detailed material. As always, a solid knowledge of normal image anatomy is a prerequisite for intelligent image evaluation. Remember that the anatomic structures are all the same—we are merely viewing them differently. Let us begin with normal image anatomy of the hand and move systematically cephalad to the shoulder girdle. This will be followed by normal image anatomy of the lower extremity from the foot to the hip.

Upper Extremity

People commonly injure their extremities because they actively encounter the environment with their arms and legs.

Consequently, you will probably order many radiographs of the extremities in your clinical practice. Thus, we need a system to evaluate upper and lower extremity images (Table 5-1). Each bone in an image must be carefully evaluated for density, variations of normal, and fracture. Also, each joint must be evaluated for width, smoothness of the articular surfaces, dislocation, arthritis, fracture, and foreign body. The soft tissues should be evaluated for edema, hemorrhage, masses, calcifications, and foreign bodies.

The hand is so complex that it is a subspecialty in both orthopedics and plastic surgery, so don't expect to conquer the anatomy overnight. When you request radiographs of the hand, the standard study usually consists of posteroanterior (PA), oblique, and lateral views (Fig. 5-1). *Remember that one of the most difficult aspects of medicine is to learn the jargon and routines, so we need to get the hand terminology correct from the beginning.* Each digit of the hand must be properly named to communicate and document information accurately. The proper terminology for each digit and the numbering system for the metacarpals are

▶ **TABLE 5-1** **Observation Checklist for Bone Radiographs**

Each bone should be evaluated for
Density
Anomaly
Fracture
Tumor
Foreign body
Infection

Each joint should be evaluated for
Articular surface smoothness
Symmetry
Fracture
Dislocation
Arthritis
Foreign body

Soft tissues should be evaluated for
Edema
Hemorrhage
Calcifications
Masses
Foreign bodies

displayed in Fig. 5-1A. Simply numbering the digits does not suffice, especially in situations where digits are missing. Would you refer to the index finger as the first or second finger when the thumb is missing? So, beginning on the radial side of the hand, the thumb is always the thumb and not the first finger. Next is the index finger (not the second finger and not the first finger as some say there are four fingers and a thumb). Then the long finger (not the third or middle finger), the ring finger (not the fourth), and the small or little finger (not the fifth).

Metacarpals (Fig. 5-1A) are numbered logically with the thumb articulating with the first metacarpal, the index finger with the second metacarpal, and so on. As a general rule, each hand digit has three phalanges except the thumb, which has only two. The phalanges are named proximal, middle, and distal. The joint between the proximal phalanx and the metacarpal is called the metacarpophalangeal (MCP) joint (Fig. 5-1A). The joint between the proximal and middle phalanges is the proximal interphalangeal (PIP) joint. The joint between the distal and middle phalanges is called the distal interphalangeal (DIP) joint. The thumb, with only two phalanges, has an interphalangeal (IP) joint. The distal-most aspect of the metacarpals and phalanges is the head, whereas the proximal portions are the bases. The central aspects of these bones are the shafts.

Commonly used bone terms such as physis, epiphysis, metaphysis, and diaphysis can be confusing to the novice, but actually they are very simple. The locations of these entities are demonstrated in Fig. 5-1C. The physis (physeal or epiphyseal plate) is the growth plate as bone formation occurs on both sides (epiphysis and metaphysis) of the physis. The physis is the weakest part of a growing bone. The epiphysis is a secondary ossification center at the end of the bone, the metaphysis is just proximal to the physis, and the diaphysis (bone shaft) is between the proximal and

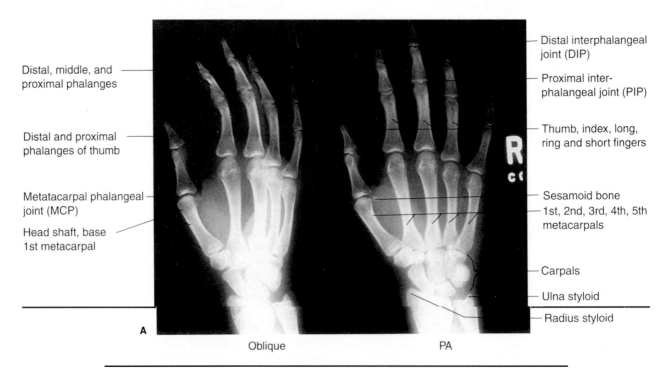

FIGURE 5-1. A: Right-hand oblique and posteroanterior (PA) radiographs. Normal. (*continued*)

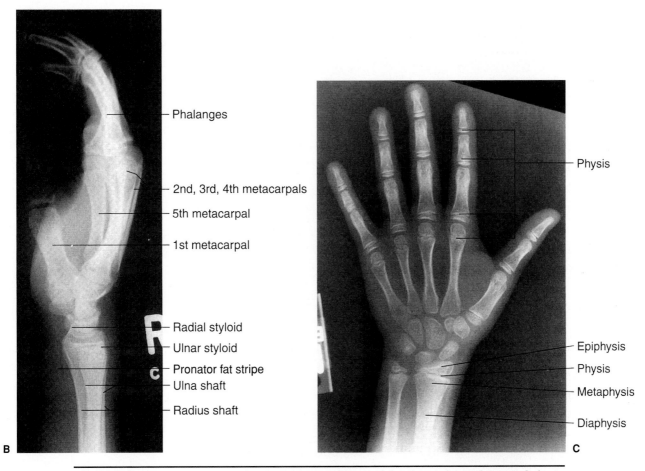

FIGURE 5-1. B: Right-hand lateral radiograph. Normal. **C:** Left-hand PA radiograph. Normal physis, epiphysis, metaphysis, and diaphysis. The cartilaginous physis is a lucent area on a radiograph.

distal metaphyses. Eventually, the epiphysis and metaphysis fuse as the physis closes. The term apophysis is confusing and merely refers to an epiphysis that does not articulate with another bone and does not contribute to bone length growth, but rather to bone contour. A typical example is the greater trochanter as seen in Fig. 5-23.

The wrist and forearm are common fracture sites, especially in children. If we are to intelligently understand and treat fractures in these areas, a thorough knowledge of wrist and forearm anatomy is very important. The appearance, location, and names of each carpal bone must be learned, as well as their relationship to the distal radius and ulna. These relationships are well visualized on standard PA, lateral, and oblique radiographic views of the wrist (Fig. 5-2).

We generally obtain anteroposterior (AP) and lateral views of the forearm in children and adults (Fig. 5-3). Routine elbow radiographs consist of AP and lateral views (Fig. 5-4), but external rotation oblique views of the elbow may be requested on occasion (Fig. 5-5A). Radiographs of the humerus usually consist of AP (see Fig. 5-5A) and lateral views. Generally, an AP radiograph is obtained to eval-

uate the shoulder (Fig. 5-5B), and this is supplemented by either an axillary or lateral view of the shoulder depending on local practice. Musculoskeletal anatomy and disease can be nicely demonstrated by computed tomography (CT) and magnetic resonance imaging (MRI) (Table 5-2). CT imaging is especially good for bone detail, whereas MRI is good for soft tissue and bone marrow imaging, which can reveal edema caused by bone contusions or subtle fractures not seen on the radiographs. MRI is especially

▌**TABLE 5-2 Musculoskeletal CT and MRI Indications**

Computed tomography
Bone detail
Fracture fragment evaluation
Bone tumor workup

Magnetic resonance imaging
Bone marrow imaging for occult fracture or metastasis
Soft tissue evaluation: ligaments, tendons, cartilages, and vessels
Bone tumor workup

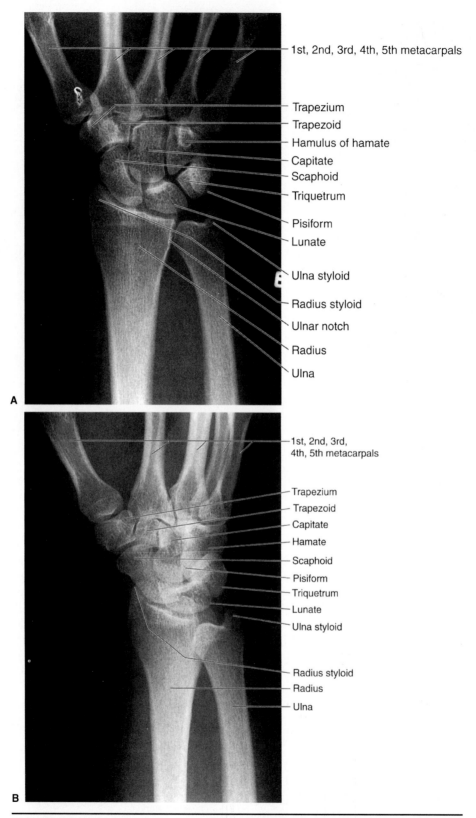

A

—1st, 2nd, 3rd, 4th, 5th metacarpals

—Trapezium
—Trapezoid
—Hamulus of hamate
—Capitate
—Scaphoid
—Triquetrum

—Pisiform
—Lunate

—Ulna styloid

—Radius styloid

—Ulnar notch

—Radius

—Ulna

B

—1st, 2nd, 3rd, 4th, 5th metacarpals

—Trapezium
—Trapezoid
—Capitate
—Hamate
—Scaphoid
—Pisiform
—Triquetrum
—Lunate
—Ulna styloid

—Radius styloid
—Radius
—Ulna

FIGURE 5-2. Right wrist PA **(A),** oblique **(B),** and lateral **(C)** radiographs. Normal. Notice that the tip of the radial styloid is distal to the tip of the ulnar styloid and the radius articulates distally with the scaphoid and lunate carpals and laterally with the ulna (ulnar or sigmoid notch). The distal radial articular surface slopes toward the ulna and anteriorly (palmar). The distal ulna articulates with the radius laterally and wrist fibrocartilage distally. The ulna does not articulate directly with a carpal. (*continued*)

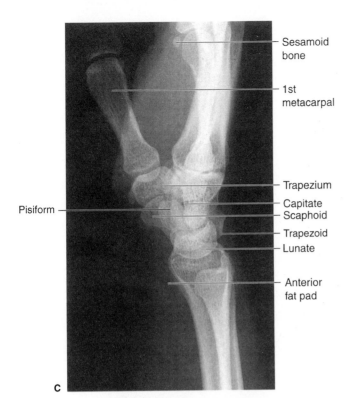

Sesamoid bone

1st metacarpal

Trapezium

Capitate

Scaphoid

Trapezoid

Lunate

Anterior fat pad

Pisiform

C

FIGURE 5-2. (*Continued*)

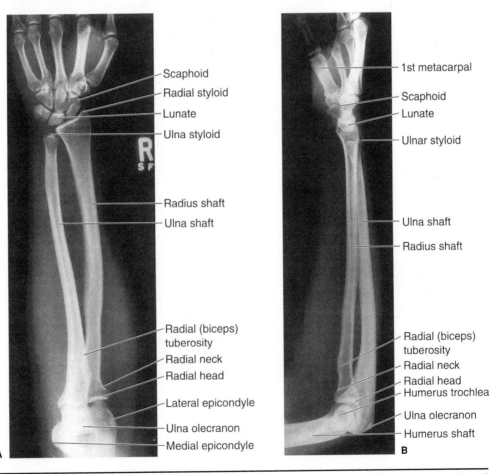

Scaphoid

Radial styloid

Lunate

Ulna styloid

Radius shaft

Ulna shaft

Radial (biceps) tuberosity

Radial neck

Radial head

Lateral epicondyle

Ulna olecranon

Medial epicondyle

A

1st metacarpal

Scaphoid

Lunate

Ulnar styloid

Ulna shaft

Radius shaft

Radial (biceps) tuberosity

Radial neck

Radial head

Humerus trochlea

Ulna olecranon

Humerus shaft

B

FIGURE 5-3. Right forearm AP (**A**) and lateral (**B**) radiographs. Normal. Note in the correct lateral of the forearm, both the elbow and wrist are in the lateral position. The distal radius is large and the proximal radius is small whereas the distal ulna is small and the proximal ulna is large. The radius is far more important than the ulna in the wrist joint whereas the ulna is more important in the elbow joint than the radius.

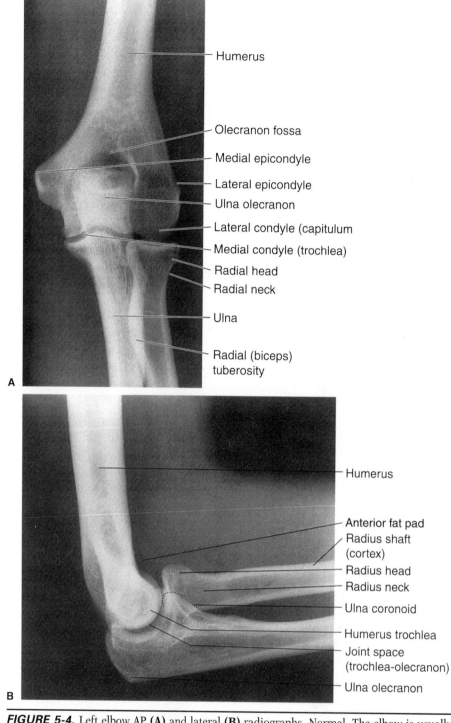

FIGURE 5-4. Left elbow AP **(A)** and lateral **(B)** radiographs. Normal. The elbow is usually flexed 90 degrees to minimize the appearance of the anterior and posterior fat pads. The *dotted line* on **B** indicates the ulna coronoid process.

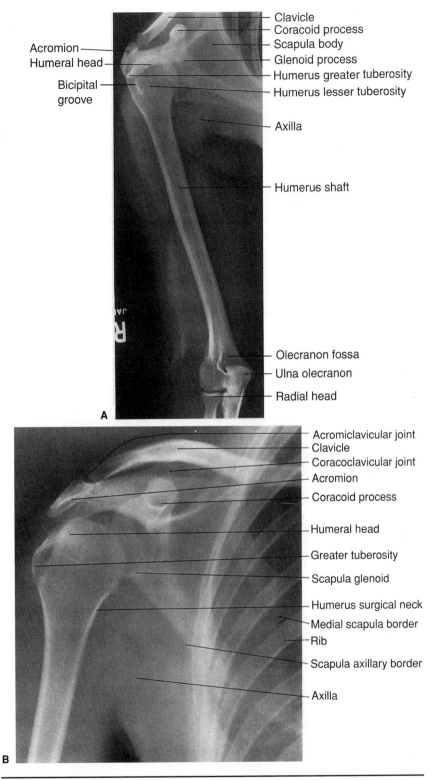

Clavicle
Coracoid process
Scapula body
Glenoid process
Humerus greater tuberosity
Humerus lesser tuberosity
Acromion
Humeral head
Bicipital groove

Axilla

Humerus shaft

Olecranon fossa
Ulna olecranon
Radial head

Acromiclavicular joint
Clavicle
Coracoclavicular joint
Acromion
Coracoid process

Humeral head

Greater tuberosity

Scapula glenoid

Humerus surgical neck
Medial scapula border
Rib
Scapula axillary border

Axilla

FIGURE 5-5. A: Right humerus AP radiograph with external rotation of the humerus. Normal. The right elbow is in an oblique position. **B:** Right shoulder AP radiograph with external rotation of the humerus. Normal. Note the prominence of the greater tuberosity.

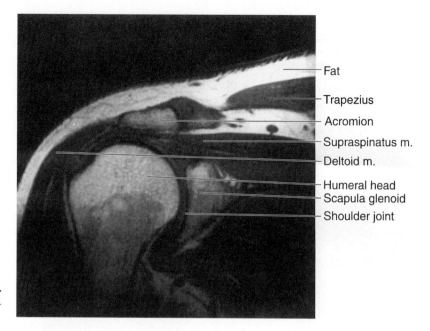

Fat

Trapezius

Acromion

Supraspinatus m.

Deltoid m.

Humeral head
Scapula glenoid
Shoulder joint

FIGURE 5-6. Right shoulder coronal T1 MR image. Normal.

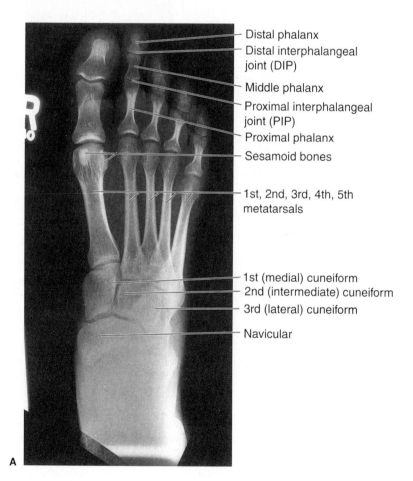

Distal phalanx
Distal interphalangeal joint (DIP)

Middle phalanx

Proximal interphalangeal joint (PIP)

Proximal phalanx

Sesamoid bones

1st, 2nd, 3rd, 4th, 5th metatarsals

1st (medial) cuneiform
2nd (intermediate) cuneiform
3rd (lateral) cuneiform

Navicular

FIGURE 5-7. Right foot AP **(A)**, oblique **(B)**, and lateral **(C)** radiographs. Normal. *(continued)*

A

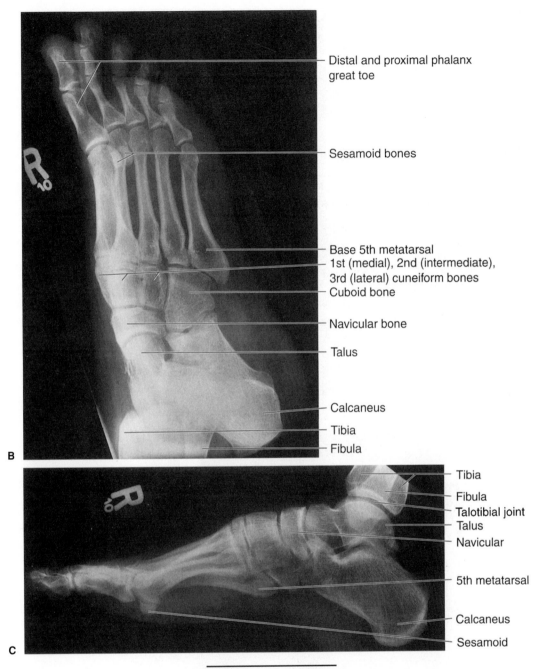

Distal and proximal phalanx great toe

Sesamoid bones

Base 5th metatarsal
1st (medial), 2nd (intermediate), 3rd (lateral) cuneiform bones
Cuboid bone

Navicular bone

Talus

Calcaneus

Tibia

Fibula

B

Tibia
Fibula
Talotibial joint
Talus
Navicular

5th metatarsal

Calcaneus

Sesamoid

C

FIGURE 5-7. (*Continued*)

helpful in displaying the soft tissue structures around joints such as shoulder rotator cuff anatomy (Fig. 5-6).

Lower Extremity

Now we approach lower extremity radiologic imaging by beginning with the foot and moving toward the hip. The standard views of the foot are AP, lateral, and oblique (Fig. 5-7). Naming of the toes is far easier than that of the fingers. The big toe or great toe may be referred to as the first toe, and the remaining toes are numbered sequentially ending with the little or fifth toe. Similarly, the metatarsals are numbered sequentially with the great toe articulating with the first metatarsal, the second toe articulating with the second metatarsal, and so forth. The ankle is usually imaged by AP, lateral, and either oblique or mortise-view (an internally rotated view) radiographs (Fig. 5-8). MRI may be used to image the ankle to detect soft tissue injury (Fig. 5-9). Radiographs of the tibia and fibula usually consist of AP and lateral views (Fig. 5-10).

Routine knee radiographs consist of AP and lateral views, and they may be supplemented by AP standing radiographs (Fig. 5-11A, B, C) and/or oblique views. Axial, coronal, and sagittal MR images of the knee (Fig. 5-12)

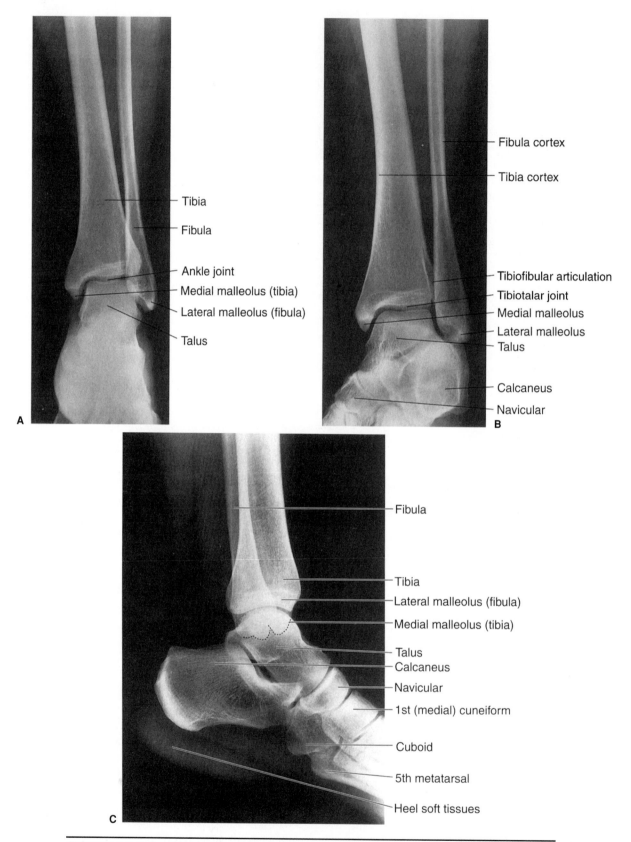

FIGURE 5-8. Left ankle AP **(A)**, oblique/mortise **(B)**, and lateral **(C)** radiographs. Normal. Note how the mortise view (B) allows improved visualization of the distal tibiofibular articulation.

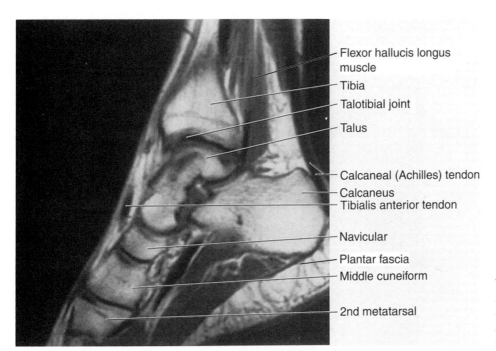

- Flexor hallucis longus muscle
- Tibia
- Talotibial joint
- Talus
- Calcaneal (Achilles) tendon
- Calcaneus
- Tibialis anterior tendon
- Navicular
- Plantar fascia
- Middle cuneiform
- 2nd metatarsal

FIGURE 5-9. Right ankle sagittal T1 MR image. Normal. Note that the calcaneal (Achilles) tendon has a homogeneous low-intensity (black) signal.

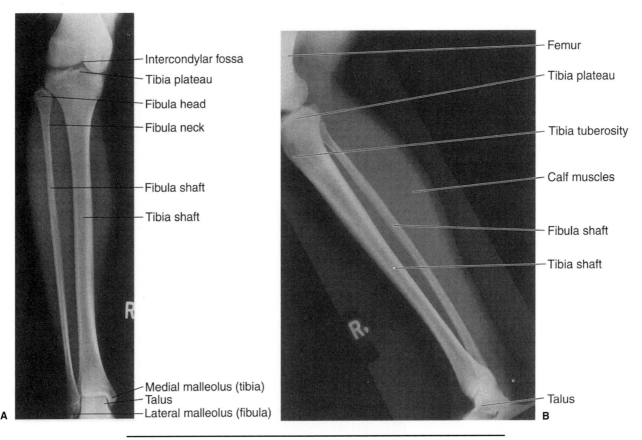

- Intercondylar fossa
- Tibia plateau
- Fibula head
- Fibula neck
- Fibula shaft
- Tibia shaft
- Medial malleolus (tibia)
- Talus
- Lateral malleolus (fibula)

A

- Femur
- Tibia plateau
- Tibia tuberosity
- Calf muscles
- Fibula shaft
- Tibia shaft
- Talus

B

FIGURE 5-10. Right tibiofibular AP (**A**) and lateral (**B**) radiographs. Normal.

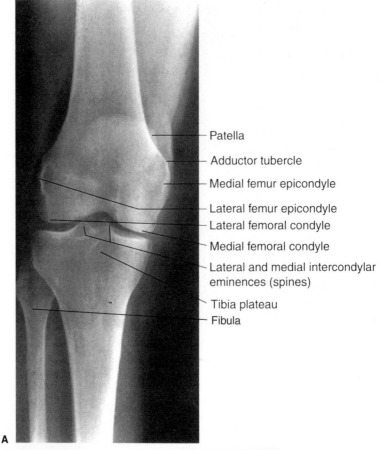

- Patella
- Adductor tubercle
- Medial femur epicondyle
- Lateral femur epicondyle
- Lateral femoral condyle
- Medial femoral condyle
- Lateral and medial intercondylar eminences (spines)
- Tibia plateau
- Fibula

A

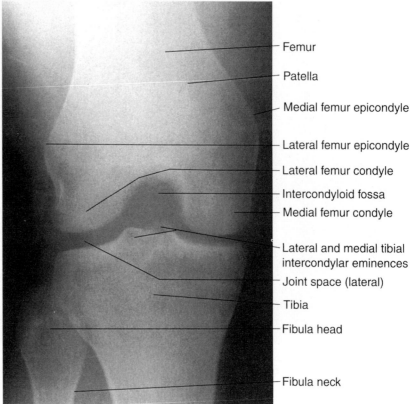

- Femur
- Patella
- Medial femur epicondyle
- Lateral femur epicondyle
- Lateral femur condyle
- Intercondyloid fossa
- Medial femur condyle
- Lateral and medial tibial intercondylar eminences
- Joint space (lateral)
- Tibia
- Fibula head
- Fibula neck

FIGURE 5-11. Right knee AP **(A)**, AP standing **(B)**, and lateral **(C)** radiographs. Normal. (*continued*)

B

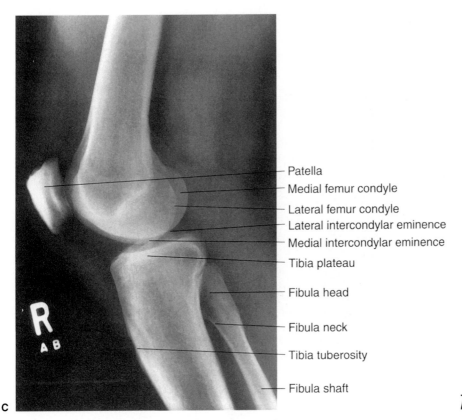

Patella
Medial femur condyle
Lateral femur condyle
Lateral intercondylar eminence
Medial intercondylar eminence
Tibia plateau
Fibula head
Fibula neck
Tibia tuberosity
Fibula shaft

C

FIGURE 5-11. (*Continued*)

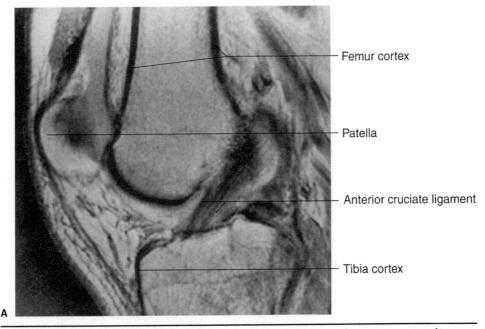

Femur cortex

Patella

Anterior cruciate ligament

Tibia cortex

A

FIGURE 5-12. A: Right knee proton-dense sagittal MR image. Normal anterior cruciate ligament in a 36-year-old man. **B:** Right knee proton-dense sagittal MR image in the same patient. Normal posterior cruciate ligament. The posterior cruciate ligament *(arrow)* is more homogeneous and has a lower intensity signal (blacker) than the anterior cruciate ligament. **C:** Right knee proton-dense medial-sagittal MR image in a 32-year-old man. Normal posterior horn *(straight arrow)* and anterior horn *(curved arrow)* of the medial meniscus.

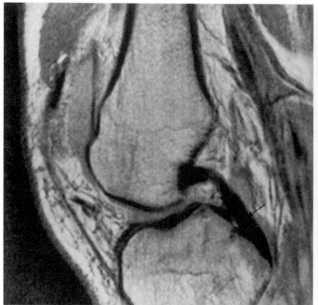

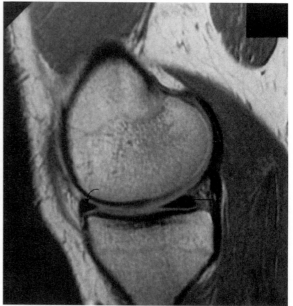

B

C

FIGURE 5-12. (*Continued*)

are commonly requested to evaluate injuries of the knee, particularly the nonosseous structures, including the medial and lateral menisci, articular cartilage, ligaments, tendons, and muscles. *Remember that ligaments, tendons, and vessels have a low-intensity signal or appear black on MR images.*

The femur and the hip joint are radiographed in the AP and lateral views (Fig. 5-13). A cross-table lateral of the hip is frequently obtained in a trauma setting as seen in Fig. 5-68B.

VARIATIONS OF NORMAL

There are several osseous variations of normal that can cause confusion for the novice (Table 5-3). One such variation of normal is the *sesamoid bone,* which is merely a normal extra bone, usually within a tendon. Sesamoids occur at numerous sites and are commonly found in the plantar aspect of the foot near the head of the first metatarsal (see Fig. 5-7), and in the palmar aspect of the hand near the head of the first metacarpal (see Figs. 5-1A and 5-14A–C),

▶ **TABLE 5-3 Normal Osseous Variations**

Sesamoid bones (located within a tendon like the patella)
Ossicles (extra small bones)
Supernumerary epiphyses
Coalitions/fusions
Bone islands

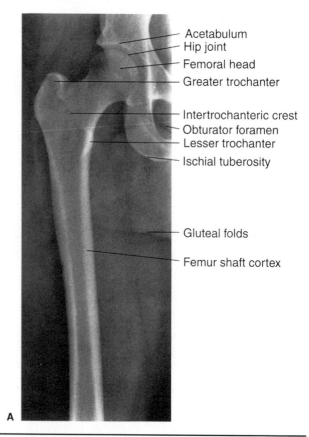

- Acetabulum
- Hip joint
- Femoral head
- Greater trochanter

- Intertrochanteric crest
- Obturator foramen
- Lesser trochanter
- Ischial tuberosity

- Gluteal folds

- Femur shaft cortex

A

FIGURE 5-13. A: Right hip and proximal femur AP radiograph. Normal. Left hip AP (**B**) and frog-leg lateral (**C**) radiographs. Normal. See Fig. 5-68B for a true lateral of the hip. (*continued*)

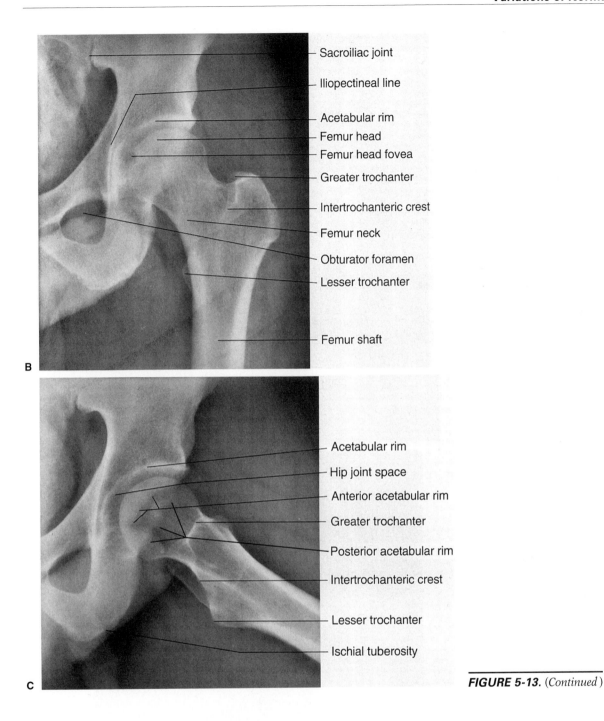

Sacroiliac joint

Iliopectineal line

Acetabular rim
Femur head
Femur head fovea

Greater trochanter

Intertrochanteric crest

Femur neck

Obturator foramen

Lesser trochanter

Femur shaft

B

Acetabular rim

Hip joint space

Anterior acetabular rim

Greater trochanter

Posterior acetabular rim

Intertrochanteric crest

Lesser trochanter

Ischial tuberosity

C

FIGURE 5-13. (*Continued*)

FIGURE 5-14. Left wrist PA **(A)**, left hand oblique **(B)** and lateral **(C)** radiographs. Multiple sesamoids (*arrows*). Bone islands (*curved arrows*) are present in the head of the 5th metacarpal and the capitate, and they have no clinical significance. **D:** Left foot AP radiograph. Os tibiale externum (*straight arrow*) and os peroneum (*curved arrow*). Right knee anterior radiograph **(E)**, tangential radiograph of right patella **(F)**, and axial fat-suppressed MR image **(G)**. Bipartite patella. Note that the patella has two sections and the accessory bone (*curved arrows*) usually lies superior and lateral to the main body of the patella. The axial image (G) shows the continuous cartilage over the ossification center (straight arrows) differentiating it from a fracture, which is rare in this superolateral position. **H:** Right wrist PA radiograph. Normal distal right radial epiphysis spur. This 21-year-old woman fell and had a painful wrist. This spur (*arrow*) is a variant of normal and must not be confused with a fracture. *I:* Right ankle AP radiograph. Accessory epiphysis near the tip of the distal tibia epiphysis in the region of the medial malleolus (*arrow*). This is a variant of normal. (*continued*)

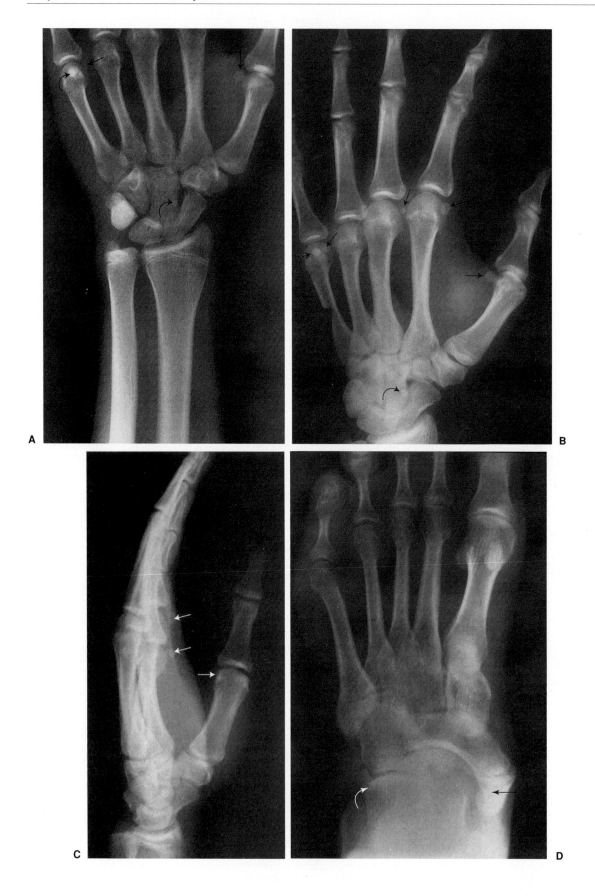

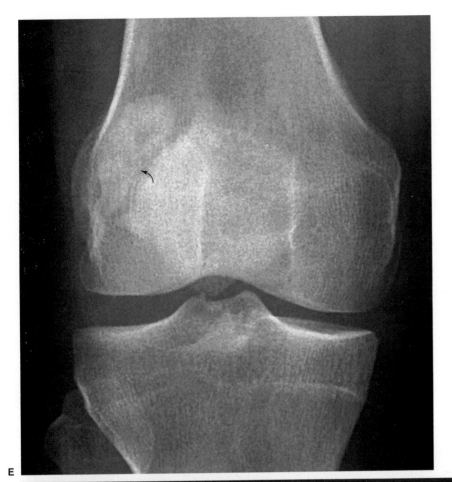

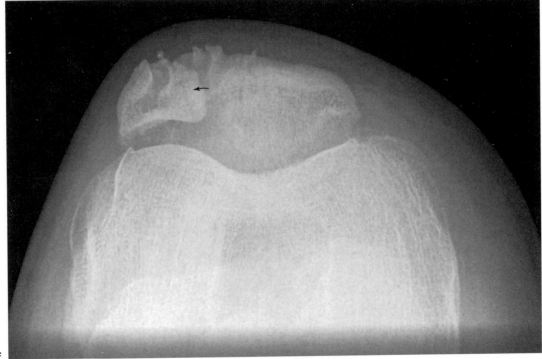

FIGURE 5-14. (*Continued*)

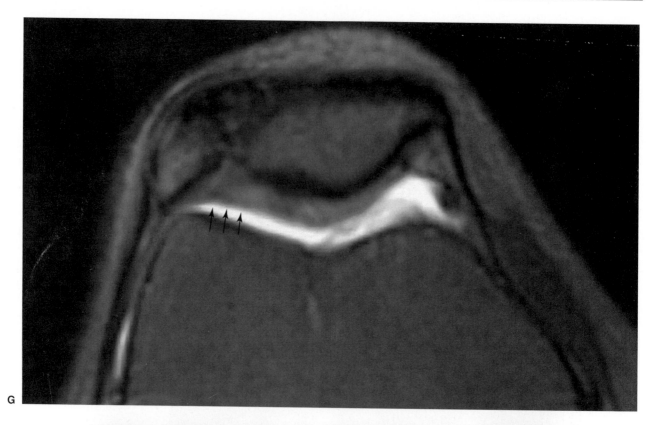

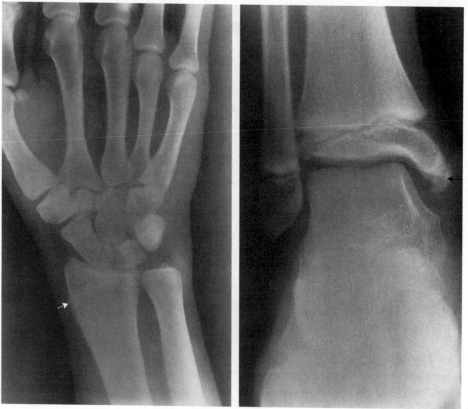

FIGURE 5-14. *(Continued)*

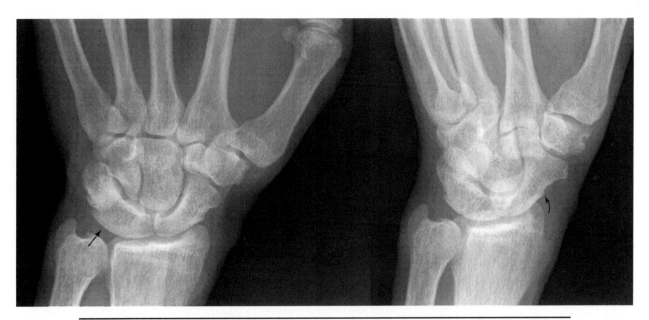

FIGURE 5-15. Left wrist PA and oblique radiographs. Congenital fusion. There is coalition of the lunate and triquetrum (*arrow*) and a prominent scaphoid tubercle (*curved arrow*). This tubercle should not be confused with a fracture. Compare to the normal carpals in Fig. 5-2.

where they are actually located in the volar plate rather than in a tendon. When you think about it, the patella is actually a sesamoid bone or a bone within a tendon. Sesamoids function to decrease the moment arm and thus the work of a muscle. The quadriceps group of muscles becomes hypertrophied to compensate for increased work following removal of the patella.

Ossicles are another variant of normal. They are small supernumerary or extra bones found in a variety of places in juxtaposition to the skeletal system and usually named after the neighboring bone (Figs. 5-14D and 6-16). The bipartite or multipartite patella (Fig. 5-14E, F, G) is another example of an accessory bone that should not be mistaken for a fracture. The condition results when one or more of the patellar ossification centers fails to fuse with the main patellar body. The result is that the patella has two or more sections, and this variant occurs superolaterally approximately 75% of the time. There is a strong male predominance.

Epiphyses can vary in appearance and in their number of ossification centers and still be normal (Fig. 5-14H, I). A sometimes confusing variant is a prominent scaphoid tubercle. This prominence can be mistaken for a fracture by even experienced clinicians (Fig. 5-15).

CONGENITAL AND DEVELOPMENTAL ANOMALIES

Osseous congenital anomalies are not uncommon, and a few of the many variations are illustrated in Figs. 5-16 to 5-19 and listed in Table 5-4.

Coalition refers to the failure of segmentation of bones during development, resulting in a congenital fusion. This fusion may be bony or fibrous. Common locations involve the lunate and triquetrum in the wrist (Fig. 5-15) and the calcaneus and navicular or calcaneus and talus in the foot (Fig. 5-16).

Osteogenesis imperfecta is a congenital, non-sex-linked, hereditary abnormality with the primary defect in collagen synthesis with deficient bone matrix. These patients have abnormal bones (Fig. 5-20) that are fragile, fracture easily, and are often deformed. Achondroplasia is a hereditary,

▶ **TABLE 5-4 Some Bone Anomalies**

Upper extremity
Supernumerary digits or polydactylism
Missing bones (fingers, radius)
Coalition (carpals)
Large digits or macrodactyly
Supracondylar process

Lower extremity
Polydactylism
Coalition (calcaneus with talus or navicular)
Developmental dysplasia hip
Slipped capital femoral epiphysis
Legg-Calvé-Perthes disease (avascular necrosis)
Talipes equinovarus (club foot)
Pes planus (flat foot)

Generalized
Osteogenesis imperfecta
Achondroplasia

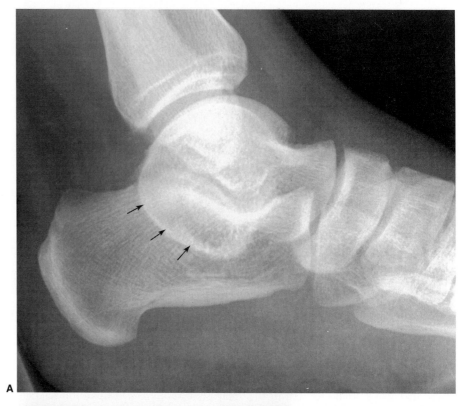

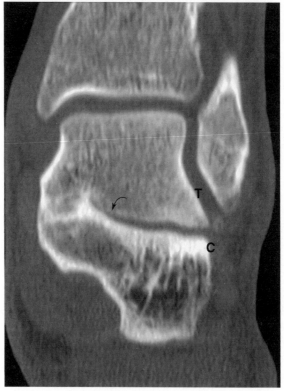

FIGURE 5-16. Lateral radiograph of the left ankle **(A)** and coronal CT image of the same patient **(B)**. There is a prominent *C* on the radiograph (*arrows*). Compare with the normal lateral in Fig. 5-8. The coronal CT clearly shows continuous bone bridging (*curved arrow*) between the talus (T) and calcaneus (C).

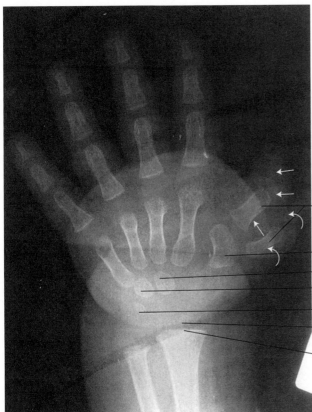

Two thumbs

1st metacarpal
Capitate
Hamate
Triquetrum
Distal radius epiphysis
Distal radius physis

FIGURE 5-17. Left-hand PA radiograph (child). Polydactylism. There are two thumbs and one first metacarpal. One thumb has three phalanges *(straight arrows)*, and the other thumb has two phalanges *(curved arrows)*.

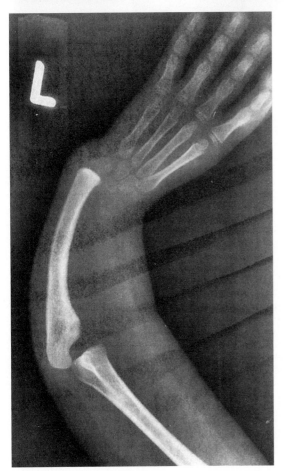

FIGURE 5-18. Left forearm pronated, oblique radiograph. Absence of the radius, 1st metacarpal, and thumb. This 6-year-old had left hand and arm deformity at birth.

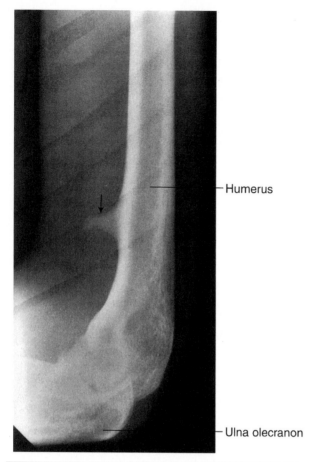

FIGURE 5-19. Right humerus lateral radiograph. Supracondylar process or spur *(arrow)*. It is usually located in the anteromedial aspect of the distal humerus.

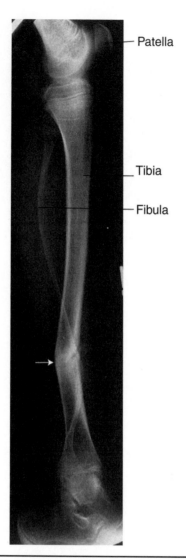

FIGURE 5-20. Left tibia and fibula lateral radiograph. Osteogenesis imperfecta. There is a healing, apex posterior, left tibia fracture *(arrow)*. Note the thin serpentine appearance of the fibula and generalized osteoporosis.

often sporadic, autosomal-dominant anomaly manifested by shortened long bones that results in this most common form of dwarfism (Fig. 5-21).

The hip joint is the most common site of congenital dislocation and has a strong female predominance. Developmental dysplasia of the hip (DDH) was formerly known as congenital dislocation of the hip (CDH) or congenital hip dysplasia (CHD). This dyplasia, shown in Fig. 5-22, is usually diagnosed in infancy. DDH is an abnormal development of the hip joint resulting in an abnormal acetabulum and femoral head. There is displacement of the femoral head referable to the acetabular cartilage. The femoral head usually displaces superiorly but can displace posteriorly. The acetabulum becomes shallow and the angle between the femoral head and shaft is widened.

Two hip problems that can cause confusion are slipped capital femoral epiphysis and Legg-Calvé-Perthes disease (Table 5-5). Slipped capital femoral epiphysis (SCFE; Fig. 5-23) is a hip problem that occurs during adolescence and is often associated with hip pain. The etiology is not understood, but there may be a history of trauma. Ap-

parently, the physis becomes weakened during the rapid growth around puberty. The radiographic findings show the femoral head slipping or displacing posteriorly, medially, and inferiorly relative to the femoral neck. The proximal epiphysis becomes widened. Mild cases may go undetected and present with an earlier-than-expected onset of osteoarthritis.

Legg-Calvé-Perthes disease (Fig. 5-24A) is a form of avascular necrosis, and the etiology is unknown. It may be referred to as osteochondrosis or coxa plana. It typically occurs in a boy between 5 and 10 years of age who complains of hip pain and walks with a limp. It occurs less frequently in females. The pain may be referred to the ipsilateral knee or the knee on the same side. Radiographic findings vary, but may include increased density

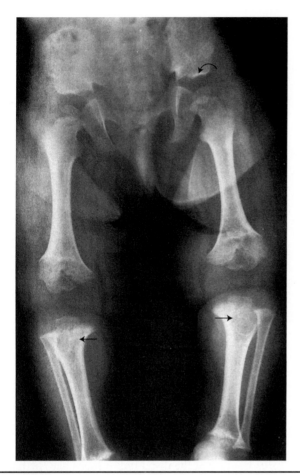

FIGURE 5-21. Pelvis and lower extremities AP radiograph. Achondroplasia. The proximal long bones are shorter and wider than normal, especially the proximal tibias *(straight arrows)*. The iliac bones are rounded *(double arrows)*, and the acetabula are flat *(curved arrow)*.

TABLE 5-6 A Partial List of Avascular Necrosis Etiologies
Steroids and antiinflammatory drugs
Trauma including fractures and dislocations
Sickle cell anemia
Hemophilia
Alcohol
Systemic lupus erythematosus
Renal transplant
Infection
Diabetes

Some of the other causes of avascular necrosis are listed in Table 5-6. The typical findings are sclerotic bone changes on one side of a joint that may go on to fragmentation and eventually to collapse or fracture. MRI (Fig. 5-24C) has proved particularly useful for the diagnosis of avascular necrosis prior to radiographic changes.

TRAUMA

Fractures and Dislocations

Extremity fractures are very common, so now is the time to discuss fractures in general. *Because a fracture or other osseous abnormality may be visible on only one of the radiographs, we obtain at least two views of a bone or joint that are 90 degrees to each other.* Give yourself every opportunity to detect a fracture or other abnormality by obtaining as many views of an area as is practical. *Never accept just one radiographic view of a bone or joint.*

In general, fractures can be conveniently divided into two major clinical categories:

1. Simple or closed fracture means that there are bone fragments and the skin is intact.
2. Compound or open fracture means the skin is not intact near the fracture. The skin has been penetrated by one or more of the bone fragments or by a penetrating foreign body.

of the femoral capital epiphysis, femoral head flattening, rarefaction (bone demineralization) of the metaphysis, and medial joint space narrowing. In general, avascular necrosis or aseptic necrosis can occur in any joint (Fig. 5-24B, C) and can result from multiple other etiologies.

TABLE 5-5 Comparison of Slipped Capital Femoral Epiphysis (SCFE) and Legg-Calvé-Perthes Disease (LCP)		
Feature	*SCFE*	*LCP*
Age	Adolescence	4–10 years
Gender	Boys more than girls (usually overweight)	Boys more than girls
Etiology	Unknown (usually during growth spurt)	Unknown
Symptoms	Hip and/or knee pain	Hip or knee pain and limping
Radiographic capital	Capital epiphysis slips posterior, medial, and inferior to the femoral neck	Flat and sclerotic epiphysis

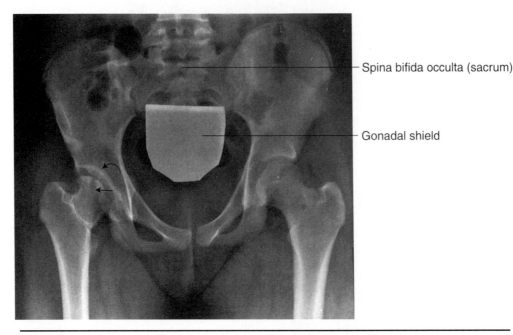

— Spina bifida occulta (sacrum)

— Gonadal shield

FIGURE 5-22. Pelvis AP radiograph. Developmental dysplasia (DDH) of the right hip in a 14-year-old. The right hip is abnormal with a flattened femoral head *(single arrow)* and a poorly formed acetabulum *(curved arrow)*. Compare the right hip to the normal left hip and note how the femoral heads remodel to conform to the shape of their corresponding acetabulum.

Many terms applied to fractures are very descriptive and quite specific (Fig. 5-25A, B). Examples of straightforward common terms for describing fractures include the following:

1. Spiral, transverse, oblique
2. Nondisplaced
3. Overriding
4. Distracted
5. Angulated
6. Offset, or displacement, usually described by the percentage of the fracture fragments abutting or touching each other

Some fracture terms (Fig. 5-25C) that are not quite so obvious include the following:

1. Torus fracture of the distal radius looks like the bump at the base of a Greek column and has nothing to do with a bull. This is an incomplete fracture that occurs in children. The bump is created by a buckling of the cortex without an obvious fracture line.
2. Greenstick fracture describes a bone that fractures by bending like a green twig and is also incomplete.
3. Comminuted or complex fracture indicates more than two bone fragments.

FIGURE 5-23. Pelvis AP radiograph. Bilateral slipped capital femoral epiphyses (SCFE) in a 15-year-old with chronic renal failure and on dialysis. The capital (proximal) femoral epiphyses *(straight arrows)* are displaced from their normal anatomic position. Usually, they are displaced inferiorly and posteromedially. There are monitoring electrodes projecting over the pelvis *(curved arrows)*.

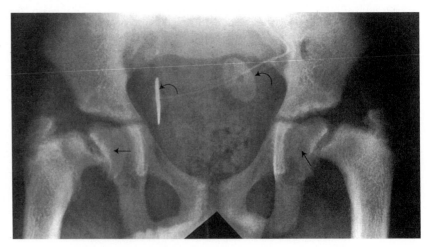

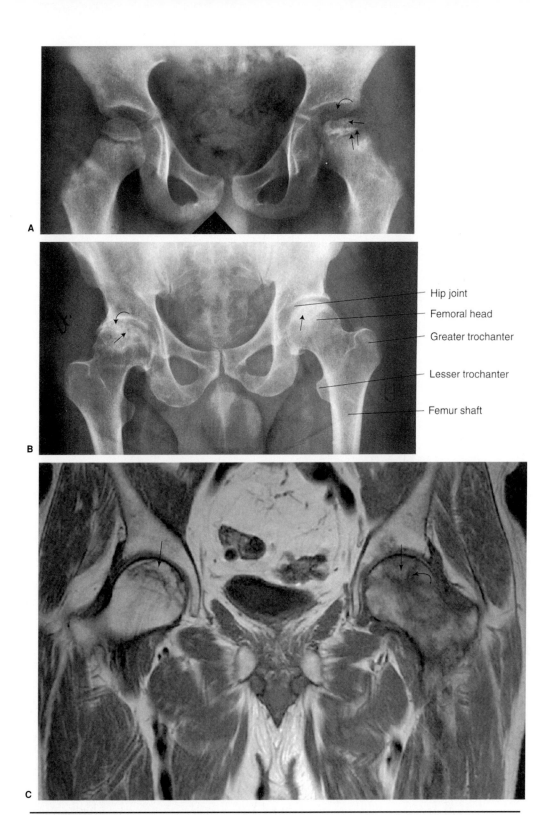

FIGURE 5-24. A: Pelvis AP radiograph. Legg-Calvé-Perthes disease. The right femoral head is normal. Note the irregular contour, flattened articular surface, and increased density of the left femoral head *(straight arrow)*. The left hip joint space is widened *(curved arrow)*. The left proximal femoral epiphysis is widened *(double arrows)*, and the metaphysis is irregular. Note that the acetabulum is normal. **B:** Pelvis AP radiograph. Bilateral femoral head avascular necrosis of unknown etiology in a 42-year-old man. Both femoral heads *(straight arrows)* are sclerotic in appearance, and the right femoral head is deformed because of mild collapse or fracture. The right hip joint is narrowed laterally *(curved arrow)*. **C:** Coronal T1-weighted MRI. Femoral head osteonecrosis in a patient on chronic steroids. The crescentic area formed by low-signal lines *(straight arrows)*, represents the infracted regions. The left hip has a large amount of low-signal edema *(curved arrows)*, suggesting a more acute infarction.

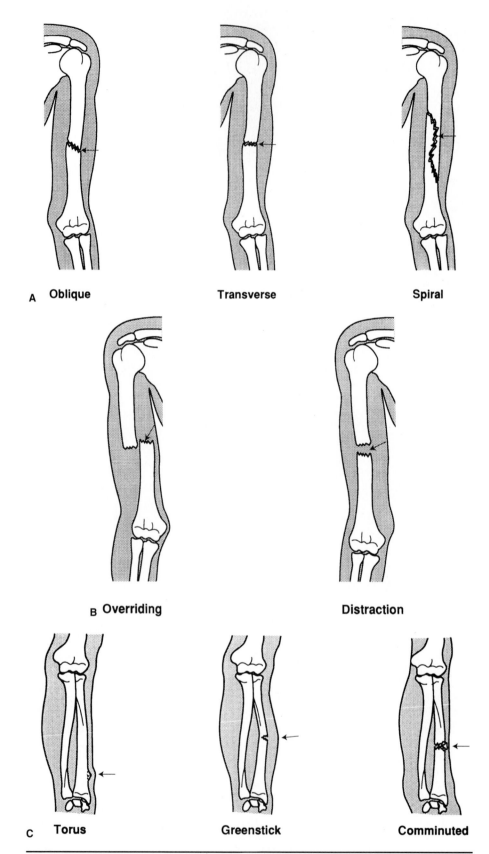

FIGURE 5-25. **A, B:** Some common fractures *(arrows)* and the terms used to describe them and their alignment. **C:** Other common terms used to describe fractures *(arrows)*. *(continued)*

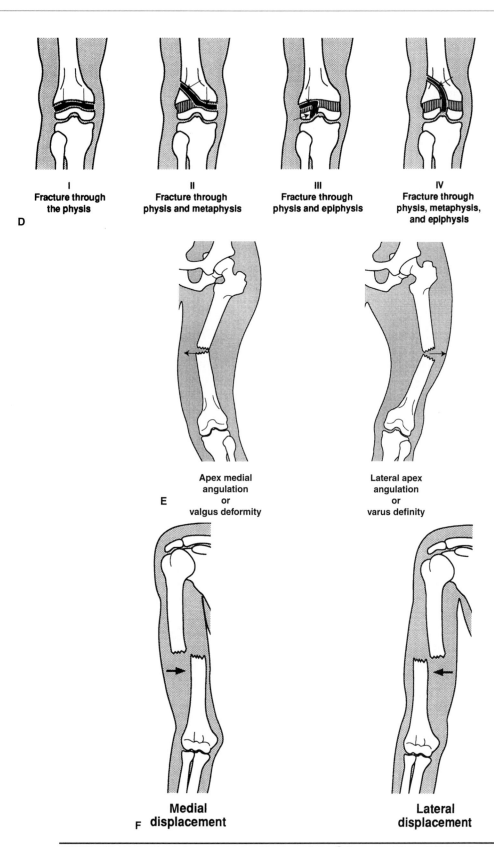

D: Fracture through the physis | I
Fracture through physis and metaphysis | II
Fracture through physis and epiphysis | III
Fracture through physis, metaphysis, and epiphysis | IV
Fracture through physis with compression | V

Apex medial angulation or valgus deformity

Lateral apex angulation or varus definity

E

Medial displacement

Lateral displacement

F

FIGURE 5-25. **D:** The Salter-Harris classification of physis fractures. The solid black line indicates the fracture *(arrows)*, whereas the physis is indicated by the vertical black and white lines. **E:** Illustrations of the nomenclature used to describe fracture angulation. **F:** Nomenclature used to describe the direction of displacement of the distal fracture fragments.

4. Pathologic fracture is one that passes through abnormal bone such as a metastasis, a primary bone tumor, or a bone cyst.
5. Stress fractures are secondary to unusual or excess stress, for example, tibial fractures in runners who overdo it.
6. Insufficiency fractures describe fractures in bone with decreased strength, for example caused by osteoporosis. Such a fracture may result from a normal stress such as merely walking across a room.
7. An avulsion fracture is usually a fracture that occurs at the site of a tendon attachment. This fracture results when the tendon and muscle remain intact while the bone gives way (avulses) at the site of the tendon attachment to the bone.

The Salter-Harris classification of fractures (Fig. 5-25D) is helpful in describing and understanding fractures around a physis. *Remember that the physis represents the weakest point in a bone.*

Type I: The fracture involves only the physis.
Type II: The fracture involves the physis and metaphysis.
Type III: The fracture involves the physis and epiphysis.
Type IV: The fracture involves the physis, metaphysis, and epiphysis.
Type V: The fracture involves only the physis, but there is compression of the physis. This type is more serious than Type 1 because there is a high risk of the physis fusing as the fracture heals. As a result, the bone stops growing and is shorter than the opposite side.

When describing the position of displaced fracture fragments, we use another set of terms. Unfortunately, much confusion can be created by the nomenclature. Traditionally, the distal fragment is described relative to the proximal fragment. An alternative nomenclature uses the apex of the angle created by the fracture fragments as the key. If the apex of the fracture fragments points lateral, the fracture is described as apex lateral. (This same fracture is described as medially angulated by the other nomenclature. You can see where confusion may arise.) I prefer using the word apex in the description so that everyone understands which system is used. If the apex of the fracture fragments points medial, then it is apex medial angulation (Fig. 5-25E). One may substitute medial with volar, dorsal, radial, ulnar, or any other appropriate direction of angulation. Varus and valgus angulation are other common terms to describe angulation and are also illustrated in Fig 5-25E. Another useful rule for describing fracture alignment describes the direction in which the distal fracture fragment is displaced (Fig. 5-25F).

Fracture Healing

The rate at which a fracture heals depends on the fracture site, type of fracture, patient age, adequacy of immobilization, nutrition, and presence or absence of infection. When a fracture occurs, there usually is an associated hemorrhage into the fracture site with subsequent hematoma formation around and between the fracture fragments. The fibrin in a hematoma serves as a framework for fibroblasts, osteoblasts, and a general inflammatory reaction. Bone matrix or osteoid appears in the repair process after a few days, and this is called soft callus or provisional callus. The soft callus is not visible on a radiograph. As calcium salts precipitate in the soft callus and new bone grows, this is called callus. As the callus gradually becomes more dense, it becomes visible on a radiograph. Eventually the callus becomes solid, and bone union is established between the fracture fragments.

In a few days following a fracture, some absorption or removal of bone occurs as a part of the repair process near the ends of the fracture fragments. Because of this bone absorption, the fracture line becomes more visible on subsequent radiographs. This explains why some subtle fractures may not be visible on radiographs obtained immediately following injury but become visible approximately 7 to 10 days postinjury.

Self-explanatory terms used to describe problems in the fracture healing process include the following:

1. Nonunion or nonhealing
2. Delayed union
3. Malunion

Upper Extremity

Fractures of the hands result from a wide variety of activities (Table 5-7). Some fractures and injuries are so obvious that the average citizen could spot them on a radiograph (Fig. 5-26). Subtle fractures can involve any bone and are common in the phalanges of the hand (Figs. 5-27 and 5-28). Joint dislocations occur in almost all joints, and the hand phalangeal joints are common dislocation sites, notably related to sports (Fig. 5-29). Metacarpal fractures are also common, and fractures of the fifth metacarpal often result from punching a solid object. These fractures are appropriately called boxer fractures although they clearly demonstrate an amateur status because professionals would strike using the second and third metacarpals (Fig. 5-30).

▶ **TABLE 5-7 Common Causes of Upper Extremity Fractures**

Work injuries
Home falls
Recreational activities
Sports
Motor vehicle accidents
Fisticuffs

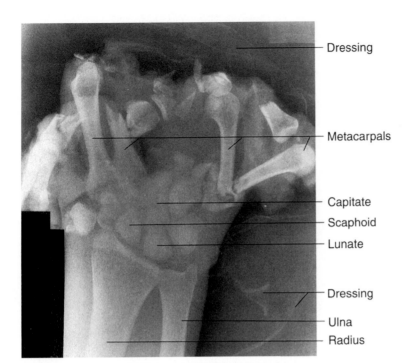

Dressing

Metacarpals

Capitate
Scaphoid
Lunate

Dressing

Ulna
Radius

FIGURE 5-26. Left hand AP radiograph. Obvious severe hand injuries secondary to a corn-picking accident. The phalanges are essentially missing, and there are fractures of the metacarpals and carpals.

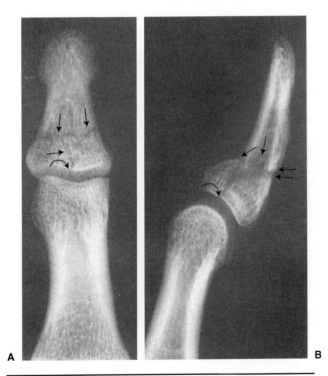

A   B

FIGURE 5-27. Left thumb PA **(A)** and lateral **(B)** radiographs. Comminuted fracture *(straight arrows)* that extends to the articular surface of the interphalangeal joint *(curved arrow)*. There is mild apex palmar angulation at the fracture site *(double arrows)*.

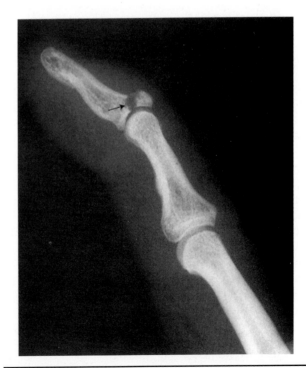

FIGURE 5-28. Right index finger lateral radiograph. Mallet finger. The distal phalanx demonstrates a slightly flexed attitude due to fracture *(arrow)* at site of the insertion of the extensor digitorum mechanism. The loss of the extensor mechanism continuity with the distal phalanx allows the distal phalanx to assume a flexed position or a mallet finger.

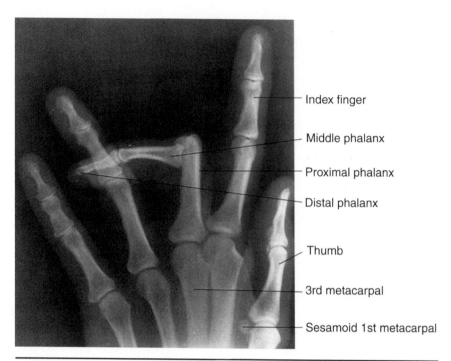

Index finger

Middle phalanx

Proximal phalanx

Distal phalanx

Thumb

3rd metacarpal

Sesamoid 1st metacarpal

FIGURE 5-29. Left hand PA radiograph. Dislocation at the Proximal interphalangeal (PIP) joint of the left long finger. The middle and distal phalanges are completely dislocated relative to the proximal phalanx. There are no fractures.

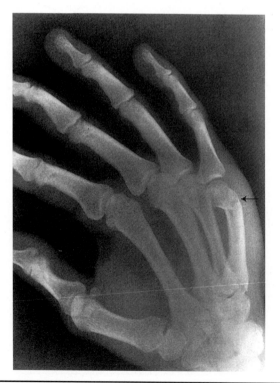

FIGURE 5-30. Right hand PA oblique radiograph. Boxer or Saturday night fracture. The apex dorsal angulated fracture *(arrow)* is through the neck of the right 5th metacarpal.

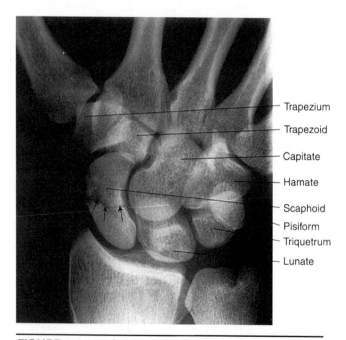

Trapezium

Trapezoid

Capitate

Hamate

Scaphoid

Pisiform

Triquetrum

Lunate

FIGURE 5-31. Right wrist PA radiograph. Essentially nondisplaced fracture *(arrows)* of the scaphoid waist.

The most commonly fractured carpal is the scaphoid (Fig. 5-31). The carpal scaphoid is occasionally referred to as the navicular (an archaic term) by clinicians, but anatomists correctly call it the scaphoid. To add to the confusion, there is a tarsal navicular. Scaphoid fractures result from the injury lines of force being transmitted along the long axis of the thumb, and the majority of these fractures are located in the scaphoid waist. Because of the location of its blood supply and variable arterial branches, scaphoid fractures may develop complications such as nonunion and avascular necrosis, which may result in secondary development of arthritis. These complications are more apt to occur when there is delayed diagnosis and delayed or inadequate treatment. If a scaphoid fracture is suspected but the initial radiographs are negative, additional radiography, CT, or MR is indicated.

Using arms and outstretched hands to cushion falls often results in fractures about the wrist. Whereas young adults typically fracture the scaphoid, children and older adults are more likely to fracture the distal radius and ulna. One such common fracture is called the Colles fracture (Fig. 5-32). It is imperative to reduce these fractured bones as close to their normal anatomic align-

▶ TABLE 5-8 Important Distal Radius Anatomic Relationships
Radius styloid tip lies 1–1.5 cm distal to the ulnar styloid tip
Distal radius articular surface slopes 15–25 degrees toward ulna (inclination)
Distal radius articular surface slopes 10–25 degrees anteriorly (volar tilt)

ment as possible, or set them, as Grandmother would say. Anything less than anatomic realignment may result in a painful and/or poorly functioning wrist. Therefore, it is important to know that the radial styloid tip is 1 to 1.5 cm distal to the ulnar styloid tip, and the distal radial articular surface slopes 15 to 25 degrees toward the ulna and 10 to 25 degrees volar or anteriorly. These important relationships are summarized in Table 5-8. Children, however, have a remarkable ability to remodel and anatomic realignment is not usually needed, depending on the age of the child. In fact, to avoid future limb length discrepancy, anatomic realignment may be purposely avoided.

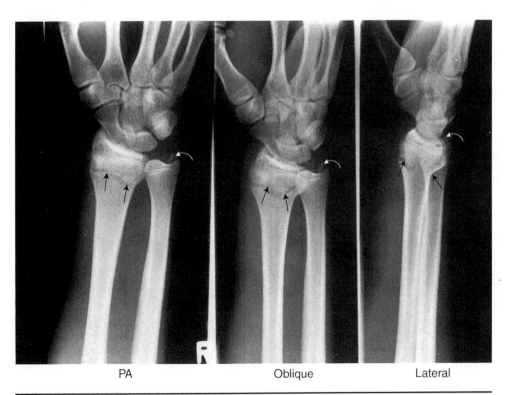

PA   Oblique   Lateral

FIGURE 5-32. Right wrist PA, oblique, and lateral radiographs. Colles fracture. There are fractures of the distal radius *(straight arrows)* and the ulna styloid *(curved arrows)* with dorsal tilting of the distal radius fracture fragment. The pronator fat stripe is obliterated when compared with Fig. 5-1B. The ulna styloid is minimally displaced radially. Note that the radial length is maintained and the distal radius articular surface slopes toward the ulna on the PA view; However, the distal radius articular surface now slopes posteriorly on the lateral view; reduction will try to bring this to neutral or restore the volar (anterior) tilt.

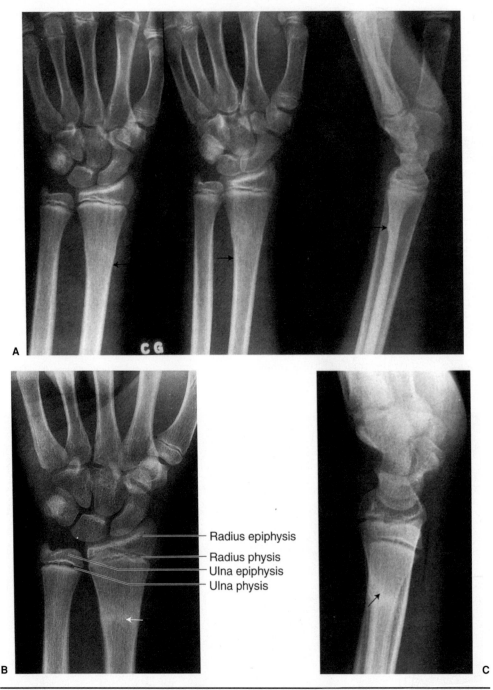

FIGURE 5-33. A: Left wrist PA, oblique, and lateral radiographs. Torus fracture *(arrows)* or a nondisplaced fracture of the distal left radius. Left wrist PA **(B)** and lateral **(C)** radiographs. Healing left radius torus fracture 6 weeks following the radiograph shown in A. The dense white zone *(arrows)* is the typical appearance of a healing fracture.

A subtle fracture in the distal forearm of children is the torus fracture (Fig. 5-33). Torus does not refer to a bull but rather the convex molding/projection (torus) located at the base of a classical column. The torus fracture on a radiograph usually appears as a minimal bump on the bone without a visible fracture line. It represents a buck-

ling of the bone cortex. However, most fractures of the radius and ulna that are encountered in practice are much more obvious (Fig. 5-34).

Elbow fractures (Figs. 5-35 to 5-37) and dislocations (Fig. 5-38A–D) can occur when children and adults fall directly on their elbow or on an extended arm or hand.

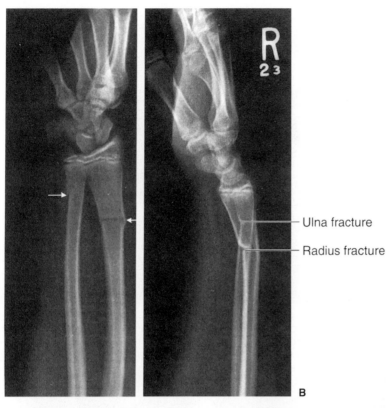

A

B

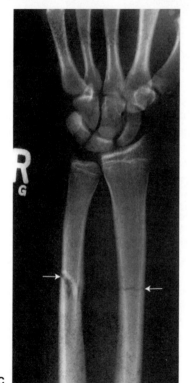

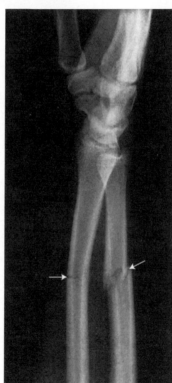

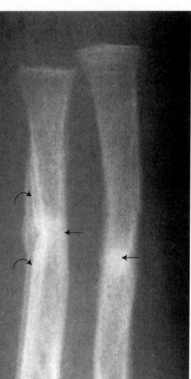

Ulna fracture

Radius fracture

FIGURE 5-34. Right forearm AP **(A)** and lateral **(B)** radiographs. Greenstick fractures *(straight arrows)* of the distal radius and ulna. The fractures simulate a broken green twig or branch wherein the twig bends or breaks but does not separate. On the lateral radiograph, the fracture lines appear to involve only the anterior cortex of both bones. There is mild apex dorsal angulation. This will probably not be reduced because of the great bone remodeling capability in a child. Right forearm AP **(C)** and lateral **(D)** radiographs. Complete transverse fractures *(arrows)* of the distal shafts of the radius and ulna in a 15-year-old. There is mild apex volar, or apex anterior, angulation at the radius fracture site. The fracture fragments in the ulna are mildly offset. **E:** Right forearm AP radiograph. Healing fractures *(straight arrows)* of the radius and ulna in a young child. The fractures are remodeling to near-anatomic alignment, and the *curved arrows* indicate periosteal reaction and new bone formation. The fracture lines are not visible, suggesting early bone union.

C

D

E

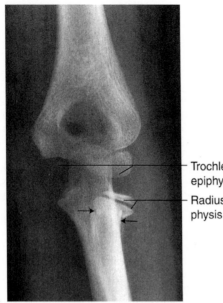

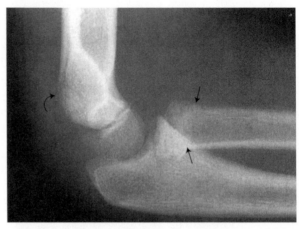

Trochlea and capitulum
epiphyses

Radius epiphysis and
physis

A

B

FIGURE 5-35. Left elbow AP **(A)** and lateral **(B)** radiographs. Radial neck fracture. The straight arrows indicate the site of the fracture, and the radial head is tilted laterally on the AP view. The fracture is very difficult to see on the lateral view *(straight arrows)*. A positive fat pad sign is faintly visible posterior to the distal humerus *(curved arrow)* on the lateral view, and this always means that one should carefully evaluate for a fracture. A visible fat pad anterior to the distal humerus is normal so long as it is not overly prominent (see Fig. 5-4).

In general, children are more likely to have a supracondylar fracture of the distal humerus and adults a radial head fracture. Dislocations of the elbow are named for the direction the radius and ulna dislocate relative to the humerus. When the radius and ulna dislocate anterior to the humerus, it is an anterior dislocation.

The radiographic anatomy of the elbow is complicated. This is especially true in children because of the presence or absence of multiple ossification centers. *When in doubt about an elbow fracture or dislocation, the noninvolved elbow may be useful for comparative purposes as seen in* Fig. 5-37A and B. This principle of comparative views applies to all areas of difficult anatomy. However, knowledge of the anatomy and ordered development of the ossification and fusion of the physes is fundamentally more important. Note that fractures and dislocations of the elbow can be a threat to the brachial artery because of its proximity to the distal humerus (Fig. 5-38E).

A very common injury to the shoulder occurs when a senior citizen trips on the rug or stairs. If they land on their extended hand and do not fracture their wrist, they may sustain a fracture of the surgical neck of the humerus (Fig. 5-39). Generally, this is very easily treated with a sling or a light hanging cast, but may require an extended time for healing due to the patient's age and the fewer stresses compared to a weight-bearing bone. A similar fracture can occur through the physis of the proximal humerus in children (Fig. 5-40).

Dislocation of the shoulder is another common injury that can occur in all age groups. In anterior dislocation of the shoulder, the humeral head becomes caudad or inferior to the glenoid cavity on an AP radiograph and an impaction fracture of the greater tuberosity, a Hill-sach's deformity, may result (Fig. 5-41A–C). Alternatively, the greater tuberosity may fracture during dislocation (Fig. 5-41D). In a posterior dislocation, the humeral head is often slightly cephalad to the glenoid cavity. However, a dislocation is often very difficult to diagnose on a single anterior view, and an axillary or scapular Y view should be obtained (Fig 5-41E). Anterior dislocation of the shoulder is much more common than a posterior dislocation. Associated fractures of the humerus or scapula and rotator cuff tears may occur. Neural and vascular injuries are much less frequent.

Occasionally, a severe fracture or other disease process of the proximal humerus necessitates a shoulder prosthesis (Fig. 5-42). Fractures of the scapula are not common and usually result from a high-force injury as in motor vehicle accidents (MVAs; Fig. 5-43). These are frequently evaluated by CT to determine if the fracture involves the glenoid or the suprascapular notch where the nerve to the supraspinatus and infraspinatus muscle travels (Fig. 5-44). Fractures of the clavicle are very common, especially in children who fall (Fig. 5-45). The most common site for clavicle fractures is at the junction of the middle and distal thirds.

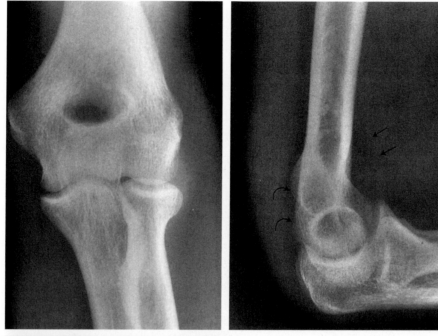

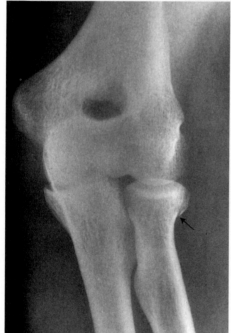

FIGURE 5-36. Left elbow AP **(A)**, lateral **(B)**, and oblique **(C)** radiographs. Fracture of the radius neck. The patient fell from a bicycle and complained of a painful elbow. A fracture is not definitely visible on the AP and lateral radiographs; however, it should be strongly suspected because the anterior fat pad *(single arrows)* is more prominent than normal and a posterior fat pad *(curved arrow)* is present. The fracture *(straight arrow)* can be clearly visualized on the oblique radiograph. This demonstrates the importance of obtaining multiple views of a suspected fracture site and reiterates the significance of a positive posterior fat pad sign and a prominent anterior fat pad.

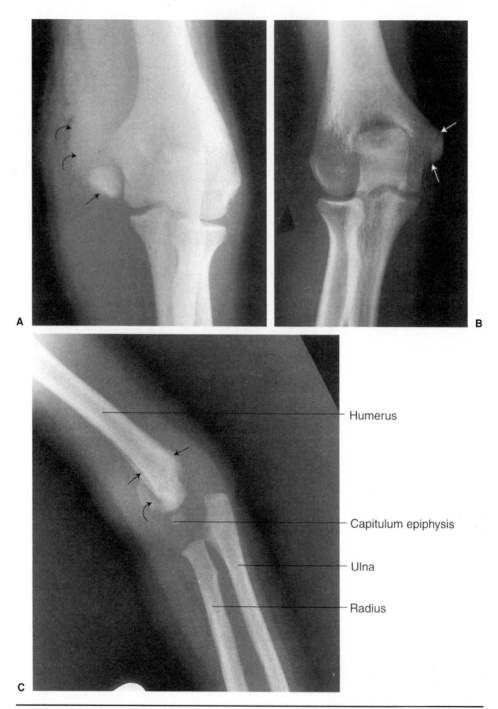

Humerus

Capitulum epiphysis

Ulna

Radius

FIGURE 5-37. A: Left elbow AP radiograph. Avulsion fracture of the medial epicondyle epiphysis *(straight arrow)*, in a 13-year-old. There is considerable soft tissue prominence *(curved arrows)*, probably due to edema and hemorrhage secondary to the avulsion fracture. Remember that the pronators and flexors of the forearm attach to the medial epicondyle and the extensors and supinators to the lateral epicondyle. **B:** Right elbow AP radiograph for comparison. Normal. The medial epicondyle epiphysis *(straight arrows)* is normal. **C:** Right elbow oblique radiograph. Bucket-handle fracture of the distal humerus *(curved arrow)* in a 14-month-old child. Bucket-handle-type fractures can be found in child abuse situations. The straight arrows indicate periosteal reaction that occurs as a part of the healing process.

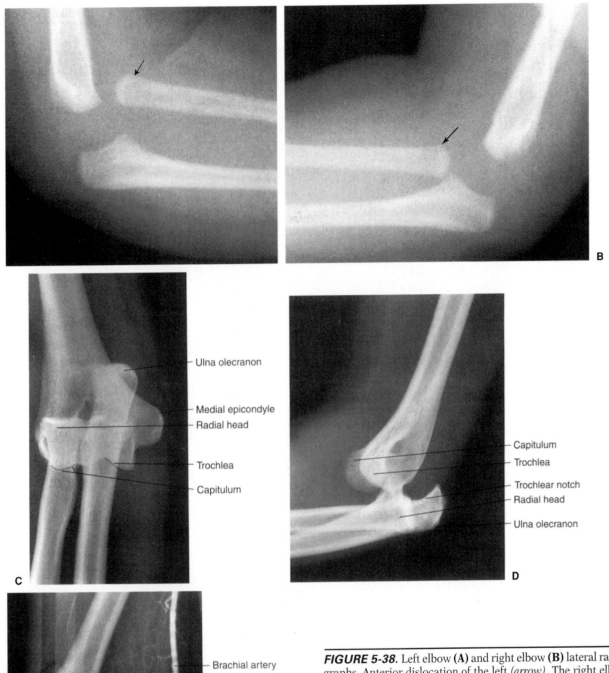

Ulna olecranon

Medial epicondyle
Radial head

Trochlea

Capitulum

Capitulum
Trochlea

Trochlear notch
Radial head

Ulna olecranon

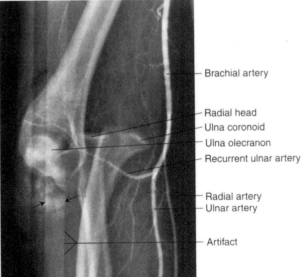

Brachial artery

Radial head
Ulna coronoid
Ulna olecranon
Recurrent ulnar artery

Radial artery
Ulnar artery

Artifact

FIGURE 5-38. Left elbow (**A**) and right elbow (**B**) lateral radiographs. Anterior dislocation of the left *(arrow)*. The right elbow lateral radiograph is normal and was obtained for comparative purposes as elbow anatomy may be especially difficult in children. Note the significant difference in position of the proximal left radius relative to the left humerus compared to the normal right proximal radius relative to the right humerus. Right elbow AP (**C**) and lateral (**D**) radiographs. Posterior dislocation of the elbow in a 23-year-old. The proximal ulna and the radial head are posterior to their normal articulations with the distal humerus, and this is best appreciated on the lateral view. There are no fractures. **E:** Left elbow lateral angiogram. Fracture-anterior dislocation of the left elbow in a different patient. The radius and ulna are dislocated anteriorly relative to the humerus, and there is a comminuted fracture of the ulna olecranon *(straight arrows)*. The brachial artery is displaced anteriorly by the dislocation and the associated soft tissue edema and hemorrhage.

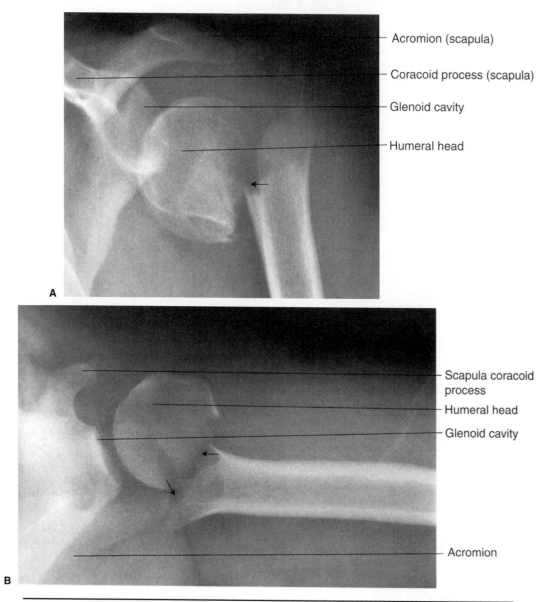

Acromion (scapula)

Coracoid process (scapula)

Glenoid cavity

Humeral head

A

Scapula coracoid process

Humeral head

Glenoid cavity

Acromion

B

FIGURE 5-39. A: Left shoulder AP radiograph. Fracture *(straight arrow)* of the humerus surgical neck with offset of the fracture fragments in a 19-year-old. The humeral head is rotated and subluxed medially on the AP view resulting in an abnormal relationship between the humerus head and the scapula glenoid cavity. **B:** Left shoulder axillary radiograph of the same patient as in A. The central x-ray beam travels through the axilla to demonstrate nicely the offset fracture fragments *(arrows)*. Note that the humeral head now is in a normal relationship with the scapula. The scapula coracoid process projects anteriorly, and the base of the scapula acromion projects posterior to the glenoid cavity on this view. Surgical internal fixation was required.

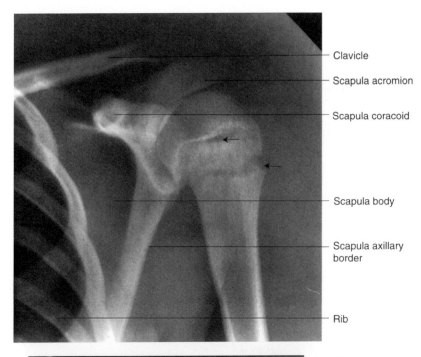

— Clavicle

— Scapula acromion

— Scapula coracoid

— Scapula body

— Scapula axillary border

— Rib

FIGURE 5-40. Left shoulder AP radiograph. Salter I fracture *(straight arrows)* through the proximal physis of the left humerus in a 15-year-old. The patient fell on an outstretched arm. The major clue to the presence of a fracture is that the physis width is greater than normal. Be careful not to overcall the normal physis a fracture—see Figs. 5-41D and 5-45.

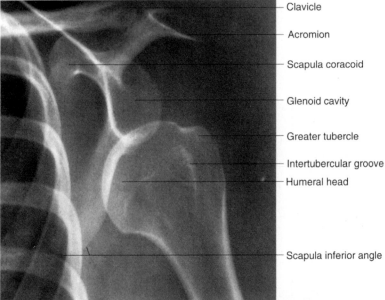

— Clavicle

— Acromion

— Scapula coracoid

— Glenoid cavity

— Greater tubercle

— Intertubercular groove

— Humeral head

— Scapula inferior angle

A

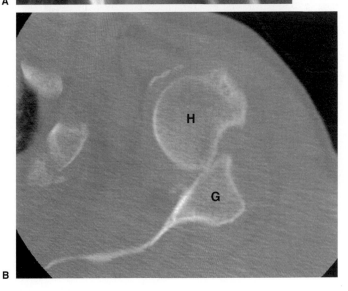

H

G

B

FIGURE 5-41. A. Left shoulder AP radiograph. Anterior dislocation of the shoulder without fracture. The humeral head is inferior to the glenoid cavity, and this is the classic position of the humeral head in an anterior dislocation. The intertubercular (bicipital) groove is well visualized and within it rests the tendon of the long head of the biceps brachii. **B.** Left shoulder axial CT of an anterior dislocation. Note how the humeral head (H) may impact the glenoid (G). **C.** Right shoulder AP radiograph. Postreduction study demonstrates a Hillsach's deformity *(arrow)* from impaction fracture. **D.** AP radiograph of left shoulder. Anterior dislocation with fracture of the greater tuberosity *(straight arrow)*. Note a fat–fluid level *(curved arrow)* on this upright study. Fat from the marrow floats in blood. **E.** Scapular Y-view. Anterior dislocation. The coracoid, acromion, and scapular body form the limbs Y. The glenoid *(dotted circle)* is located at the intersection. The humeral head should contact this intersection.

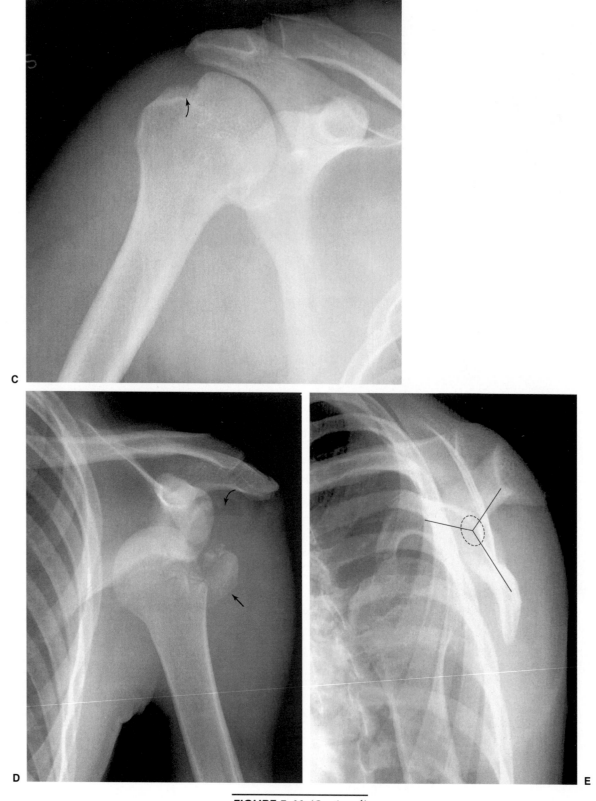

FIGURE 5-41. (*Continued*)

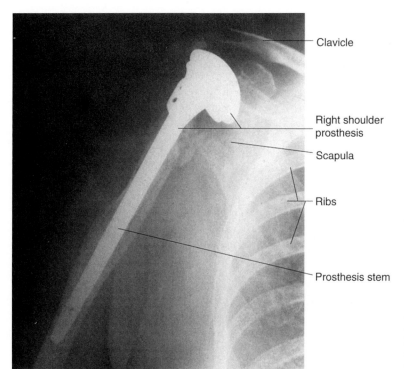

Clavicle

Right shoulder prosthesis

Scapula

Ribs

Prosthesis stem

FIGURE 5-42. Right shoulder AP radiograph. Right shoulder prosthesis. The prosthesis was necessitated by a severe old fracture deformity of the proximal humerus.

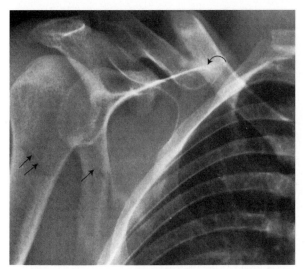

FIGURE 5-43. Right shoulder AP radiograph. Acute fracture *(straight arrow)* of the scapula body and an old healed fracture *(curved arrow)* of the right midclavicle with deformity (malunion). The radiolucent line, or pseudofracture *(double arrows)*, in the proximal right humerus is secondary to overlying soft tissues.

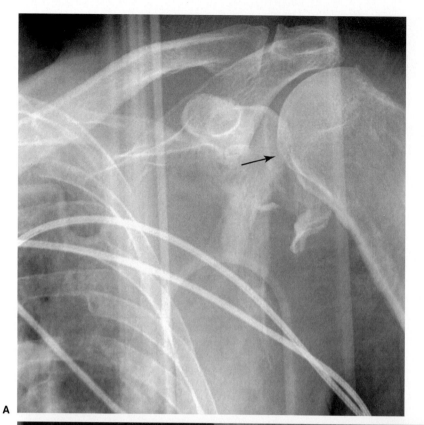

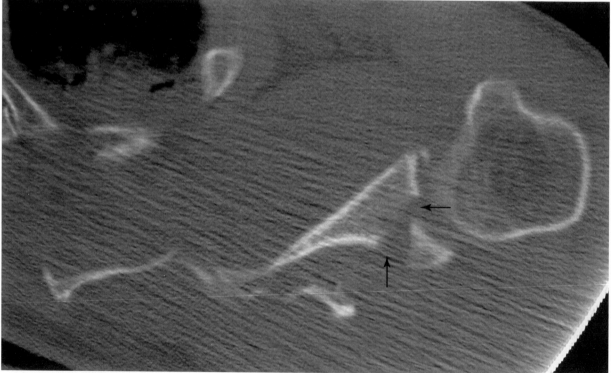

FIGURE 5-44. Left shoulder AP radiograph **(A)** and axial CT **(B)**. Scapular fracture. The most important finding is involvement of the glenoid *(arrows)*, which can lead to arthritis.

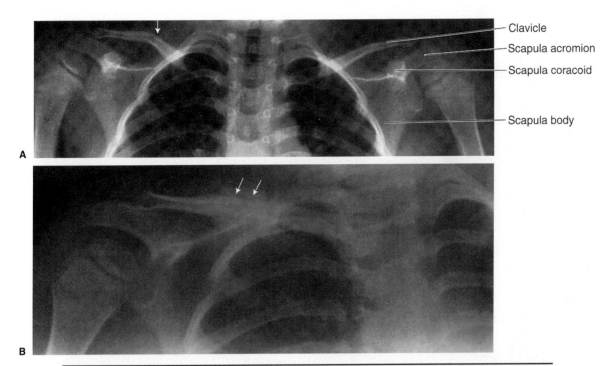

Clavicle
Scapula acromion
Scapula coracoid
Scapula body

A

B

FIGURE 5-45. A: Right and left clavicles AP radiograph. Subtle greenstick fracture of the middle third of the right clavicle *(arrow)* in a 3-year-old child. There is minimal apex cephalad angulation at the fracture site. The fracture is more apparent when compared to the normal left clavicle. **B:** Right clavicle AP radiograph in the same patient 4 weeks later. Healing fracture. The white material surrounding the fracture site in the middle third of the right clavicle *(arrows)* is callus. The bone has remodeled the angulation, and the clavicle alignment is normal.

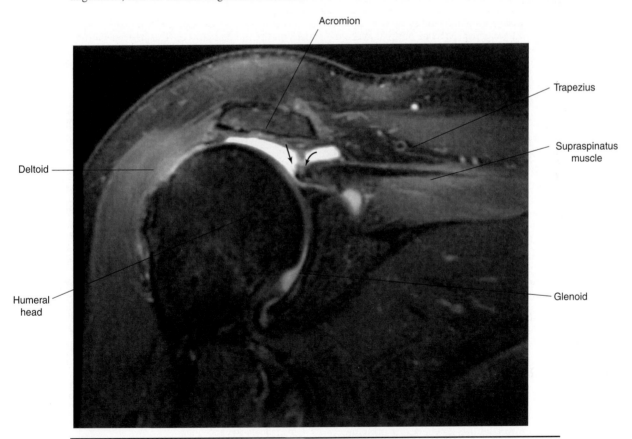

Acromion

Trapezius

Supraspinatus muscle

Deltoid

Humeral head

Glenoid

FIGURE 5-46. Right shoulder fat-suppressed T2 coronal MR image. Rotator cuff complete tear in a 55-year-old man. The area of high intensity or white signal *(straight arrow)* represents blood, edema, and joint fluid in the laceration of the supraspinatus tendon. The free margin of the torn supraspinatus tendon is indicated by the curved arrow. Note that the bone cortex is black on the MR image. Note the edema (brighter signal) in the supraspinatus muscle.

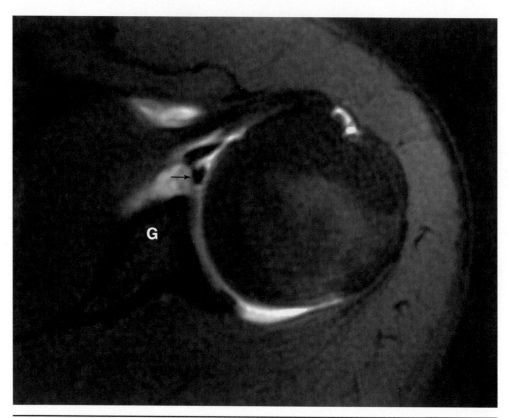

FIGURE 5-47. Axial fat-suppressed T1 MR shoulder arthrogram. Labral tear. MR contrast is bright on the T1-weighted sequence (normal joint fluid is dark on the same sequence). The anterior labrum *(arrow)* is detached from the glenoid (G).

MRI is a powerful tool for evaluating shoulder rotator cuff integrity, and a complete interruption of the rotator cuff is shown in Fig. 5-46. An arthrogram is performed by distending a joint, usually with fluid that will provide contrast to the structures of interest. MR arthrograms are especially helpful for evaluating tears of the glenoid labrum (Fig. 5-47). Remember that MRI is excellent for demonstrating the bone marrow and soft tissue detail, whereas CT imaging is better for trabecular and cortical detail.

Sudeck's atrophy, or reflex sympathetic dystrophy or chronic regional pain syndrome (Fig. 5-48), is a poorly understood phenomenon that can be the result of a fracture or almost any type of mild or severe injury. It is frequently associated with pain, swelling, and stiffness.

Lower Extremity

The etiologies of lower extremity injuries are similar to those in upper extremity injuries (see Table 5-7). Injuries to the feet are very common, as this is where our body meets mother earth (see Figs. 5-49 to 5-54 for a gallery of common foot injuries). CT is often used to evaluate complex ankle and calcaneal fractures (Fig. 5-54). Remember that a lateral radiolucent line near the base of the fifth metatarsal

that runs parallel to the long axis of the metatarsal in a growing person represents a normal apophysis (Fig. 5-50C), whereas *a transverse lucent line at the base of the fifth metatarsal always represents a fracture* (Fig. 5-50D). An apophysis is a growth center (like the epiphysis) that does not contribute to bone length. It alters bone contour and usually is not located in a joint but typically has tendons attached to it.

The ankle is frequently injured, and the injuries vary from minor sprains to severe trimalleolar fracture-dislocations (Figs. 5-55 to 5-58). Fractures of the shafts of the tibia and fibula are common in sports, especially contact sports and skiing. A fracture that fails to heal and has persistent motion about it is called a nonunion fracture. Nonunion fractures have a variety of causes, some of which are listed in Table 5-9. Nonunions are

▌TABLE 5-9 Causes of Fracture Nonunion

Infection and osteomyelitis
Inadequate immobilization
Poor blood supply
Interposition of muscle or other structure between the fracture
  fragments
Combinations of the above

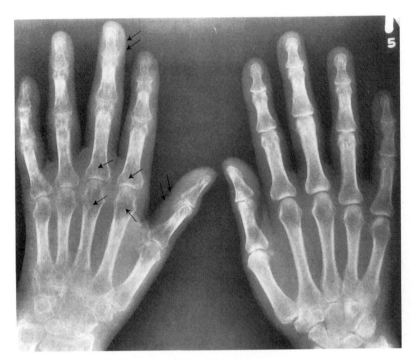

FIGURE 5-48. Right and left hand PA radiographs. Sudeck's atrophy of the left hand compared to the normal right hand. This patient's left upper extremity had been immobilized in a cast for 3 weeks. Sudeck's atrophy typically has patchy osteoporosis *(single arrows)* accompanied by soft tissue swelling *(double arrows)*, and the latter is minimal in this 58-year-old patient. Disuse from immobilization may also lead to osteoporosis, and clinical information is necessary in this case.

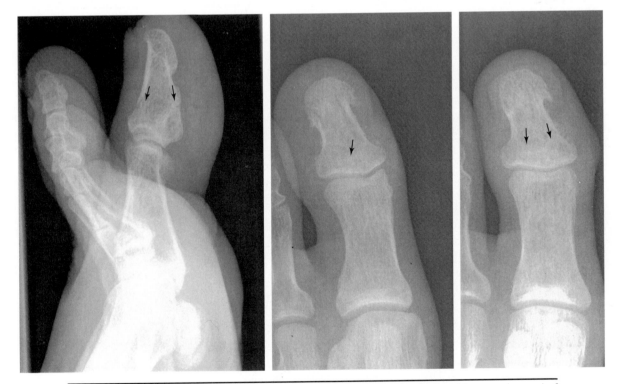

FIGURE 5-49. Left great toe lateral, oblique, and AP radiographs. Nondisplaced fracture *(arrows)* of the distal phalanx. As is commonly the case, this patient dropped a heavy object on the great, or big, toe.

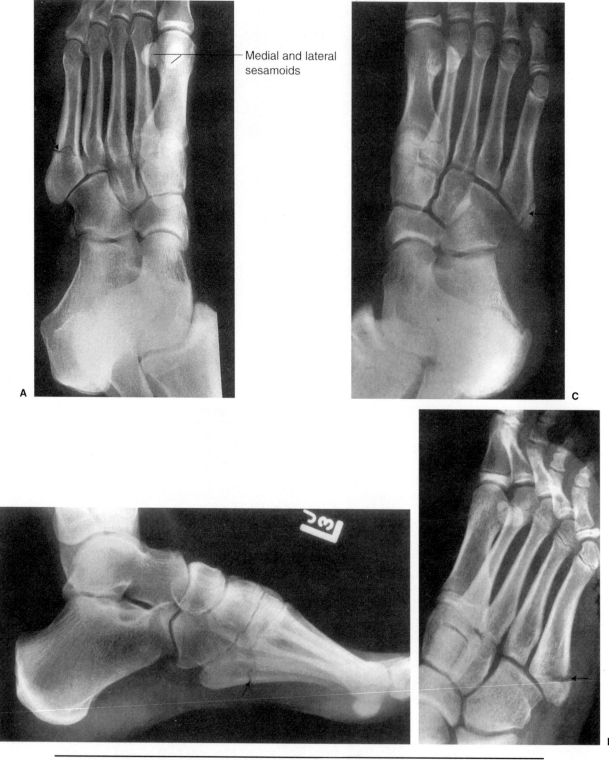

Medial and lateral sesamoids

FIGURE 5-50. Left foot oblique (**A**) and lateral (**B**) radiographs. Nondisplaced transverse fracture of the proximal left 5th metatarsal shaft *(arrows)*. **C:** Right foot AP radiograph. Normal in a 14-year-old boy. The normal apophysis *(arrow)* at the base of the 5th metatarsal appears as a longitudinal radiolucent or black line and should not be confused with a fracture. **D:** Right foot oblique radiograph. Transverse nondisplaced fracture *(straight arrow)* involving the 5th metatarsal base. This injury usually results from an inversion stress on the peroneus brevis that attaches to the base of the 5th metatarsal.

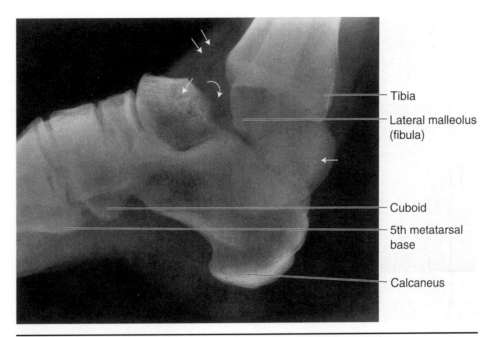

FIGURE 5-51. Right ankle lateral radiograph. Midtalus distracted fracture *(curved arrow)*. The fracture fragments *(straight arrows)* are markedly distracted, and the soft tissue edema and/or blood is indicated by the double arrows. The fracture resulted from a dorsiflexion injury

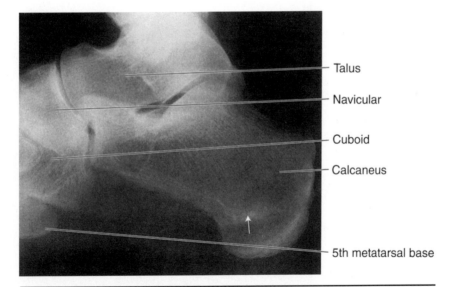

FIGURE 5-52. Right calcaneus lateral radiograph. Calcaneus insufficiency fracture in a 53-year-old woman. The white line *(arrow)* indicates a healing mildly impacted fracture that was not visible on radiographs 2 months prior to this study. The shape and height of the calcaneus are fairly well maintained. She had been on steroids for inflammatory bowel disease, and the steroids caused osteoporosis. As a consequence of the osteoporosis, the bone was not strong enough to prevent fracture.

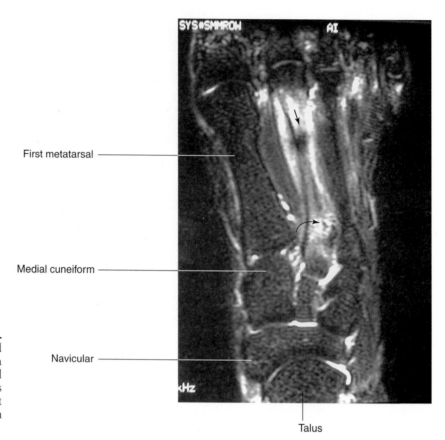

First metatarsal ————————

Medial cuneiform ————————

Navicular ————————

Talus

FIGURE 5-53. Long axis fat-suppressed T2-weighted MR of the right foot in a runner. Stress fracture. Second metatarsal stress fracture has some callus, which is black *(straight arrow)*, and a large amount of edema in the bone and soft tissues, which is white *(curved arrows)*.

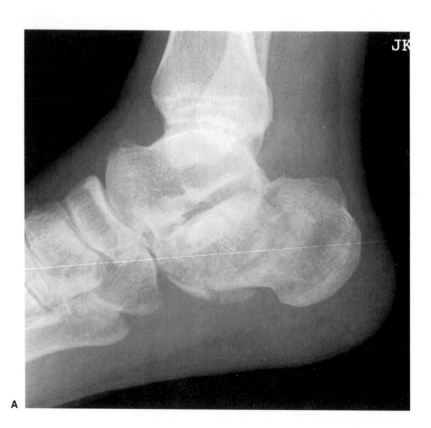

FIGURE 5-54. A. Right calcaneus lateral radiograph. Calcaneus fracture *(arrow)* with impaction and collapse of the vertical height of the calcaneus. Compare the shape of the calcaneus in this patient to the calcaneus in Fig. 5-52. Axial *(continued)*

A

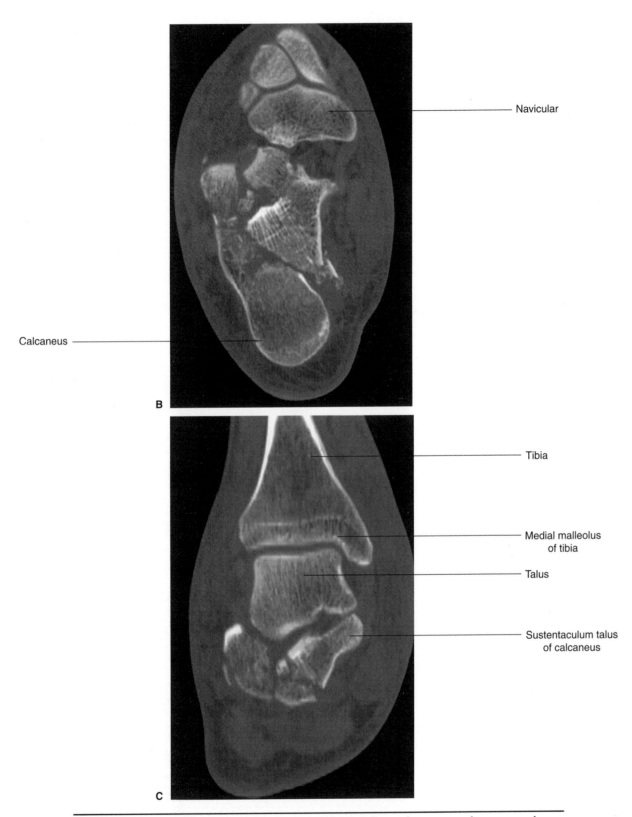

FIGURE 5-54. **(B)** and coronal reformatted **(C)** CT images better demonstrate the extent and comminution of the fracture.

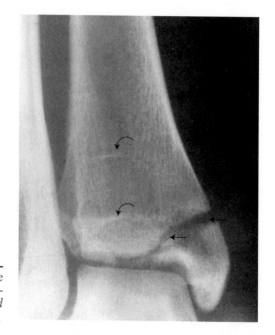

FIGURE 5-55. Right ankle oblique radiograph. Mildly distracted fracture *(straight arrows)* through the base of the medial malleolus in an adult. The fracture extends onto the articular surface of the distal tibia. The white lines *(curved arrows)* represent previous physis location and arrested growth lines.

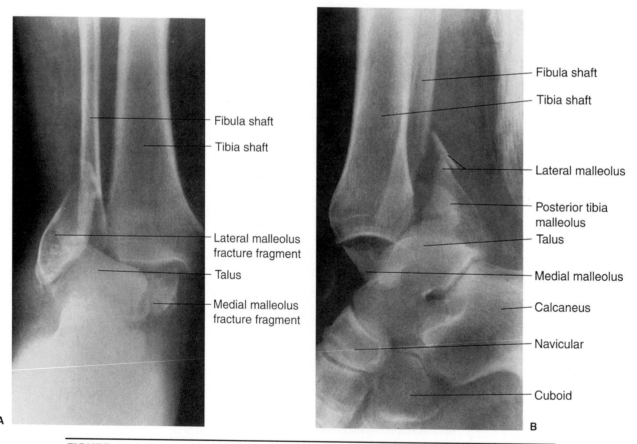

FIGURE 5-56. Right ankle AP (**A**) and lateral (**B**) radiographs. Displaced trimalleolar fractures and talotibial dislocation. The medial and posterior tibial malleoli fracture fragments and the fibula lateral malleolus fracture fragments are all displaced. The talus is severely displaced laterally and posteriorly relative to the tibia. This is an eversion injury.

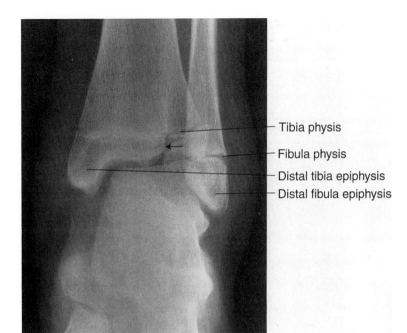

— Tibia physis

— Fibula physis

— Distal tibia epiphysis

— Distal fibula epiphysis

FIGURE 5-57. Left ankle AP radiograph. Salter III fracture of the left distal tibia in a 12-year-old. The fracture line *(arrow)* extends from the physis through the distal tibial epiphysis to the articular surface.

frequently found in the mid- and distal tibia where the blood supply can be a problem (Fig. 5-59). Severe fractures of the tibia may require internal fixation to facilitate immobilization and healing (Fig. 5-60). The tibia is also the site of stress fractures in all age groups, especially in runners (Fig. 5-61).

A wide variety of fractures occur in and around the knee, and examples are demonstrated in Figs. 5-62 to 5-64. These figures demonstrate that not all fractures are visible on the initial radiographs around the time of injury. Whenever symptoms persist following an injury and the original radiographs were negative, you must consider follow-up imaging that might include radiographs, MRI, CT, or radionuclide scans. CT scans are often used for obvious tibial plateau fractures (Fig. 5-63) to better demonstrate the number and position of fragments and depth of depression of articular surface.

Although 90% of child abuse deaths are secondary to head injuries, child abuse can involve all parts of the skeletal system. The metaphyseal fractures demonstrated in Fig. 5-65A are typical of the findings in some child abuse cases, and these metaphyseal fractures are probably due to a twisting mechanism. Subperiosteal hemorrhage on a radiograph is another twisting type of injury that should make you highly suspicious of child abuse (Fig. 5-65B). Bucket-handle fractures (Fig. 5-37C) are also associated with child abuse. Skeletal injuries and fractures that should make the observer highly suspicious for child abuse

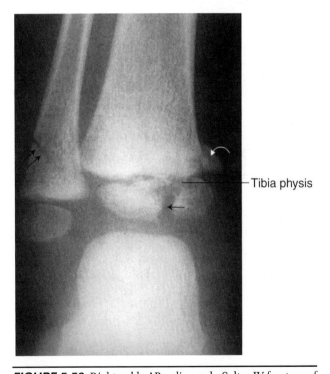

— Tibia physis

FIGURE 5-58. Right ankle AP radiograph. Salter IV fracture of the distal tibia. The fracture line *(straight arrow)* extends from the distal tibial physis through the epiphysis to the tibial articular surface. The fracture also involves the medial tibia metaphysis *(curved arrow)*. There is an associated fracture of the distal fibula *(double arrows)*.

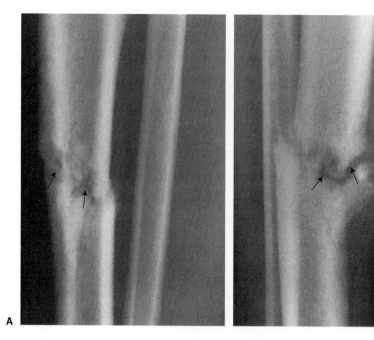

A

B

FIGURE 5-59. Left tibia and fibula AP **(A)** and lateral **(B)** radiographs. Osteomyelitis and nonunion of a tibia fracture. The fracture line *(arrows)* is clearly visible 3 months following the injury, and this indicates a nonunion or nonhealing fracture. Infection at the fracture site caused the nonunion.

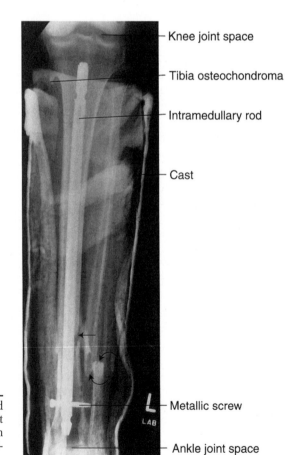

- Knee joint space
- Tibia osteochondroma
- Intramedullary rod
- Cast
- Metallic screw
- Ankle joint space

FIGURE 5-60. Left tibia and fibula AP radiograph. Intramedullary rod internally fixating a transverse fracture in the distal one-third of the left tibia *(straight arrow)*. There is an offset overriding transverse fracture in the distal one-third of the fibula *(curved arrows)*. The fibula is non-weight-bearing so the displacement is not important to a good functional outcome.

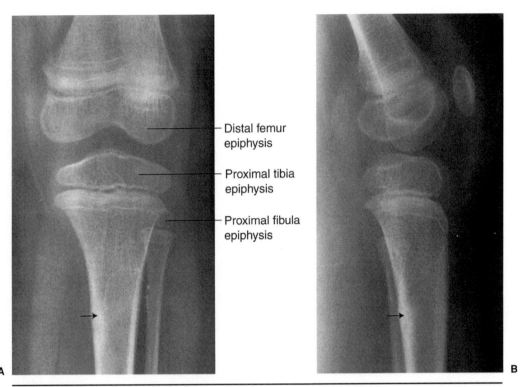

FIGURE 5-61. Left knee AP **(A)** and lateral **(B)** radiographs. A healing stress fracture in this 5-year-old is indicated by the zone of increased density in the posteromedial proximal tibia *(arrows)*. The fracture resulted from excessive usage or stress.

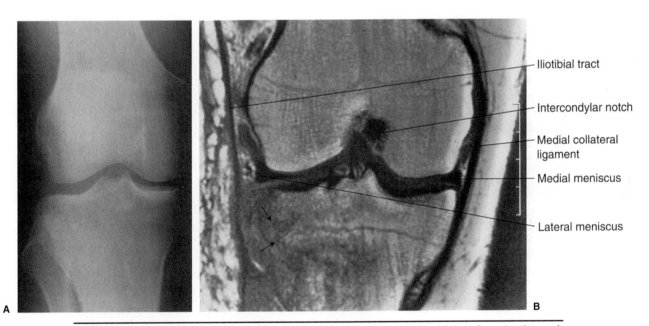

FIGURE 5-62. A: Right knee AP radiograph. This AP radiograph and a lateral *(not shown)* radiograph were interpreted as normal. The radiographs were obtained because of right knee pain immediately following knee trauma in a 31-year-old man. **B:** Right knee coronal T1 MR image. Lateral tibial plateau fracture. This study was obtained 2 weeks following the initial radiograph in A because of persistent knee pain and a clinical suspicion of an anterior cruciate ligament injury. The *arrows* indicate an area of low-intensity signal (dark) caused by blood and edema replacing the bone marrow fat (white) in the tibial plateau fracture site. The anterior cruciate ligament was intact. The fracture eventually became apparent on subsequent radiographs.

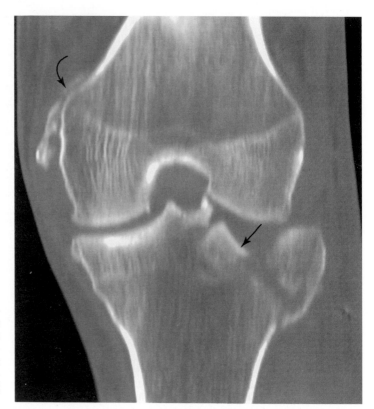

FIGURE 5-63. Coronal CT of the knee reformatted from axial images. Lateral tibial plateau fracture. CT is often used to better evaluate the amount of depression of the articular surface *(straight arrow)* and number and location of fragments. The irregular bone formation along the medial femur *(curved arrow)* is the result of a prior medial collateral ligament injury.

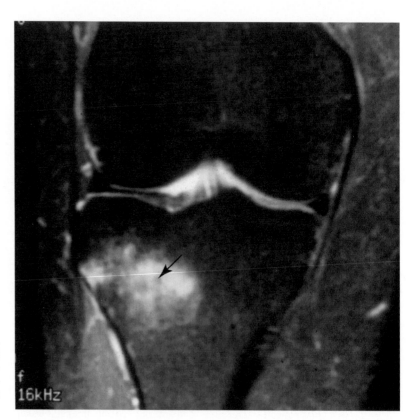

FIGURE 5-64. Coronal inversion recovery MRI of the right knee. Insufficiency fracture of the medial tibia in an elderly patient with pain. The fracture line *(arrow)* is white on this sequence from blood and edema.

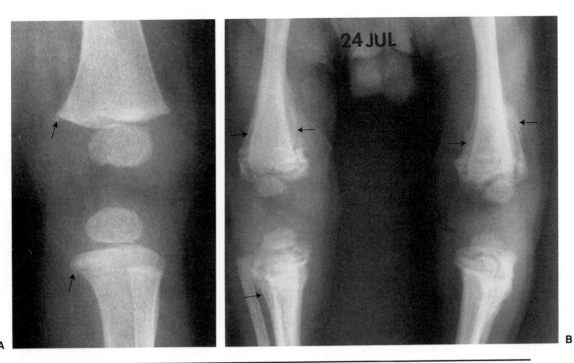

A   B

FIGURE 5-65. A: Left knee AP radiograph. Metaphyseal corner fractures *(arrows)*. This battered child complained of knee pain and had an obvious limp. **B:** Right and left lower extremities radiograph. Subperiosteal hemorrhage. The *straight arrows* indicate the appearance of blood beneath the periosteum secondary to severe squeezing and twisting of the extremities. This appearance is highly suspicious for child abuse and should be investigated further.

are summarized in Table 5-10, and the common child abuse fracture sites outside the skull are shown in Table 5-11.

The patella is a large, superficial sesamoid bone. It is not uncommonly fractured in falls and MVAs (Fig. 5-66).

Osteochondritis dissecans (Fig. 5-67A, B) is a common abnormality involving the knee in adolescents and young adults. It occurs most frequently along the lateral aspect of the medial femoral condyle, but it can be found elsewhere in the knee and in other joints including the hip, shoulder, ankle, and elbow. It is thought to be a localized ischemic or avascular necrosis that often occurs after injury and results in a button of necrotic bone that may or may not detach from the donor site. When it becomes detached, it is a joint loose body. In middle-aged to older adults, the abnormality is typically the weight-bearing aspect of the medial femoral

condyle and the term spontaneous osteonecrosis (SONC) is often used (Fig. 5-67C, D). In the older age group, these lesions may be due to subchondral insufficiency fractures. Avascular necrosis is bone ischemia and localized bone death. The clinical presentations of bone ischemia (Table 5-12) vary with the bone site and size as well as bone age (Fig. 5-24). Osteonecrosis has a variety of causes. The term infarct is used when the dead bone is not near a joint (Fig 5-99C).

As a general rule, femoral shaft fractures are easy to detect both clinically and radiographically, as the patient experiences severe pain at the fracture site and is usually unable to bear weight (Fig. 5-68). This is an uncommon area for stress fractures, but they may occur here in young athletes.

The hip is another area commonly injured in MVAs and falls, especially in the elderly (Fig. 5-69). MRI has become

▶ **TABLE 5-10 Osseous Injuries Suspicious for Child Abuse**

Corner fractures
Periosteal hemorrhage
Bucket-handle fractures

▶ **TABLE 5-11 Common Fracture Sites in Abused Children**

Lower extremity: femur (commonest), tibia
Elbow
Shoulder
Ribs

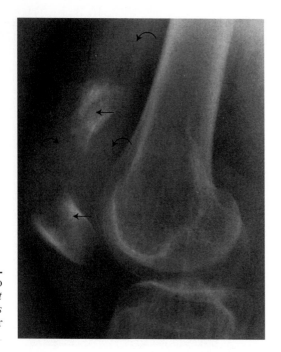

FIGURE 5-66. Right knee lateral radiograph. Midpatella fracture secondary to a motor vehicle accident. There are two distracted fracture fragments *(straight arrows)* secondary to the fracture through the midpatella. The *curved arrows* indicate blood and increased synovial fluid in the supra-, pre-, and retropatellar spaces of the knee.

the standard in evaluating for hip fracture with seemingly normal radiographs (Fig. 5-70). Dislocations of the hip are not common and require violent trauma as in MVAs (Fig. 5-71). As opposed to the shoulder, posterior dislocations of the hip are much more frequent than anterior. CT is quite useful in the assessment of complex pelvic and acetabular fractures (see figures in Chapter 6). However, patients with a hip prosthesis may on occasion dislocate the prosthetic head with a minimal amount of stress (Fig. 5-72).

Soft Tissue Injury

One of the commonest injuries of the lower extremity is the sprained ankle. A sprain is simply an injury to a ligament around the ankle (or any other joint), and it varies in severity from a strain or stretching of the ligament to a complete disruption. Sprains usually result from a turning or twisting of the ankle joint while walking or running. When the foot turns outward, there is an eversion or abduction injury. When the foot turns inward, there is an inversion or

▶ **TABLE 5-12 Some Clinical Presentations of Bone Ischemia**

Osteochondritis dissecans
Legg-Calvé-Perthes disease
Avascular necrosis
Aseptic necrosis
Bone infarcts

adduction injury. Sprains occur with and without associated fractures. A dramatic example of a severe sprain is demonstrated in Fig. 5-73.

Because ankle sprains are usually treated by casting in the United States, MRI is not commonly used to image ankle sprains, and the imaging usually is limited to radiographs; one exception is high-performance athletes. However, MRI of the ankle is used for specific problems such as Achilles tendon tears. The Achilles tendon or calcaneal tendon is a common injury site (Fig. 5-74). This injury can result from violent sport activities or simply stepping in a hole, and the diagnosis usually is made by the history of pain in the Achilles tendon. When there is a complete tear or disruption of the Achilles tendon, physical examination often shows pinpoint tenderness at the site of injury and inability to plantarflex the foot. An MRI is usually requested to confirm a clinical diagnosis or suspicion and evaluate the degree of separation. This will aid in the decision for casting versus surgical intervention. Alternatively, ultrasound has also been used to evaluate the Achilles tendon (Fig. 5-75).

Following injury to muscles there may be subsequent calcification and/or ossification at the injury site called *myositis ossificans.* Common locations include the quadriceps and brachialis muscles.

MRI is a wonderful imaging tool for evaluating cartilage, tendons, and ligaments in and around the knee. Usually the radiographs are negative in such injuries, but based on the physical findings and the patient's symptoms, an MR image is requested for a more definitive evaluation of these soft tissue structures (Figs. 5-76 to 5-81).

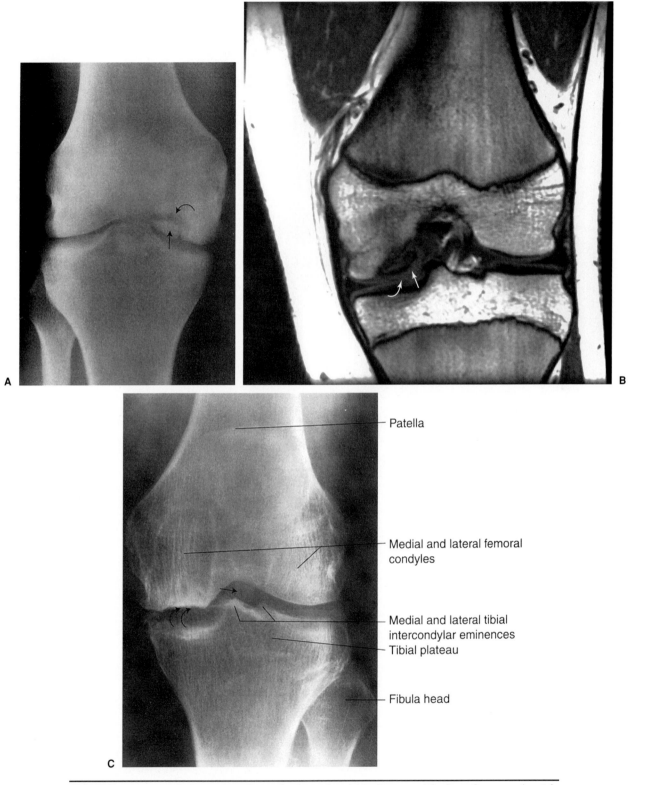

Patella

Medial and lateral femoral
condyles

Medial and lateral tibial
intercondylar eminences
Tibial plateau

Fibula head

FIGURE 5-67. A: Right knee AP radiograph. Osteochondritis dissecans. The bone fragment *(straight arrow)* is not displaced from the donor site *(curved arrow)* on the lateral aspect of the medial femoral condyle. **B:** Coronal T1-wieghted MR right knee in a different patient. The fragment *(straight arrow)* is clearly seen and cartilage covers it *(curved arrow)*. Left knee AP **(C)** and lateral **(D)** radiographs in a different patient. Spontaneous osteonecrosis. There is a displaced bone fragment or loose body *(straight arrow)* in the joint space. The radiolucent defect surrounded by the sclerotic zone *(curved arrow)* in the weight-bearing portion of the medial femoral condyle is the donor site of the loose body.

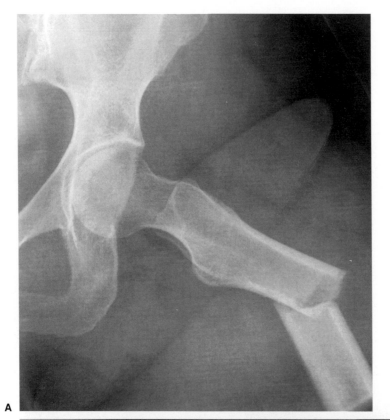

A

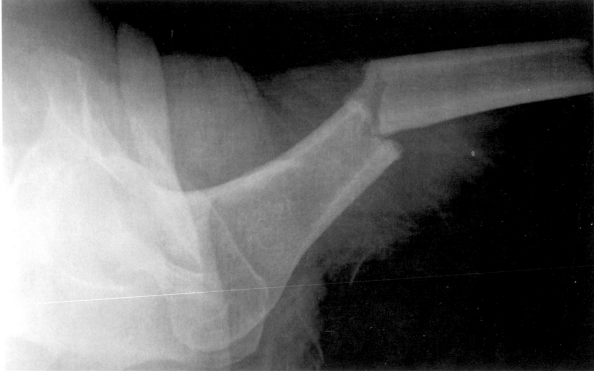

B

FIGURE 5-68. Left femur frog-leg (**A**) and true (**B**) lateral radiographs. Transverse fracture of the femur in a 26-year old automobile accident victim. There is apex anterior angulation. Note how the fracture fragments can change when the patient is moved. Displacement is posterior in the frog-leg lateral, but was anterior on the true lateral. The patient is supine and the x-ray beam horizontal on the true lateral.

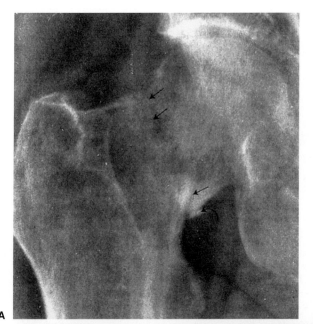

A

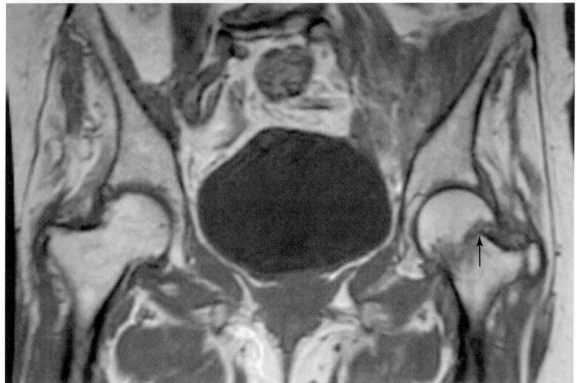

B

FIGURE 5-69. **A:** Right hip AP radiograph. Femoral neck fracture. There is a mildly impacted fracture *(arrow)* through the midfemoral neck. The *curved arrow* denotes a small fracture fragment. The patient complained of right hip pain and inability to bear weight on the right leg following a minor fall. **B:** Coronal T1-weighted MR in a different patient. A left subcapital fracture is easily seen *(arrow)*.

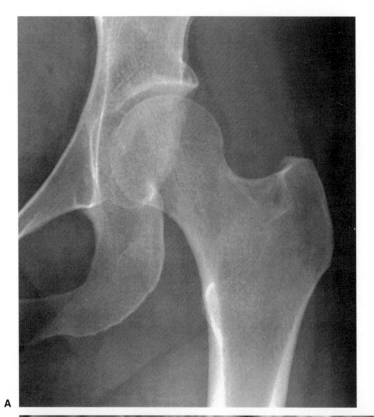

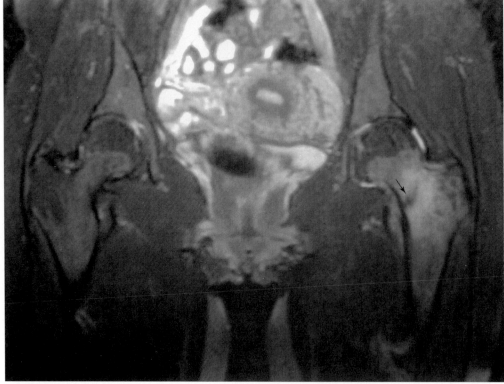

FIGURE 5-70. AP radiograph **(A)** of the left hip was interpreted as normal. This avid runner complained of persistent pain and an MR was obtained. Coronal fat-suppressed T2-weighted image **(B)** demonstrates edema (white) around the developing stress fracture *(arrow)*. Left untreated, this might well progress to a complete fracture.

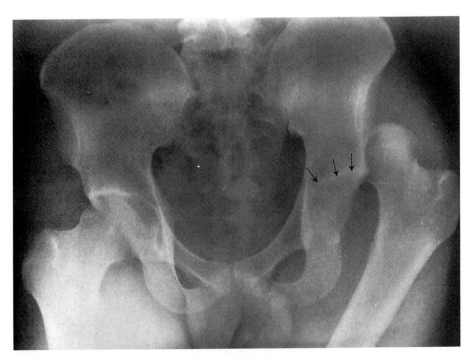

FIGURE 5-71. Pelvis AP radiograph. Posterior dislocation of the left hip without fracture secondary to a motor vehicle accident. The left femoral head is displaced cephalad and lateral relative to the acetabulum *(straight arrows)*. The right hip is normal and makes an excellent comparison.

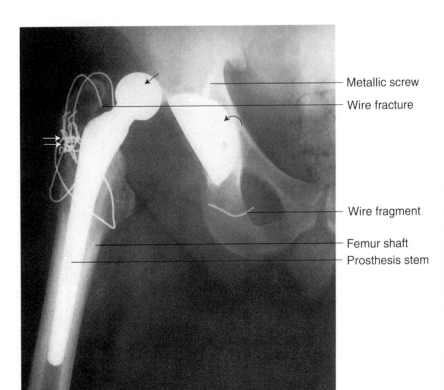

— Metallic screw

— Wire fracture

— Wire fragment

— Femur shaft
— Prosthesis stem

A

FIGURE 5-72. **A:** AP radiographs of the right hip. There is posterior dislocation of the right hip prosthesis head *(straight arrow)* in relation to the acetabular component *(curved arrow)*. The dislocation occurred while bending over to pick up a grandchild. Wires *(double arrows)* anchor the greater trochanter to the femur, and at least one of the wires is fractured. A fragment of loose wire lies inferior to the prosthesis acetabular component. **B:** Following closed reduction (no surgery) under general anesthesia, the prosthetic head has been returned to its proper position relative to the acetabular prosthetic component.

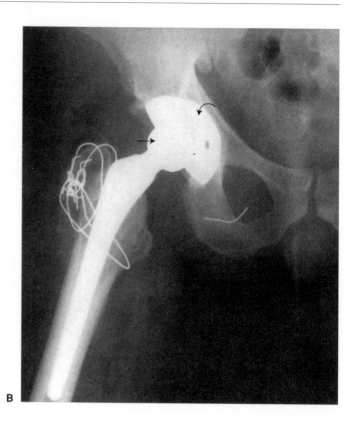

FIGURE 5-72. (*Continued*)   **B**

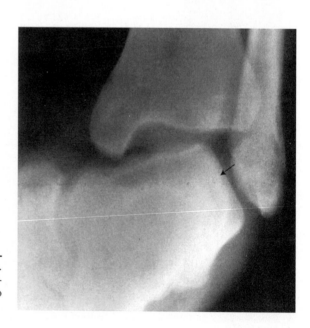

FIGURE 5-73. Left ankle inversion stress AP radiograph. Ankle sprain. The talus is tilted laterally *(arrow)* secondary to disruption of the lateral collateral ligament in an inversion or adduction injury. There are no fractures.

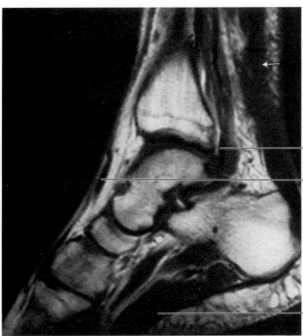

Flexor hallucis longus tendon

Tibialis anterior tendon

Flexor digitorum brevis muscle

FIGURE 5-74. Right ankle midsagittal T1 MR image. Calcaneal (Achilles) tendon tear. The tear site is manifest by a high-intensity signal due to blood and edema within the tear *(arrow)*.

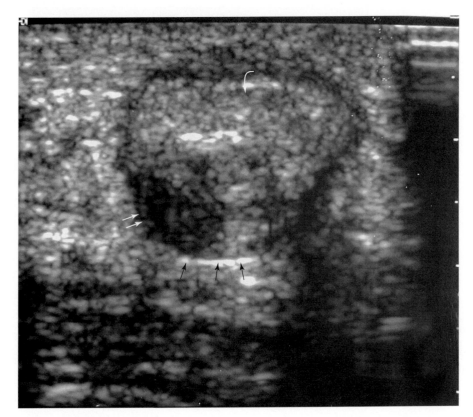

FIGURE 5-75. Transverse ultrasound image of an Achilles tendon. Partial tear. The normal portion of the tendon is echogenic *(curved arrow)*. The anterior portion, which is normally flat or concave, is rounded *(arrows)* and has low echogenicity *(double arrow)* due to edema and blood.

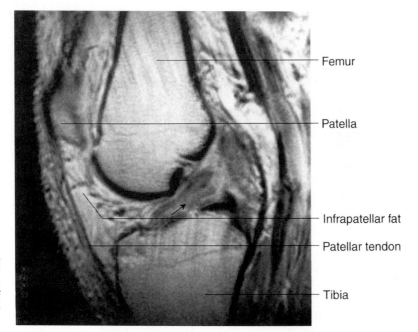

Femur

Patella

Infrapatellar fat

Patellar tendon

Tibia

FIGURE 5-76. Right knee sagittal proton-density MR image. Anterior cruciate ligament tear in a 41-year-old man. The arrow indicates the site of the anterior cruciate ligament tear manifested by a wavy high-intensity (white) signal.

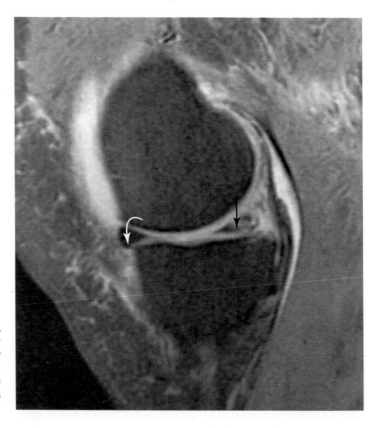

FIGURE 5-77. Sagittal fat-suppressed proton-density MR image through medial meniscus. Tear of the posterior horn in a 45-year-old woman. The high-intensity signal *(arrow)* likely represents edema and synovial fluid within the tear. The anterior horn of the meniscus *(curved arrow)* is normal.

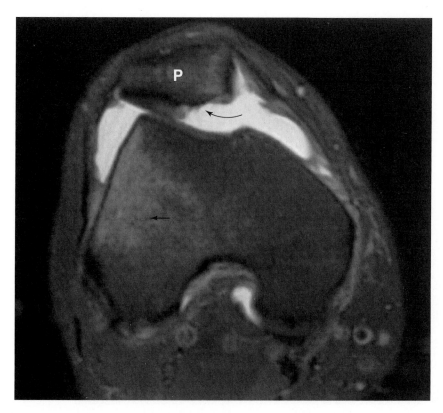

FIGURE 5-78. Axial fat-suppressed T2 MR right knee. Post patellar dislocation. The patella (P) is laterally subluxed: It should closely articulate with the trochlea of the femur. There is edema of the lateral femur *(arrow)* where the patella impacted. A cartilage defect *(curved arrow)* was created in the patella during the dislocation or relocation.

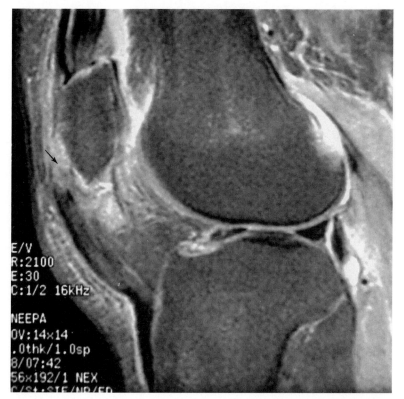

FIGURE 5-79. Sagittal proton-density MR right knee. Patellar tendon tear. There is disruption of the patellar tendon (ligament) at its patellar attachment *(arrow).*

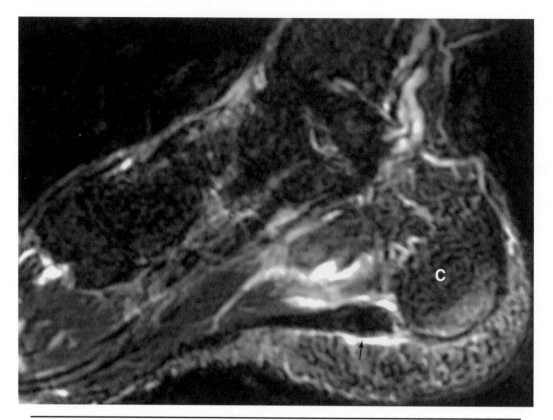

FIGURE 5-80. Sagittal inversion recovery MRI of left foot. Plantar fasciitis. The plantar fascia is thickened *(arrow)* and has surrounding edema (white). Mild edema is also seen in the adjacent calcaneus (C).

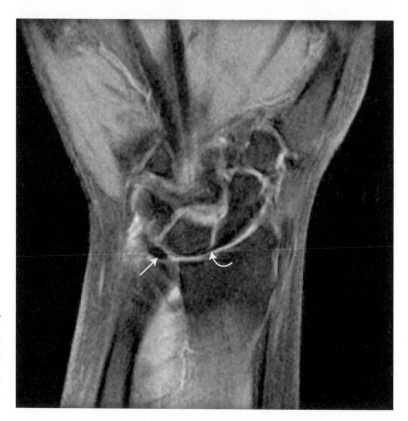

FIGURE 5-81. Coronal fat-suppressed proton-density MRI of left wrist. Triangular fibrocartilage (TFC) tear. There is disruption and slight retraction of the TFC from its radial attachment *(straight arrow)*. Wrist MRIs are also useful in evaluating the scapholunate ligament *(curved arrow)*, which is normal in this patient.

Many foreign bodies in soft tissue and bone are radiopaque and readily identified on radiographs (Fig. 5-82A, B). Occasionally, a nonopaque foreign body in an extremity is suspected. If a foreign body is not visible on a radiograph, an ultrasound, CT, or MR study can be requested to assist in the detection and location of the foreign body (Fig. 5-82C).

ARTHRITIDES

Osteoarthritis

Osteoarthritis (degenerative arthritis) is the most common form of arthritis. You can categorize osteoarthritis into two types. Secondary osteoarthritis, or degenerative joint disease (DJD), can occur at all ages, but tends to appear with increasing age as a result of wearing-out processes. It may involve almost all of the joints of the extremities and spine (Figs. 5-83 to 5-85), but favors the DIP joints and thumb carpometacarpal joint in the hand, hips, and knees. In younger individuals, secondary arthritis may result from trauma, infection, or any other process that may disrupt the normal joint. Primary osteoarthritis is probably familial and involves the DIP joints of the hands, hips, and the first metacarpal–carpal joint. Another frequent location of arthritis is the great toe (MTP) joint. A bunion may develop from a familial predisposition or related to shoeware, particularly high heels. The apex at the metatarsophalangeal MTP joint is medial and becomes more prominent. Overlying soft tissue irritation may develop or osteoarthritis may result form the now incongruent joint (Fig. 5-86).

The radiograph is the primary tool for evaluating osteoarthritis as well as all other arthritides. Some important facts and radiographic findings of osteoarthritis are listed in Table 5-13 and include asymmetric, irregular joint narrowing because of articular cartilage destruction, osteosclerosis, and osteophyte formation. When advanced osteoarthritis involves the medial knee compartment, a genu varus deformity or bowed leg usually results. When advanced osteoarthritis involves the lateral knee compartment, a genu valgus deformity or knock-knee often results. When advanced osteoarthritis involves the hip, the femoral head migrates cephalad because of asymmetric cartilage destruction, whereas in rheumatoid arthritis the femoral head tends to drift centrally from uniform cartilage loss. Acetabular protrusion may result from softening of the bones due to osteoporosis.

Rheumatoid Arthritis

Rheumatoid is another type of arthritis that is frequently encountered in the everyday practice of medicine (Figs. 5-87 to 5-90). It is an inflammatory arthritis of unknown etiology that involves synovial joints and is charac-

▶ **TABLE 5-13** Typical Symptoms and Radiographic Findings in Osteoarthritis and Rheumatoid Arthritis
Osteoarthritis
Pain, deformity, and limitation of joint motion
Involves all joints of the extremities and spine
Typically involves the hand distal interphalangeal (DIP) joints and the 1st metacarpophalangeal (MCP) joint
Irregular joint narrowing
Sclerotic bone changes
Cysts or pseudocysts
Osteophyte formation
Usually absence of osteoporosis
Genu valgus and varus deformities
Cephalad and sometimes lateral migration of the femoral head
Rheumatoid arthritis
Pain, stiffness, limitation of motion, especially in the hands and feet
Involves all joints of the extremities and spine and all synovial joints
Typically involves the hand MCP joints
Symmetric joint narrowing
Periarticular osteoporosis (prominent feature)
Periarticular soft tissue thickening and swelling
Marginal and central osseous erosions
MCP subluxation and ulnar deviation
Medial migration of the femoral head and acetabular protrusio
Pencil appearance of the distal clavicle

terized by symmetric joint narrowing secondary to articular cartilage destruction by pannus, which is granulation tissue derived from the synovium. Some important facts and radiographic findings are listed in Table 5-13. As in osteoarthritis, any or all of the joints in the extremities and spine can be involved. The most commonly affected joints, in decreasing frequency, are the MCP, wrist, PIP, knee, MTP, shoulder, ankle, cervical spine, hip, elbow, and temporomandibular joints. Often the initial symptoms of rheumatoid arthritis are stiffness, pain, limitation of movement, and swelling in the hands and/or feet. Usually, the first joints involved are the MP joints, and this tends to be symmetric. Potentially the earliest abnormality detectable on a radiograph is periarticular soft tissue thickening. Additional radiographic findings include periarticular osteoporosis due to hyperemia, symmetric joint narrowing, and marginal central erosions. As the disease progresses, joint deformity may develop due to subluxation and ulnar deviation of the fingers at the MCP joints. This later finding is quite characteristic of rheumatoid arthritis. When joint cartilage destruction becomes far advanced, bony ankylosis of the joint may result. The differential diagnosis of rheumatoid arthritis is shown in Table 5-14.

In gout, osteoporosis is usually absent, and articular and juxtaarticular erosions are more sharply defined. In osteomyelitis and infectious arthritis, the osteoporosis is greatest near the infection site. In Sudeck's atrophy, the

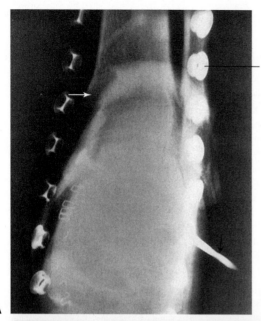

A

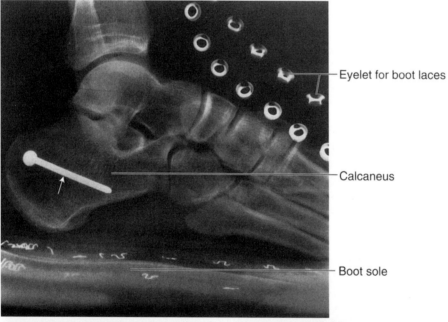

B

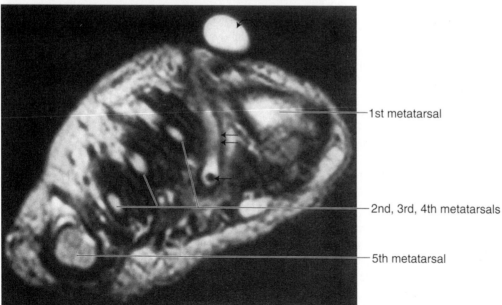

C

Eyelets for
boot laces

Eyelet for boot laces

Calcaneus

Boot sole

1st metatarsal

2nd, 3rd, 4th metatarsals

5th metatarsal

FIGURE 5-82. Left foot AP **(A)** and lateral **(B)** radiographs taken through the boot. Metallic nail *(arrows)* piercing the boot and lodged in the calcaneus. The nail was driven into its present location by a power tool. **C:** Left foot axial T2 MR image. Foreign body *(straight arrow)* in a different patient. The site of the foreign body entry wound *(curved arrow)* is marked by the white pill containing fat. The foreign body tract *(double arrows)* is white, probably because it is filled with edema, blood, granulation tissue, or inflammatory cells.

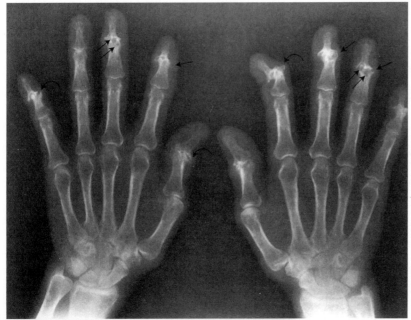

A

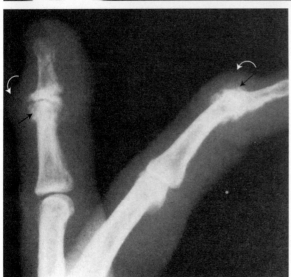

B

FIGURE 5-83. A: Right and left hand PA radiograph. Osteoarthritis or erosive osteoarthritis. This 63-year-old woman worked as a typist for 20 years. Note the advanced osteoarthritic changes *(straight arrows)* involving the distal interphalangeal (DIP) joints of both hands. The DIP joints are markedly narrowed and osteophytes *(curved arrows)* are present. Erosions are also present *(double arrows)*. **B:** Left index and long finger lateral radiograph. Osteoarthritis DIP joints. For many years this 60-year-old woman operated an adding machine with her left hand. There is narrowing of the DIP joint spaces due to articular cartilage destruction. There are soft tissue prominences *(curved arrows)* overlying bone excrescences near the DIP joints. These bone excrescences or protuberances are called Heberden nodes *(straight arrows)*.

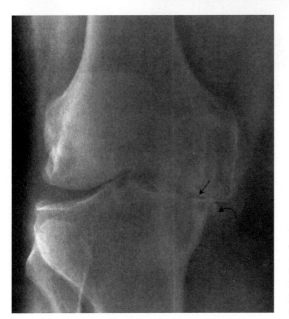

FIGURE 5-84. Right knee AP radiograph. Osteoarthritis. The medial joint space or medial knee compartment is markedly narrowed, the articular surfaces are irregular *(straight arrow)*, osteophyte formation *(curved arrow)* is present, and there is varus deformity. Note that the medial joint space has all but disappeared compared to the lateral joint space.

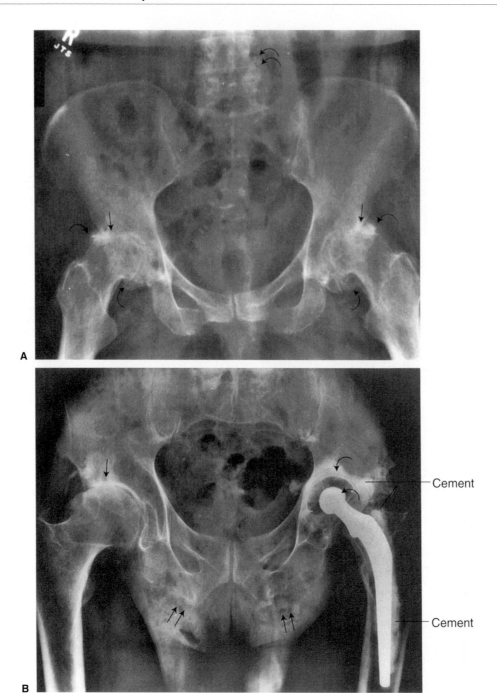

FIGURE 5-85. A: Pelvis AP radiograph. Bilateral hip osteoarthritis in a 61-year-old. The hip joint spaces are irregularly narrowed, and the femoral heads are typically migrating in a cephalad direction *(straight arrows)*. The femoral heads are cystic and sclerotic in appearance. Osteophyte formation is present along the periphery of the joints *(curved arrows)*. Osteophyte formation is also present in the lower lumbar spine *(double curved arrows)*. **B:** Pelvis AP radiograph. Osteoarthritis of the right hip, left hip prosthesis, and bilateral inguinal hernias. There is irregular narrowing of the right hip joint and cephalad migration of the femoral head *(straight arrow)*. A left hip prosthesis is in place. The curved arrows indicate the prosthetic femoral head and acetabular components. Large bilateral inguinal hernias contain air-filled loops of bowel *(double arrows)*.

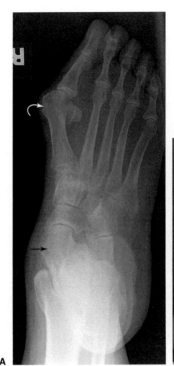

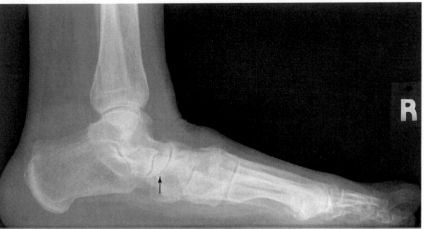

A

B

FIGURE 5-86. Anterior **(A)** and lateral **(B)** radiographs of the right foot in a 64-year old woman. Hallux valgus. The head of the first metatarsal is uncovered as the great toe is directed laterally *(curved arrow)*. The great toe is also pronated and the sesamoids of the first metatarsal are subluxed laterally. This person also has a flat foot deformity (pes planus). The head of the talus is directed medially and plantar *(arrows)*.

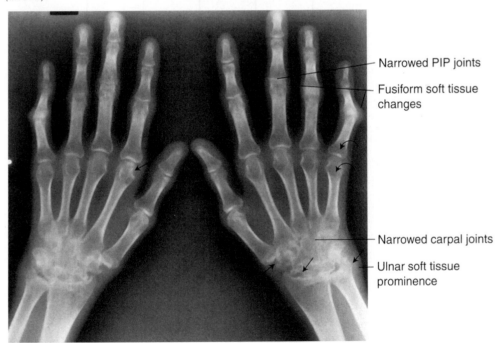

Narrowed PIP joints

Fusiform soft tissue changes

Narrowed carpal joints

Ulnar soft tissue prominence

FIGURE 5-87. Right and left hand PA radiograph. Rheumatoid arthritis. The radiographic findings include periarticular osteoporosis *(curved arrows)*, swan neck deformities of the little fingers, narrowing of the proximal interphalangeal (PIP) joints with associated fusiform soft tissue swelling, narrowing of the carpal and PIP joints, and soft tissue thickening or prominence around the distal ulna. Also, there are erosions involving the carpals, ulnar styloids, and metacarpal heads *(straight arrows)*. The fusiform soft tissue swelling surrounding the joints represents edema and effusion. The soft tissue prominence around the distal ulna is secondary to edema and thickening around the external carpi ulnaris.

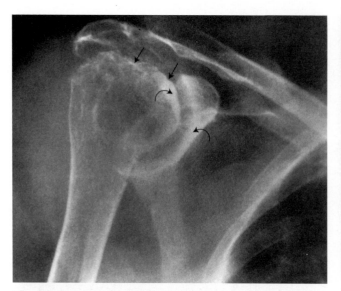

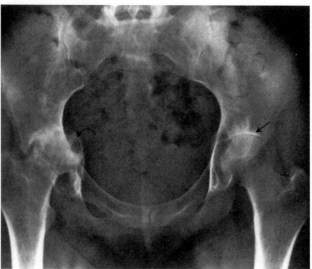

FIGURE 5-88. Right shoulder AP radiograph. Rheumatoid arthritis. There is characteristic osteoporosis, a pointed distal clavicle, and mild cephalad drift of the humeral head. The cephalad drift of the humeral head suggests rotator cuff damage that is common in this disease. There are articular bone erosions *(straight arrows)* and sclerosis *(curved arrows)*.

FIGURE 5-90. Pelvis AP radiograph. Rheumatoid arthritis in a 27-year-old. There is generalized osteoporosis. The entire left hip joint space is symmetrically narrowed *(straight arrow)*. There is characteristic medial drift of the right femoral head and acetabular protrusio *(curved arrow)*. Note that the sacroiliac joints are not involved.

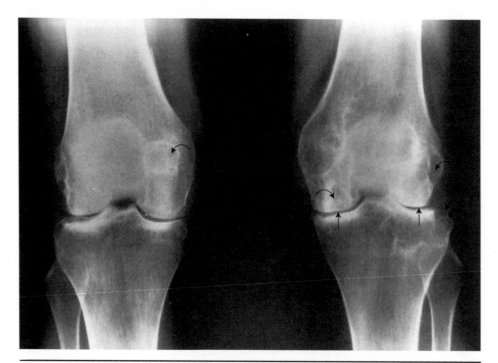

FIGURE 5-89. Right and left knees AP radiograph. Rheumatoid arthritis in a 27-year-old. There are symmetric narrowing of the knee joints *(straight arrows)*, periarticular cysts *(curved arrows)*, erosions *(double arrows)*, and osteoporosis.

▶ **TABLE 5-14 The Differential Diagnosis of Rheumatoid Arthritis**

Gouty arthritis
Infectious arthritis
Sudeck's atrophy
Sarcoid
Osteoarthritis
Ankylosing spondylitis
Scleroderma
Systemic lupus erythematosus

osteoporosis is severe but the articular margins remain sharp. In osteoarthritis, osteoporosis is usually absent and osteophytes are often present.

Gout, Pseudogout, and Hemophilic Arthritis

Some arthritides that are associated with metabolic diseases and blood dyscrasias are listed in Table 5-15. Gout arthritis (Fig. 5-91) is secondary to hyperuricemia or elevated serum uric acid levels, and it is characterized by exacerbations and remissions. The patients classically present with podagra or pain and inflammatory changes near the medial aspect of the first MTP joint. The disease usually is present for a number of years before it is detectable on a radiograph; the radiographic findings of gout are listed in Table 5-16.

Chondrocalcinosis means calcification of cartilage, and it is most often noted in the knee. It can be associated with a number of conditions that are listed in Table 5-17. The arthritis of calcium pyrophosphate deposition (CPPD), or the clinical exacerbation termed pseudogout, is found in middle-aged or older people and is caused by the deposition of calcium pyrophosphate dihydrate crystals in the soft tissues of a joint, including menisci, ligaments, articular cartilage, and the joint capsule (Fig. 5-92).

The joints in patients with hemophilia are gradually injured by repeated bleeding into the joints. Cystic changes develop in the bones neighboring the injured joints, and osteoporosis is a common feature (Fig. 5-93). In general, osteoporosis is a common feature in rheumatoid arthritis, blood dyscrasias, and osteomyelitis, but not in osteoarthritis and gout.

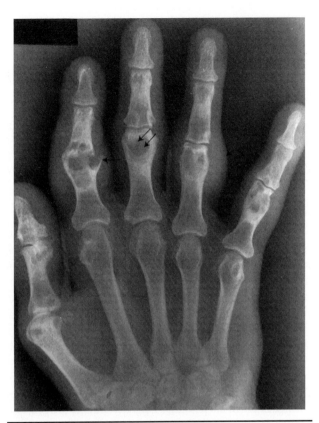

FIGURE 5-91. Right-hand PA radiograph. Gout arthritis. The proximal interphalangeal (PIP) joint spaces are at least partially preserved, and the lucent areas *(double arrows)* are typical of the sharply marginated periarticular erosions. Erosions that extend into the joint often have an overhanging edge *(single straight arrow)*. Note the classic appearance of a tophus *(curved arrow)*. A tophus is an asymmetric swelling about the joint that may or may not be calcified.

Neuropathic Joints

Chronic trauma to a joint that has lost pain sensation can result in a neuropathic or Charcot's joint (Fig. 5-94). Some common causes are shown in Table 5-18. Diabetic neuropathic joints are most common in the lower extremity whereas syringomyelia-related neuropathic joints are usually found in the shoulders and upper extremities. The radiographic findings include joint space narrowing, fragmentation of sclerotic subchondral bone, articular bone cortex destruction, joint loose bodies, and bone mass formation at the articular margins. Some of the neuropathic joint findings are similar to those found in osteoarthritis.

▶ **TABLE 5-15 Arthritides Associated with Metabolic Diseases and Blood Dyscrasias**

Gout
Calcium pyrophosphate deposition (CPPD) disease
Hemophilia

▶ **TABLE 5-16 Radiographic Features of Gout**

Sharply marginated and sometimes sclerotic bordered erosions with overhanging edges near a joint
Tophus formation or soft tissue nodules
Usually osteoporosis is absent
Occasionally joint deformity

▶ **TABLE 5-17** **Causes of Chondrocalcinosis**

Calcium pyrophosphate deposition (CPPD)
Gout
Aging
Hyperparathyroidism

It is generally not true that patients do not feel pain in their neuropathic joints; rather, the degree of pain is disproportionate to the amount of damage.

Other

Periarticular calcifications can result from acute and chronic trauma (Fig. 5-95). Although they do not involve joints, bone spurs are sometimes considered a form of arthritis. Bone spurs cause pain and may be clinically difficult to differentiate from arthritis. Also, bursitis may cause periarticular pain and can sometimes be demonstrated radiographically. Scleroderma is a connective tissue disorder that potentially involves the musculoskeletal system. Multiple soft tissue calcifications are commonly seen in these patients (Fig. 5-96). Other radiographic changes in scleroderma include atrophy of the finger tips and loss of bone at the tips of the distal phalanges. If joint changes are present, they may simulate rheumatoid arthritis.

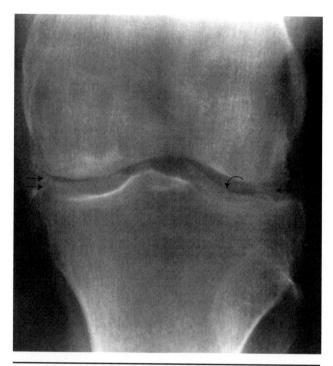

FIGURE 5-92. Left knee AP radiograph. Calcium pyrophosphate deposition (CPPD) disease or pseudogout. There are calcifications in the lateral meniscus *(single straight arrow)* and the medial meniscus *(double straight arrows)*. There is also calcification of the articular cartilage *(curved arrow)*.

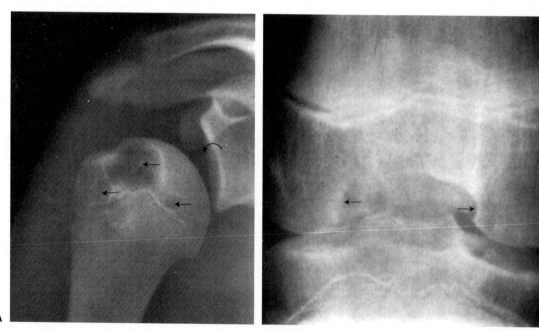

FIGURE 5-93. A: Right shoulder AP radiograph. Hemophilia in a 15-year-old boy. There are cystic changes *(straight arrows)* in the humeral head secondary to repeated bleeds, and there is widening of the shoulder joint *(curved arrow)* due to hemarthrosis. **B:** Knee AP radiograph. Hemophilia in the same patient as in A. He has a widened intercondylar notch *(arrows)* secondary to repeated episodes of hemarthrosis. There is osteoporosis.

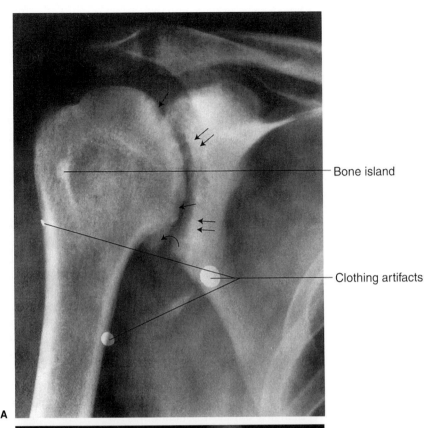

Bone island

Clothing artifacts

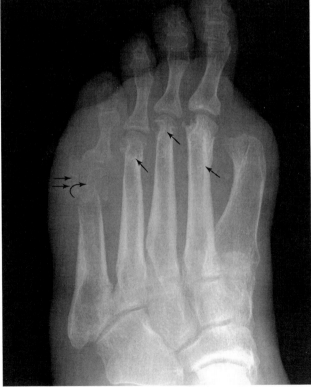

FIGURE 5-94. **A:** Right shoulder AP radiograph. Neuropathic joint or Charcot's joint in a patient with syringomyelia. There is characteristic irregularity of the articular surfaces secondary to destruction of bone and joint cartilage *(single arrows)*. There are sclerotic changes or increased density *(double arrows)* of the bone surrounding the joint and an osteophyte *(curved arrow)*. **B:** Oblique radiograph of the left foot in a diabetic. Neuropathic joints. There are healed fracture deformities of the metatarsal heads *(arrows)*. The great toe has been amputated because of infection. Note destruction of the 5th metatarsal head *(curved arrow)* and adjacent ulcer *(double arrow)* from current osteomyelitis.

▶ **TABLE 5-18** **Causes of Neuropathic or Charcot's Joints**

Diabetes mellitus
Syringomyelia
Congenital indifference to pain
Meningomyelocele
Peripheral nerve injury

▶ **TABLE 5-19** **Some Benign Bone Lesions**

Bone island
Nonossifying fibroma/fibrous cortical defect
Osteochondroma
Osteoma
Osteoid osteoma
Enchondroma
Bone cyst
Fibrous dysplasia
Chondroblastoma
Osteoblastoma
Hemangioma

TUMORS

Benign

There are a number of benign bone lesions, and it is important to recognize them as such (Table 5-19). A bone island, or enostosis, is the most common bone lesion. It is essentially cortical bone that is found in the medullary cavity and appears as a small sclerotic focus. It blends with the surrounding trabeculae and has no aggressive features (Figs. 5-14 and 5-104D). Fibrous cortical defects or nonossifying fibroma may appear similarly in adults, but are closely related to the cortex. These are fibroosseous lesions that are lucent and may expand the cortex in children and adolescents. They are typically small and found incidentally, but are occasionally large and may focally weaken the cortex where fractures may occur. They heal or involute as the child matures (Fig. 5-97). An osteochondroma or osteocartilaginous exostosis is a common benign bone lesion and can occur in nearly all bones. They are bony projections from the external surface of a bone with a cartilage cap and are most commonly found in the metaphysis of long bones, especially around the knee and shoulder. These lesions can result in bone deformities and/or cause pressure on surrounding structures. The cartilaginous cap of osteochondromas undergoes malignant transformation to chondrosarcoma in less than 1% of the cases. Multiple osteochondromas or multiple or familial multiple exostoses is a hereditary autosomal-dominant disorder (Fig. 5-98). Growth abnormalities and malignant transformation (5% to 15%) are more common in multiple osteochondromas than in a single osteochondroma.

Another benign bone lesion is the enchondroma (Fig. 5-99A, B). It is a slow-growing cartilaginous tumor usually found in the hand phalanges and in the distal metacarpals. Small calcifications may be present within the lesions, and they may be difficult to differentiate from bone infarcts. Bone infarcts (Fig. 5-99C) are most commonly present in long bones, and they may or may not be symptomatic. Bone infarcts usually have a well-defined and sclerotic border, whereas enchondromas do not. On occasion, infarcts may have a more permeative appearance, mimicking a malignant primary bone tumor that necessitates a bone biopsy. Some etiologies of bone infarcts include steroid use, sickle cell anemia, systemic lupus erythematosus, Caisson's disease, and pancreatitis.

A simple benign bone cyst (Fig. 5-100) is commonly found in the metaphysis of the proximal humerus and femur, but it can occur in almost any bone. Usually this lesion occurs in patients before the age of 25, and a common complication is a pathologic fracture.

Fibrous dysplasia is a benign fibrous-osseous lesion that arises centrally in the bone, and it can affect one bone (monostotic) or multiple bones (polyostotic). The exact etiology is unknown, and these lesions may or may not be symptomatic. The radiographic features include expansive bone lesions, bone cortex thinning, radiolucent lesions of variable density, and pathologic fractures. The differential diagnosis includes Paget's disease, hyperparathyroidism, and simple bone cyst.

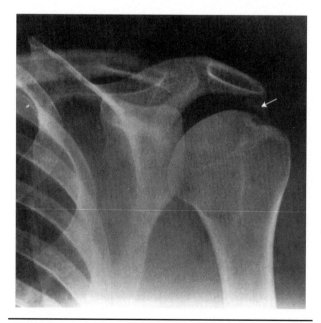

FIGURE 5-95. Left shoulder AP radiograph with the humerus in external rotation. Calcific tendinitis. There is posttraumatic calcification *(arrow)* in the region of the supraspinatus mechanism.

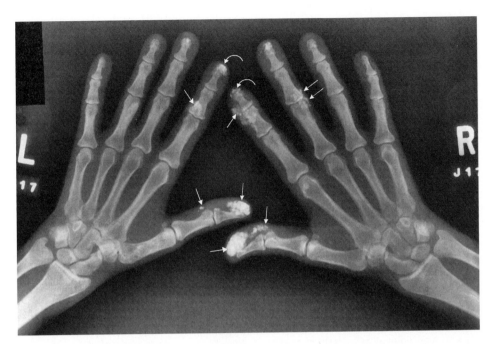

FIGURE 5-96. Right and left hands PA radiograph. Scleroderma. Scleroderma is a connective tissue disease that may involve the musculoskeletal system. There are soft tissue calcifications *(straight arrows)*, and the soft tissues at the tip of the fingers are atrophic *(curved arrows)*. The joints are normal.

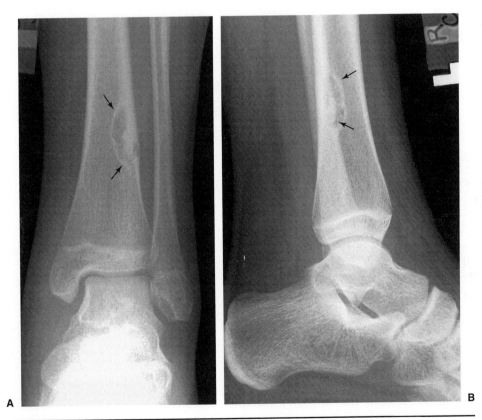

FIGURE 5-97. Anterior **(A)** and lateral **(B)** left ankle radiographs in a 12-year-old girl. Nonossifying fibroma (NOF). The bony lesion has a sclerotic margin *(arrows)*, is slightly lobulated, and arises form the cortex. This benign fibroosseous lesion will eventually become sclerotic and appear as a focal area of cortical thickening when she is an adult.

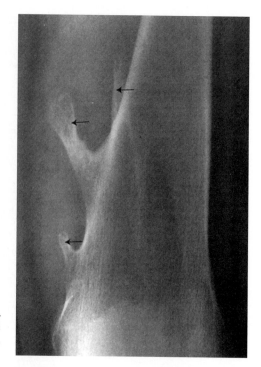

FIGURE 5-98. Left femur AP radiograph. Multiple osteochondromas or familial multiple exostoses. The osteochondromas *(arrows)* point away from the knee joint, simulating a coat hook.

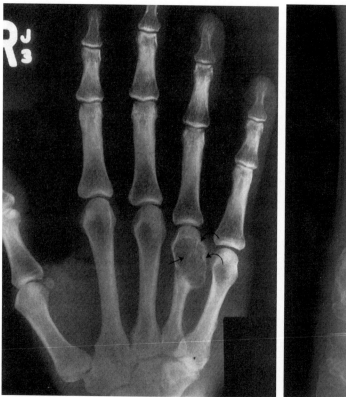

A

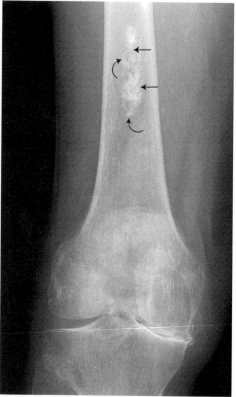

B

FIGURE 5-99. A: Right-hand PA radiograph. Enchondroma of the distal 4th metacarpal *(straight arrow)*. This slow-growing tumor typically causes thinning and scalloping *(curved arrows)* of the inner bone cortex. **B:** Right knee radiograph. Enchondroma. In a large bone, scalloping of the cortex is less common. The calcification of cartilage often appears as small balls *(straight arrows)* or as arcs *(curved arrows)* and rings. Note osteoarthritis predominantly in the medial compartment of the knee. *(continued)*

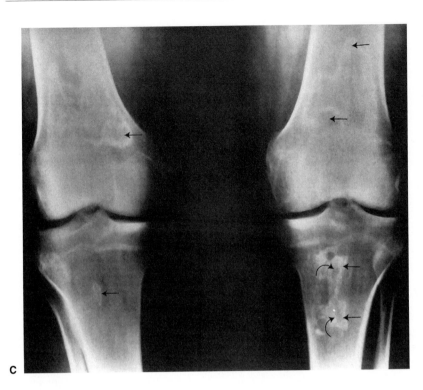

c

FIGURE 5-99. C: Right and left knees AP radiograph. Multiple bone infarcts. The multiple infarcts are manifested by thin zones of sclerosis surrounding lucencies *(straight arrows)* and marrow calcifications *(curved arrows)*. The etiology in this patient is unknown.

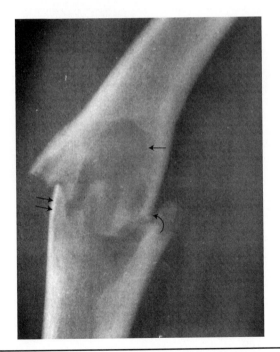

FIGURE 5-100. Right femur AP radiograph. Benign cyst *(straight arrow)* with pathologic fracture *(curved arrow)* in a 10-year-old child. There is apex lateral angulation and mild offset of the fracture fragments. Note the thinning of the bone cortex *(double straight arrows)* caused by the expanding benign cyst.

Osteoid osteoma (Fig. 5-101) is a benign bone lesion of unknown etiology, and the typical symptom is night pain relieved by aspirin. It can occur in almost every bone, but is most often found in the femoral neck and the tibia. Approximately 75% to 80% of these lesions are intracortical and have multiple radiographic appearances, but the classical appearance is sclerosis surrounding a radiolucent center or nidus. In some instances, there may be calcifications within this lucent zone mimicking a sequestra of osteomyelitis. The differential diagnosis would also include stress fracture, bone island, infection, and metastatic disease.

Osteoid osteoma has intense activity on a radionuclide bone scan (Fig. 101B), whereas bone islands have none, or very little activity (Table 5-20). CT is usually diagnostic, demonstrating the classic nidus (Fig. 5-101C). MRI may

▶ TABLE 5-20 Using the Radionuclide Bone Scan to Differentiate Bone Lesions

| **Positive bone scans** |
| Osteoid osteoma |
| Primary bone tumors |
| Metastases |
| Paget's disease |
| **Negative bone scans** |
| Multiple myeloma |
| Bone island |
| Enchondroma |

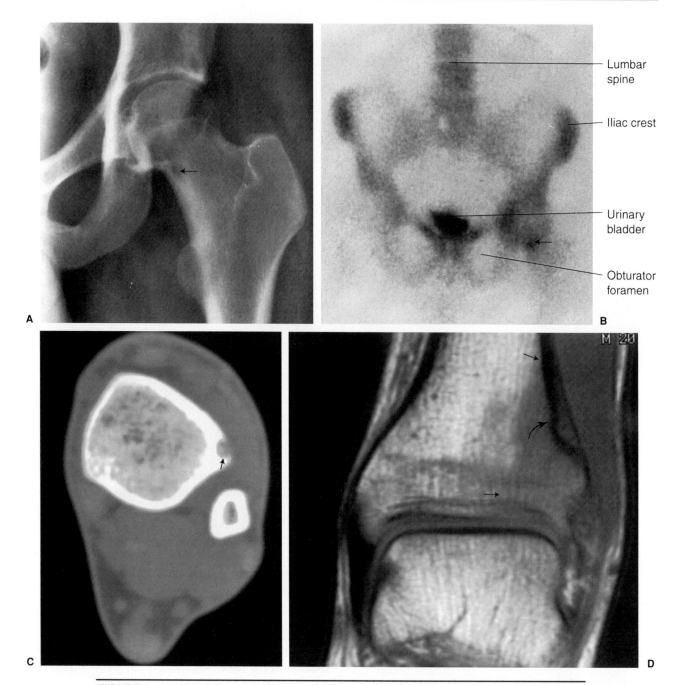

FIGURE 5-101. A: Left hip AP radiograph. Osteoid osteoma in a 20-year-old. The patient experienced left hip night pain that was typically relieved by aspirin. The lucent zone *(arrow)* in the inferior aspect of the left femur subcapital region is the osteoid osteoma. **B:** Anterior pelvis radionuclide scan on the same patient. The single area of increased radionuclide uptake *(arrow)* in the left femoral neck corresponds to the radiolucent abnormality visualized in A. The bone scan is otherwise normal. **C:** Axial CT distal tibia. Osteoid osteoma. The cortical lucent nidus *(arrow)* is nicely demonstrated by CT. Rarely, there is a central dot of calcification in the lucency. **D:** Coronal T1 MR in the same patient does not show the nidus as well as CT *(curved arrow)*, but the large amount of edema (gray) is easy to see *(straight arrows)*.

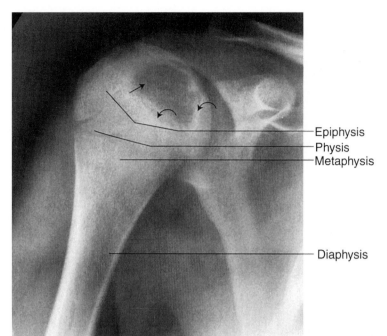

Epiphysis
Physis
Metaphysis

Diaphysis

FIGURE 5-102. Right shoulder AP radiograph. Benign chondroblastoma *(straight arrow)* of the proximal humerus epiphysis in a 14-year-old. The typical sclerotic border is present *(curved arrows)*.

also show the nidus, but may be confusing because of the large amount of bone edema surrounding it (Fig. 5-101D).

A chondroblastoma (Fig. 5-102) is an uncommon benign bone lesion found in the epiphysis, usually before skeletal maturity. These radiolucent lesions generally have sclerotic borders and sometimes contain scattered calcifications. The differential diagnosis should include infection, giant cell tumor, osteoid osteoma, and metastatic disease.

Giant cell tumors occur in young adults following skeletal maturity (Fig. 5-103). These lesions are eccentrically located in the end of long bones such as the tibia, femur, radius, and humerus. They usually have sharp nonsclerotic borders without periosteal reaction and usually abut the articular surface. Based on their radiographic appearance, it is difficult to determine if they are benign or malignant. Approximately 15% will recur following simple curettage and packing of the defect. They are rarely malignant, if metastases are considered as a malignant indicator.

Malignant

Metastatic lesions (Fig. 5-104 A–C) are the most common malignant bone tumors and represent spread from a wide variety of primary neoplasms. Bone metastases may be single, multiple, osteolytic (radiolucent or black), osteoblastic (white), or mixed. The majority of metastases are osteolytic radiolucent, but osteoblastic metastases frequently result from cancers of the prostate and breast (Table 5-21). A bone island (Fig. 5-104D) should not be confused with an osteoblastic metastatic lesion. Bone

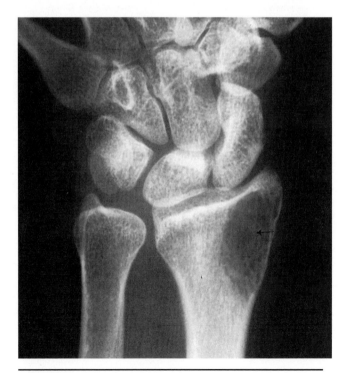

FIGURE 5-103. Left wrist PA radiograph. Giant cell tumor *(arrow)* of the distal radius. This is the classic appearance and common location of this tumor.

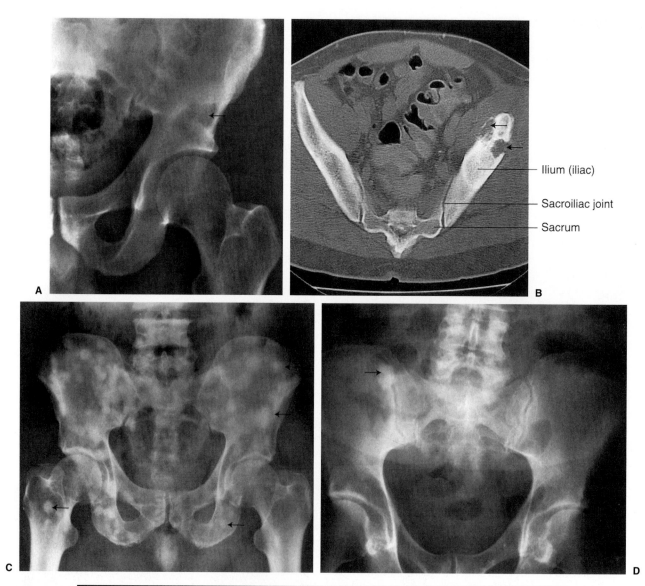

FIGURE 5-104. A: Left hip AP radiograph. Metastatic carcinoma of the lung. The radiolucent area in the left iliac bone *(arrow)* represents a suspected osteolytic metastasis. **B:** Pelvis axial CT image in the same patient. Two osteolytic metastases *(arrows)* in the left iliac bone. The CT image confirmed the presence and extent of two bone lesions. **C:** Pelvis AP radiograph. Osteoblastic metastases from carcinoma of the prostate. The arrows indicate multiple bilateral osteoblastic (white) metastatic lesions *(arrows)*. **D:** Pelvis AP radiograph. Bone island *(straight arrow)*. Bone islands are usually ovoid or oblong with a spiculated contour. They are benign and generally asymptomatic.

▌**TABLE 5-21** Radiographic Appearance of Bone Metastases

Osteoblastic or sclerotic
Prostate
Breast
Carcinoid
Neuroblastoma

Mixed (lytic and blastic)
Breast
Cervix
Bladder

Osteolytic
Nearly all neoplasms

▌**TABLE 5-22** Some Malignant Bone Lesions

Primary
Multiple myeloma
Osteosarcoma
Ewing's sarcoma
Chondrosarcoma

Secondary
Metastases

islands are benign, asymptomatic, and distributed widely and usually sparingly in the skeletal system.

Multiple myeloma originates in the bone marrow and is the most common primary malignant bone tumor (Table 5-22). The patient usually complains of pain in the involved area. Although any bone can be involved, the most commonly affected sites include the skull, spine, ribs, and pelvis. Unlike Ewing's sarcoma, this disease occurs in the over-40 age group. The typical radiographic appearance (Fig. 5-105) consists of multiple osteolytic areas with a punched-out appearance. At times it is difficult to differentiate multiple myeloma from osteolytic metastatic disease. *Urine and serum protein electrophoresis is important in the diagnosis of multiple myeloma.*

Osteosarcoma is a primary malignant bone tumor that commonly occurs during the second decade of life. It can occur in many locations, but is usually found in the

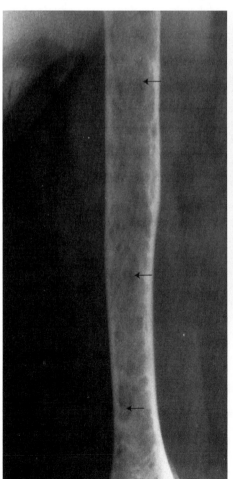

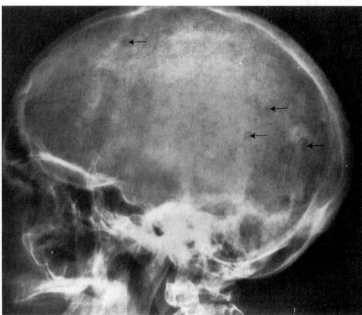

FIGURE 5-105. Left humerus AP radiograph **(A)** and lateral skull radiograph **(B)**. Multiple myeloma. The lucent or black areas indicated by the *arrows* represent the classic appearance of multiple myeloma in bone.

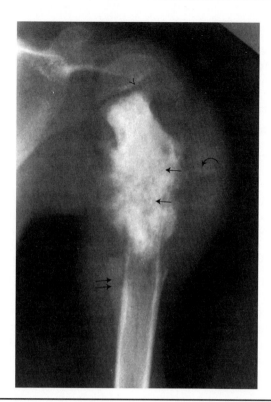

FIGURE 5-106. Left humerus AP radiograph in a 6-year-old. Large osteosarcoma of the humerus metaphysis and diaphysis. The tumor *(single straight arrows)* has not crossed the physis *(arrow head)*. Codman's triangle *(double straight arrows)* represents periosteal new bone formation reacting to the tumor growth, and the sunburst or ray appearance *(curved arrow)* represents tumor bone.

metaphysis of a long bone. It has a wide variety of radiographic appearances, but classically produces an abundance of new, irregular bone (Fig. 5-106). In some primary bone tumors a Codman's triangle may be identified, and the triangle represents periosteal new bone formation reacting to the growing tumor. Osteosarcomas may have a Codman's triangle as well as a sunburst or ray appearance that is secondary to bone formation in the tumor (Fig. 5-106). On occasion, it can be difficult to differentiate osteosarcomas from metastatic disease and other primary bone tumors, especially Ewing's sarcoma.

Ewing's sarcoma usually occurs in children and young adults (Fig. 5-107). The classic appearance is a permeative or moth-eaten pattern, but it may have a variety of other associated bone changes such as sclerosis. Occasionally, Ewing's sarcoma has a layered periosteal reaction secondary to the tumor's presence that looks like onion skin. Other lesions in children with periosteal reaction include osteomyelitis, fracture, eosinophilic granuloma, neuroblastoma, and osteosarcoma. The soft tissue extension of Ewing's sarcoma usually will not contain bone or cartilage calcification, whereas the soft tissue extensions of osteosarcomas tend to produce bone.

▶ **TABLE 5-23   Some Metabolic Diseases That May Affect Bones**

Paget's disease
Hypothyroidism
Scurvy
Acromegaly
Rickets
Diabetes mellitus
Hyperparathyroidism

METABOLIC DISEASES

Some metabolic diseases have the potential to affect bones significantly. A few examples are listed in Table 5-23.

Paget's Disease

Paget's disease is a common, chronic, and progressive metabolic bone disease of unknown etiology that occurs in adults over the age of 40. This disease can involve all bones (Figs. 5-108 and 6-53). The radiographic features of Paget's disease are listed in Table 5-24. On radiographs, the bone cortices are thick and sclerotic in appearance and the trabecular pattern is thickened and prominent. Rarefaction and bone destruction may occur. Occurring secondary to bone softening are bone deformities such as bowing of long bones and protrusio acetabula. The two most significant complications are pathologic fractures and sarcomatous degeneration. The differential diagnosis should include osteoblastic metastatic disease, fibrous dysplasia, lymphoma, and osteosclerosis.

Osteoporosis and Osteomalacia

Osteoporosis (Figs. 5-20, 5-48, 5-87 to 5-90, 5-93B) is secondary to a reduced amount of bone matrix (osteoid) with normal mineralization, whereas osteomalacia is a normal bone matrix (osteoid) with a reduced amount of mineralization. Osteoporosis has become a major public health problem with countless related fractures per year and probably costing billions of dollars per year. There is a long list of osteoporosis etiologies, and a partial list of etiologies is shown in Table 5-25. Radiographs are insensitive

▶ **TABLE 5-24   Radiographic Features of Paget's Disease**

Thick and sclerotic bone cortices
Thick and prominent trabecular pattern
Long bone bowing
Acetabular protrusio
Pathologic fractures

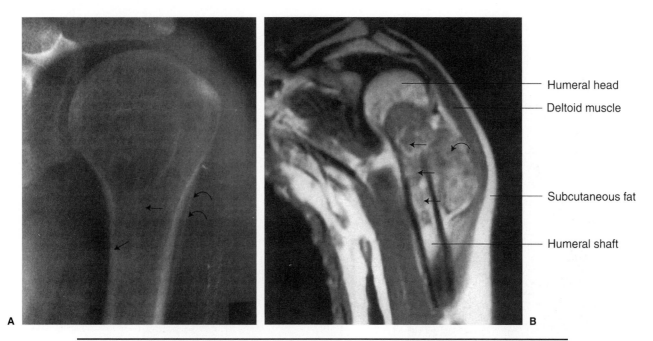

Humeral head
Deltoid muscle
Subcutaneous fat
Humeral shaft

A

B

FIGURE 5-107. **A:** Left humerus AP radiograph. Ewing's sarcoma. This 27-year-old presented with left arm and shoulder pain, and the radiographic appearance is typical: a permeative or moth-eaten appearance *(straight arrows)*, ill-defined borders, and periosteal reaction *(curved arrows)*. **B:** Left humerus coronal T1 MR image on the same patient. Ewing's sarcoma. The tumor replaces nearly all the proximal humerus bone marrow *(straight arrows)*. Note how much of the tumor extends into the soft tissue surrounding the proximal humerus *(curved arrow)*. This latter finding cannot be fully appreciated on the radiograph. An osteosarcoma could have this same appearance.

for evaluation of osteoporosis. Dual x-ray absorptiometry (DEXA) is currently the standard screening method.

Rickets

Rickets is a good example of osteomalacia and osteopenia in children. It is found in the growing portions of infant bones and is caused by poor calcification of the osteoid matrix that may result from vitamin D deficiency, renal disease, or intestinal malabsorption diseases. The radiographic findings include widened and irregular physes,

cupping of the metaphyses, bowing of the legs, and osteopenia (Fig. 5-109). When this disease occurs in adults, it does not affect the growth plates and is termed osteomalacia.

INFECTION

Osteomyelitis (Fig. 5-110) can occur in all age groups, and the classic clinical presentation is bone or joint pain and fever. There are multiple etiologies including trauma and hematogenous spread of infection (Fig. 5-111). In adults, particularly diabetics, the bone destruction is usually adjacent to a soft tissue ulcer and known infection (See Fig. 5-94B). However, the radiographic appearance of osteomyelitis can be similar to a bone tumor with bone and joint destruction, periosteal reaction, and a soft tissue component. It can be especially confusing when found in the center of bone, such as at a site of prior fracture. Unlike tumors, infections may occasionally have gas in the soft tissues secondary to gas-forming organisms. MRI is a very useful tool for the demonstration of bone and soft tissue involvement by infection. However, it can be a confusing picture in a diabetic foot, which may also have abnormalities and fractures due to neuropathic changes (Fig. 5-94B).

▶ **TABLE 5-25 Some Etiologies of Osteoporosis**

Immobilization
Sudek's atrophy
Estrogen deficiency or postmenopausel
Steroid therapy
Cushing's disease
Hyperparathyroidism
Diabetes mellitus
Anemias
Paget's disease
Malnutrition
Osteogenesis imperfecta

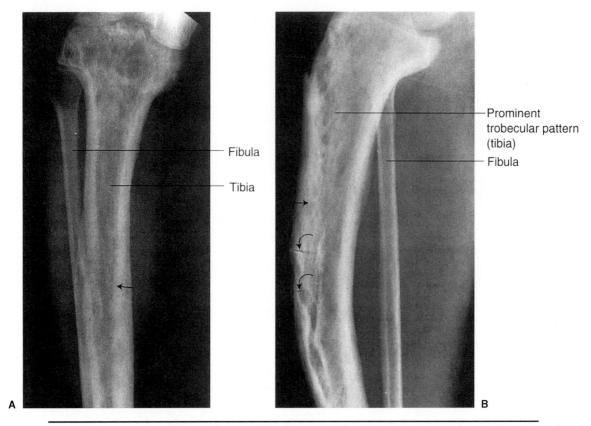

Fibula

Tibia

Prominent trobecular pattern (tibia)

Fibula

A

B

FIGURE 5-108. Right tibia and fibula AP **(A)** and lateral **(B)** radiographs. Paget's disease. The tibia cortices are sclerotic in appearance *(straight arrows)* because of widening and thickening of the cortices and a prominent trabecular pattern. The tibia is bowed anterolaterally. The fibula is spared. The typical transverse pathologic fractures are best visualized on the lateral radiograph *(curved arrows)*, and they are the most common complication of this disease. There is osteoporosis.

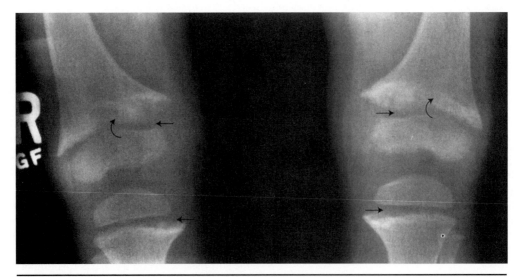

FIGURE 5-109. Right and left knees AP radiographs. Rickets. The physes are widened *(straight arrows)*, and the metaphases are cupped *(curved arrows)*.

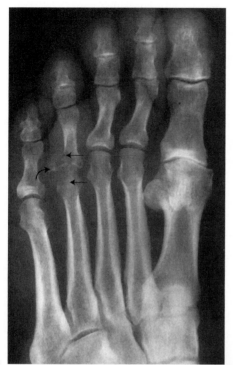

A

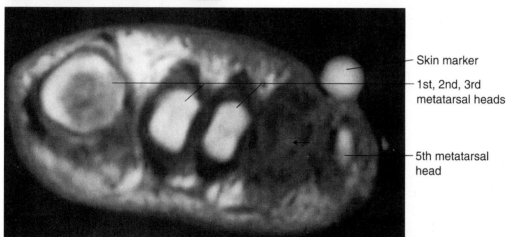

B

- Skin marker
- 1st, 2nd, 3rd metatarsal heads

- 5th metatarsal head

FIGURE 5-110. **A:** Left foot AP radiograph. Osteomyelitis in a patient with diabetes mellitus. There are destructive changes *(straight arrows)* involving the base of the proximal phalanx of the 4th toe as well as the 4th metatarsal head. Also, there are destructive changes in the 4th metatarsophalangeal joint manifested by narrowing of the joint space. The infection has characteristically caused destructive joint changes as well as bone destruction on both sides of the joint. Loose bone fragments have resulted from the osteomyelitis *(curved arrows)*. **B:** Left foot axial T1 MR image in the same patient. When compared to the other metatarsal heads, the 4th metatarsal head is not visible because the infection *(arrow)* has destroyed and replaced the bone marrow.

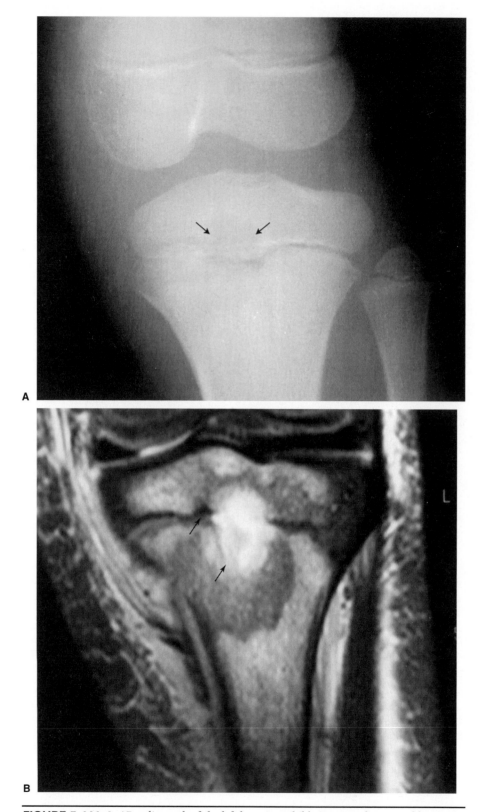

FIGURE 5-111. A: AP radiograph of the left knee in a child. Osteomyelitis. Focal lucency is noted in the epiphysis *(arrows)*. **B:** Coronal fat-suppressed T2 MR in the same patient shows the abscess crosses the physis and involves the metaphysic as well *(arrows)*.

APPROACH TO COMMON CLINICAL PROBLEMS

When evaluating the musculoskeletal system, a thorough physical examination should dictate the next appropriate steps in imaging. Radiographs are typically the initial screening tool, but should be used appropriately. For example, if a patient presents with pain after falling on an outstretched arm, one would not order a radiograph of the upper arm. Nor should one order radiographs of the humerus and forearm in an attempt to screen for injuries to the shoulder, humerus, elbow, forearm, and wrist. A bone is best imaged when the x-ray beam is centered at that bone or joint. Elbow joint effusions are typically not seen on films of the humerus and forearm. Similarly, radial head fractures or scaphoid fractures may be seen only on specialized dedicated views. If our hypothetical patient has focal tenderness over the radial head, or has pain with pronation and supination, a dedicated elbow radiographic series is the appropriate choice. If a shoulder dislocation is suspect, a shoulder series to include an axillary or transcapular Y-view is the appropriate study of choice.

When the radiographs are normal, the clinical setting and degree of suspicion of injury will dictate how to proceed. Often, immobilization with repeat radiographs in one week is sufficient to evaluate for an occult fracture. This is not appropriate, however, for a potential hip fracture in an elderly person as immobilization could have devastating effects. An emergent MRI has been shown to be the imaging procedure of choice in this circumstance.

KEY POINTS

- It is important to recognize sesamoid bones and ossicles as normal variants. Sesamoids are bones within a tendon. Ossicles are extra or supernumerary bones next to the skeleton and usually named after the neighboring bone.
- MRI is useful for injuries to the shoulder rotator cuff, knee ligaments and menisci, ankle ligaments, and Achilles tendon. CT imaging is good for bone detail, fracture diagnosis, locating fracture fragments, and evaluating matrix formation in bone tumors.

- The Salter-Harris classification describes fractures around the physis, which is considered the weakest point in a growing bone.
- Because fractures and other abnormalities may not be visualized on all radiographic views, always insist on at least two views of an injured or diseased area that are 90 degrees to each other.
- Fractures may not be visible on the first radiographs but may become visible after time (7 days) because of bone resorption at the ends of the fracture fragments.
- A transverse lucent line at the base of the fifth metatarsal always represents a fracture, whereas the normal apophysis in this area is lateral and parallel to the long axis of the metatarsal.
- Osteoarthritis is the most common form of arthritis and often results from asymmetric cartilage wear.
- The radiographic features of osteoarthritis include irregular joint narrowing, sclerosis, absence of osteoporosis, and osteophyte formation.
- The radiographic features of rheumatoid arthritis include periarticular thickening, symmetric joint narrowing, marginal erosions, periarticular osteoporosis, and joint deformity.
- Metastatic cancer is the most common malignant bone tumor. The majority of metastatic lesions are osteolytic or radiolucent. Osteoblastic metastatic lesions most commonly are secondary to prostate and breast neoplasms.
- Multiple myeloma is the most common primary malignant bone tumor, and it originates in the bone marrow.
- Ewing's sarcoma usually occurs in children and young adults. They may have a permeative type of lesion and an onion-skin-like periosteal reaction.
- Osteomyelitis and septic joints typically present with localized pain and fever. The radiographic features include bone and joint destruction, periosteal reaction, and occasionally, a soft tissue component.

FURTHER READINGS

El-Khoury GY, Bergman RA, Montgomery WJ. *Sectional anatomy by MRI*, 2nd ed. New York: Churchill Livingstone, 1995.

El-Khoury GY. *Essentials of musculoskeletal imaging.* New York: Churchill Livingstone, 2003.

Chew FS, Kline MJ, Bui-Mansfield LT. *Core curriculum: musculoskeletal imaging*, Philadelphia: Lippincott Williams & Wilkins, 2003.

Spine and Pelvis

Carol A. Boles

The axial skeleton is the next focus for our consideration. It consists of the skull (which is covered separately), the spine, and the pelvis. It is the main structural support for the body and, as a result, is subjected to many stresses. The spine consists of cervical, thoracic, lumbar, and sacral divisions composed of bones, joints, ligaments, muscular attachments, and nerves. The pelvis articulates with the sacrum on each side, supports many soft tissue structures, articulates with the femurs, and is the proximal attachment for many muscles involved in locomotion.

Back pain is a problem for the majority of our patients at some time in their lives. Most people recover from their back pain with little or no medical care. Occupation-related back injuries are common, and other common etiologies of back pain are listed in Table 6-1. When patients do seek medical care for back pain, radiologic imaging often becomes an important diagnostic tool. Following a thorough history and physical examination, routine anteroposterior (AP) and lateral radiographs often are the first radiologic consultation to be requested to evaluate the symptomatic region of the spine. These images may be supplemented with oblique and coned-down views to better visualize an area, and occasionally lateral flexion and extension views are requested to document spine motion and stability.

Computed tomography (CT) and magnetic resonance imaging (MRI) are extremely useful noninvasive diagnostic tools in visualizing the spine, and their use is increasing while use of the invasive myelogram is decreasing. CT delineates anatomy and pathology more clearly than does myelography. One significant shortcoming of myelography is its inability to demonstrate lateral disc herniations and lateral stenosis. For this reason, CT is obtained following myelography to better delineate the contrast distribution in the dural sac and visualize the intervertebral discs. CT is excellent for bone detail and is useful for diagnosing fractures not visible on plain radiographs as well as better defining the extent of injury. CT is helpful for localizing the exact position of vertebral fracture fragments, particularly important when the fracture fragments are displaced into the spinal canal. CT is also useful in screening for disc disease and degenerative disease, but has largely been

▶ **TABLE 6-1 Back Pain Etiologies**

Congenital
Meningocele and myelomeningocele
Scoliosis
Transitional vertebra with pseudarthrosis

Acquired
Arthritis—degenerative, rheumatoid, ankylosing spondylitis
Infection—staphylococcus, tuberculosis
Metabolic—osteoporosis, osteomalacia, Paget's disease, sickle cell
    anemia
Neoplasm—benign and malignant primary bone tumors, metastases
Trauma—fracture, muscle and ligament injury, spondylolysis, and
    spondylolisthesis

Extraspinal
Cardiovascular system—referred myocardial pain, aortic aneurysm
Gastrointestinal disease
Genitourinary system—renal and ureteral pain
Muscle strain
Psychosomatic or functional

replaced by MRI for this purpose. MRI is very good for imaging soft tissues and the bone marrow, and allows a wonderful view of the spinal cord and the intervertebral discs. MRI is also used when a spine fracture is present and an associated cord injury is suspected. However, MRI costs approximately twice as much as CT imaging (Table 6-2). In addition, some patients may not be able to

▶ **TABLE 6-2 Indications for the Use of Imaging
            Modalities in the Spine and Pelvis**

Radiographs
Routine
Cervical spine—AP and lateral
Thoracic spine—AP and lateral
Lumbar spine—AP and lateral
Pelvis—AP

Optional when indicated
Cervical spine—AP open mouth view and/or swimmer's view in
    trauma, flexion, and extension views for mobility and stability,
    oblique views for the neural foramina
Lumbar spine—flexion and extension views for stability and mobility,
    oblique views for spondylolysis
Sacroiliac joints—oblique views, modified outlet view

CT
Fractures and disc disease

MRI
Soft tissues and bone marrow
Spinal cord and disc disease
Fractures with suspected cord injury

Myelogram
Disc disease, spinal stenosis, cord, and extradural tumors

have an MRI because the strong magnetic field may disrupt a pacemaker or displace an aneurysm clip, or the patient may not tolerate the relatively confined space.

NORMAL IMAGES

Cervical Spine

As previously emphasized in other anatomic regions, a systematic approach for evaluating the spine is needed. You will eventually develop your own system, but the following one will work until you do (Table 6-3). Start with the lateral radiograph (Fig. 6-1A) as it is the most important cervical spine radiograph. Glance at the entire image to see if something obvious jumps out at you. If it does, put that aside and force yourself to look at the entire study. It is not uncommon to stop looking once one abnormality is found. This can lead to serious consequences! On the lateral radiograph, the normal cervical curve should be mildly convex anteriorly (lordotic). When the patient has pain, straightening of the spine may occur secondary to muscle spasm. A patient in a hard cervical collar also has a straightened curvature. Make note of the normal lines that should be intact on this view (Fig. 6-1B). Now simply count the cervical vertebrae. Things you must see include all seven cervical vertebrae, the entire C7 and T1 intervertebral disc space, and, ideally, the T1 vertebral body. This is especially important in trauma situations as a fracture could be lurking in nonvisualized areas of the spine, and the result could be catastrophic. For example, if the C7 vertebra is not included on the lateral cervical spine radiograph, a fracture of C7 might go unrecognized. An unrecognized and displaced fracture has the potential to cause a serious cord injury. *Always* gauge the vertical heights of the vertebral bodies and the intervertebral disc spaces. The vertical heights of each vertebral body and intervertebral disc space should be approximately equal to those

▶ **TABLE 6-3 Checklist for Spinal Radiograph
            Observations**

Lateral radiograph
Alignment (3 lines in cervical spine)
Must visualize 7 cervical vertebrae
Vertebral body heights
Disc space heights
Osseous density

AP radiograph
Alignment
Vertebral body heights
Disc space heights
Bone density
Pedicles (lower cervical)

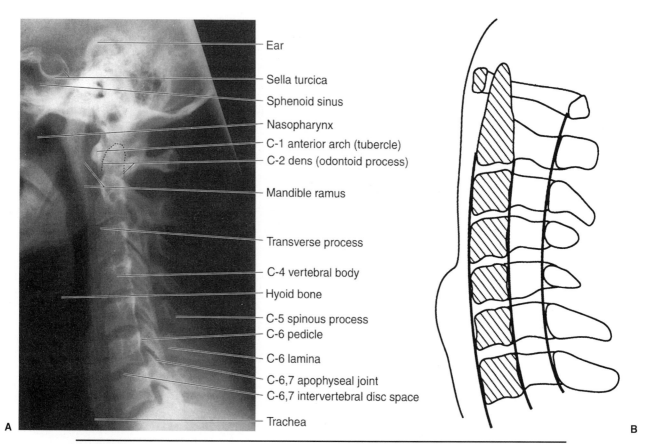

Ear
Sella turcica
Sphenoid sinus
Nasopharynx
C-1 anterior arch (tubercle)
C-2 dens (odontoid process)
Mandible ramus
Transverse process
C-4 vertebral body
Hyoid bone
C-5 spinous process
C-6 pedicle
C-6 lamina
C-6,7 apophyseal joint
C-6,7 intervertebral disc space
Trachea

A

B

FIGURE 6-1. A: Cervical spine lateral radiograph. Normal. **B:** Cervical spine lateral illustration. Normal lines found on the normal lateral radiograph.

immediately above and below. Note the osseous densities in general. Some common causes for decreased (osteopenia) and increased bone density are shown in Table 6-4. Metastatic bone disease from prostate, breast, and other malignancies can result in an increased bone density or osteosclerotic appearance.

Next look at the AP radiograph (Fig. 6-2A) and again check the alignment of the cervical spine. The spine should be straight on this view. Again note the heights of the vertebral bodies and intervertebral disc spaces. When disease or injury is suspected at the C1 and C2 levels, an AP radiograph of the upper cervical spine is obtained by directing the central x-ray beam through the patient's open mouth. This is called the *open mouth view* (Fig. 6-2B), and it allows visualization of the dens, or odontoid process, of the C2 vertebra and the C1 and C2 alignments and joints. An extremely important observation to make is the presence or absence of the vertebral pedicles. Pedicles look like the headlights of the vertebrae in the low cervical, thoracic, and lumbar regions, but are obliquely oriented in the upper and mid cervical spine and best seen on cervical oblique views. They are often involved by metastatic disease because of their abundant blood supply. *If one or more pedicles are absent, metastatic involvement or some*

▶ **TABLE 6-4 Some Common Causes for Increased and Decreased Bone Density**

Decreased
Osteolytic metastases
Osteomalacia
Osteomyelitis
Osteoporosis
Primary bone tumor, especially multiple myeloma
Rheumatoid arthritis, ankylosing spondylitis

Increased
Bone infarcts
Bone island
Callus formation—fractures
Endplate sclerosis—disc degeneration
Fibrous dysplasia
Lymphoma
Osteoblastic metastases (prostate and breast)
Osteopetrosis
Paget's disease
Primary bone tumors (<5% of multiple myeloma)

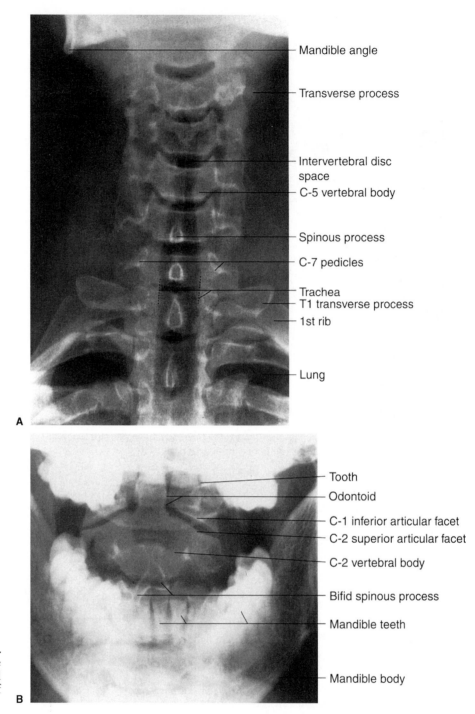

Mandible angle

Transverse process

Intervertebral disc space
C-5 vertebral body

Spinous process

C-7 pedicles

Trachea
T1 transverse process
1st rib

Lung

A

Tooth
Odontoid

C-1 inferior articular facet
C-2 superior articular facet

C-2 vertebral body

Bifid spinous process

Mandible teeth

Mandible body

B

FIGURE 6-2. **A:** Cervical spine AP radiograph. Normal. **B:** Cervical spine AP open-mouth radiograph of the upper cervical spine. Normal.

other destructive process must be strongly suspected. There are benign causes such as a meningocele or congenital absence of the pedicle, but these need to be proven rather than assumed.

Occasionally, oblique views (Fig. 6-3) are obtained and the same observations are made as on the other views. The intervertebral foramina, through which the spinal nerves pass, are well seen on these views. Any disease process that narrows the foramina could potentially cause pressure on

the nerve exiting through that neural foramen, resulting in radiculopathy, or pain along the distribution of the involved nerve. Some processes that can impinge on the intervertebral foramina include intervertebral disc disease, arthritis, and primary and secondary neoplasms. In the trauma setting, these oblique views allow for evaluation of the facet joints to look for fractures or dislocations.

Lateral flexion and extension views may be necessary to evaluate stability of the spine and assess for ligamentous

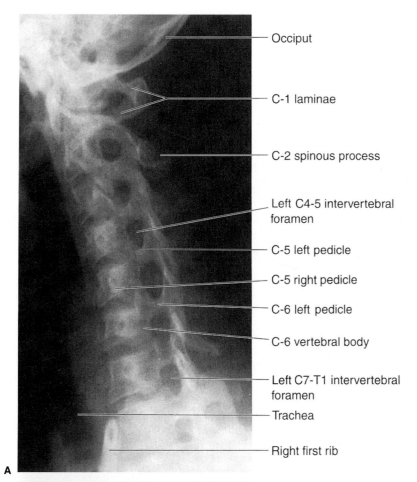

Occiput

C-1 laminae

C-2 spinous process

Left C4-5 intervertebral foramen

C-5 left pedicle

C-5 right pedicle

C-6 left pedicle

C-6 vertebral body

Left C7-T1 intervertebral foramen

Trachea

Right first rib

A

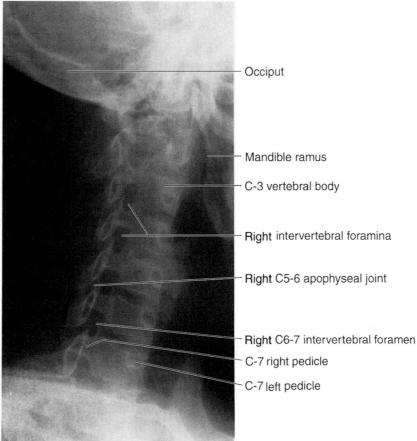

Occiput

Mandible ramus

C-3 vertebral body

Right intervertebral foramina

Right C5-6 apophyseal joint

Right C6-7 intervertebral foramen

C-7 right pedicle

C-7 left pedicle

B

FIGURE 6-3. Cervical spine right **(A)** and left **(B)** oblique radiographs. Normal.

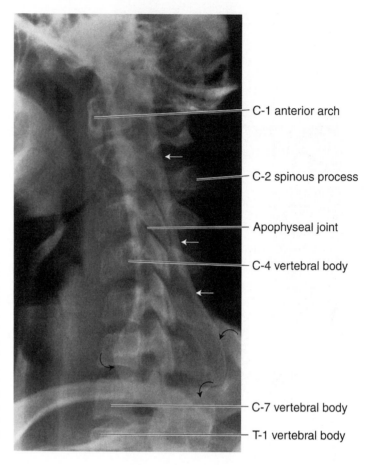

C-1 anterior arch

C-2 spinous process

Apophyseal joint

C-4 vertebral body

C-7 vertebral body

T-1 vertebral body

FIGURE 6-4. Cervical spine lateral swimmer's view. Normal. The patient is almost always radiographed supine with one arm, usually the left, abducted upward alongside the head whereas the other arm is lowered. This position makes patients appear as if they are swimming the backstroke. The central x-ray beam is directed to the C7-T1 level from the patient's side on which the arm is lowered, usually the right. The *straight arrows* indicate the raised arm humerus projecting over the spine. The *curved arrows* outline the humeral head. Note how well the C7 vertebra is visualized as well as a portion of the T1 vertebra and the apophyseal joints. In this view, it is considered good technique when you can see the entire C7 vertebra and at least the upper one-third of the T1 vertebral body.

injury. They should not routinely be obtained when a fracture is present. The majority of motion occurs in the upper cervical spine. When the lower cervical vertebrae cannot be visualized on the lateral view, a swimmer's view is indicated (Fig. 6-4). CT is often used to diagnose occult cervical spine fractures, determine the extent of fractures, and localize fracture fragments. At many medical centers, severe trauma patients are routinely screened with a CT of the entire cervical spine. The CT data can then be reformatted into coronal and sagittal plane images (Fig. 6-29B) As already mentioned, MRI is especially useful for evaluating the spinal cord and the intervertebral discs and for assessing ligamentous injury (Fig. 6-5).

Thoracic (Dorsal) Spine

Routine radiographic study of the thoracic spine consists of AP and lateral radiographs (Fig. 6-6). When viewing the thoracic spine, it is easiest to begin with the lateral view and follow the same method of evaluation as used for the lateral cervical spine radiograph. The normal dorsal curve should be mildly convex posterior (kyphotic). Again, assess the vertical heights of the dorsal vertebral bodies and intervertebral disc spaces. As always, check the overall densities of the bones. The lamina and spinous processes are not well seen because the ribs project over them (Fig. 6-6B).

It is difficult to number the vertebral bodies without using the anterior view to determine the size of the twelfth ribs.

Next, evaluate the AP thoracic spine radiograph; the spinal alignment should be straight. Assess the vertical height of each dorsal vertebral body and each dorsal intervertebral disc space. The paraspinal line along the left side of the vertebra should be narrow and straight. A focal bulge may be your first indication of a fracture. The pedicles look like headlights on the vertebral bodies, and every attempt should be made to visualize all of them. On AP radiographs, the spinous processes project over the midvertebral bodies at all levels in the spine. Assess the number of rib-bearing vertebra. T12 typically has two short ribs, but transverse processes may instead be present. Similarly, L1 may have rudimentary ribs, so it is important to count from the top down. Occasionally, C7 will have short ribs, but these do not have the typical curved appearance of the true first rib and are usually not a cause of mislabeling. MRI and CT (Fig. 6-7) imaging are useful in the dorsal spine for the same indications as in the cervical spine.

Lumbar Spine

Pain in the lumbar spine region is a major cause of disability, lost work time, and health dollar expenditure. The

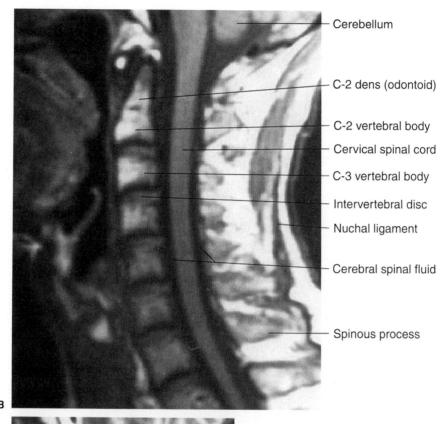

Cerebellum

C-2 dens (odontoid)

C-2 vertebral body
Cervical spinal cord
C-3 vertebral body
Intervertebral disc
Nuchal ligament

Cerebral spinal fluid

Spinous process

B

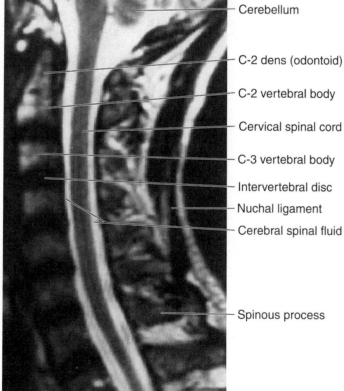

Cerebellum

C-2 dens (odontoid)

C-2 vertebral body

Cervical spinal cord

C-3 vertebral body

Intervertebral disc

Nuchal ligament

Cerebral spinal fluid

Spinous process

B

FIGURE 6-5. **A:** Cervical spine sagittal T1 MR image. Normal. The cerebral spinal fluid is black on a T1 image and white on a T2 image. The bone marrow fat appears whiter (high-intensity signal) on a T1 image than on a T2 image. **B:** Cervical spine sagittal T2 MR image. Normal.

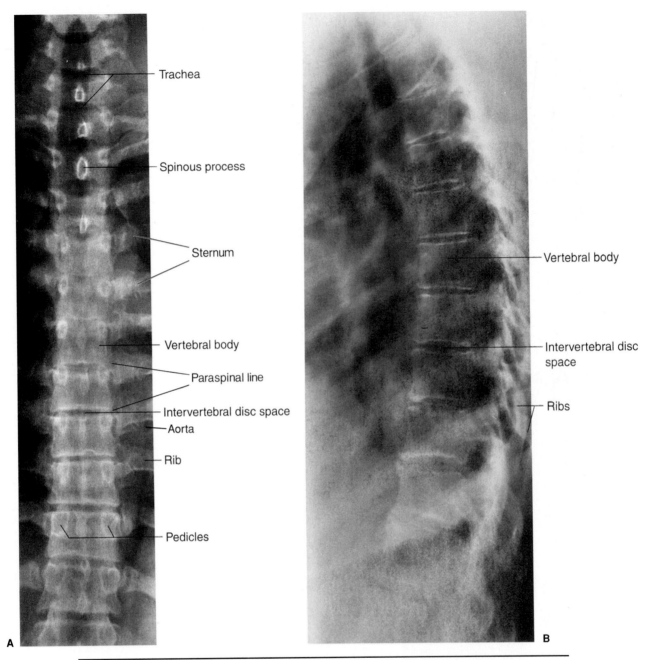

FIGURE 6-6. A: Thoracic spine AP radiograph. Normal. The pedicles on each vertebra have an appearance similar to automobile headlights. **B:** Thoracic spine lateral radiograph. Normal.

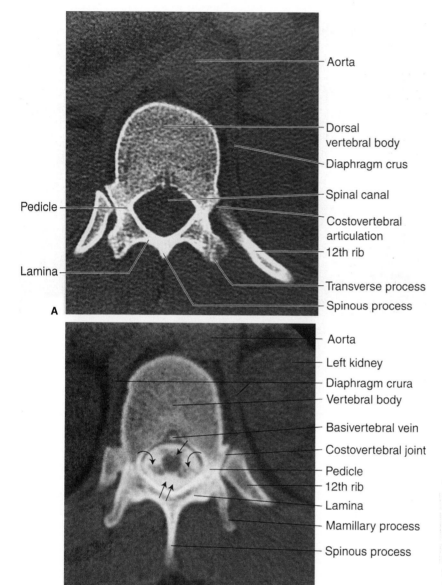

A: Aorta

Dorsal vertebral body

Diaphragm crus

Spinal canal

Costovertebral articulation

12th rib

Transverse process

Spinous process

Pedicle

Lamina

A

B: Aorta

Left kidney

Diaphragm crura

Vertebral body

Basivertebral vein

Costovertebral joint

Pedicle

12th rib

Lamina

Mamillary process

Spinous process

B

FIGURE 6-7. A: Thoracic spine axial CT image at the T-12 level. Normal. **B:** Thoracic spine axial CT image at the T-12 level. Normal. The spinal cord *(straight arrow)*, nerve roots *(curved arrows)*, and the contrast-filled subarachnoid space *(double arrows)* are well visualized. The contrast media was introduced into the subarachnoid space as part of a myelogram while the CT imaging followed the myelogram. Note how well the osseous structures of the spine are demonstrated.

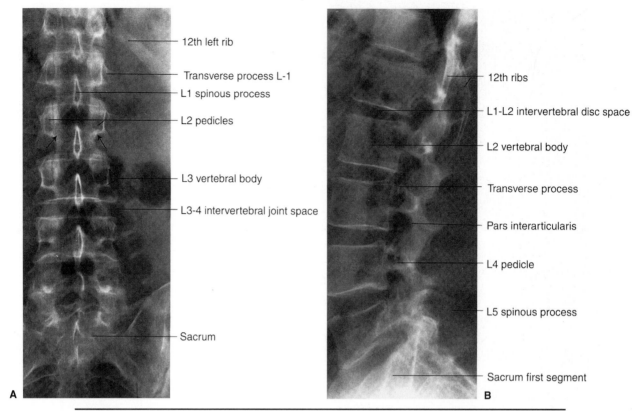

FIGURE 6-8. Lumbar spine AP **(A)** and lateral **(B)** radiographs. Normal. The *arrows* on the AP radiograph indicate the pars interarticularis region.

etiology of back pain is complicated, varied, and poorly understood. Following a careful history and physical examination of the lower back, the next step in the evaluation process usually includes radiographs. Routine lumbar radiographs generally consist of AP and lateral views (Fig. 6-8). As previously noted, look first at the lateral view using the same system as described for the lateral cervical and dorsal spine radiographs. In general, note the lumbar spine alignment, which is normally convex anterior (lordotic). When muscle spasm or disease processes are present, this normal curvature may be lost and the spine may appear straight. In addition, observe the overall osseous densities. Next, carefully evaluate the vertical heights of the lumbar vertebral bodies and the intervertebral disc spaces; they should be approximately equal to those immediately above and below, but gradually become taller as you progress distally. As a general rule, the L4-5 intervertebral disc space height is greater than the other lumbar disc spaces. If the L4-5 disc space is the same height as those above or below, you should suspect L4-5 disc disease. This also means that the L5-S1 disc level is typically narrower than that at L4-5 and should not be considered abnormal because of decreased height alone. Approximately 15% of the population will have variability in the appearance at the lumbosacral junction.

There may be partial or complete lumbarization of S1 or sacralization of L5. Numbering of the lumbar spine can be very difficult, and every attempt should be made to number correctly using chest radiographs if needed to count the number of ribs. It is incorrect to assume that the first non-rib-bearing vertebra on the anterior view is L1 and the vertebra above the sacrum on lateral view is L5. I have seen the same vertebral body numbered differently on the AP and lateral views!

Always observe the pars interarticularis region of each vertebra for a possible defect; an interruption of bone continuity in the pars interarticularis is abnormal and called *spondylolysis*. The pars can be seen on lateral view, but is difficult on the anterior projection. It is easiest to see on the oblique view. Similar observations are made on the AP radiograph regarding alignment, density, vertical heights of the lumbar vertebral bodies and the lumbar intervertebral disc spaces. Again, be certain that all of the pedicles are present. Depending on the angulation at L5-S1, it may be difficult to see the L5 pedicles. Occasionally, an angled anterior view is obtained to better evaluate L5 (Fig. 6-9). This view also nicely displays the SI joints. Note also that oblique radiographs (Fig. 6-10) are sometimes necessary to better assess the pars interarticularis when spondylolysis is suspected. Once again, the

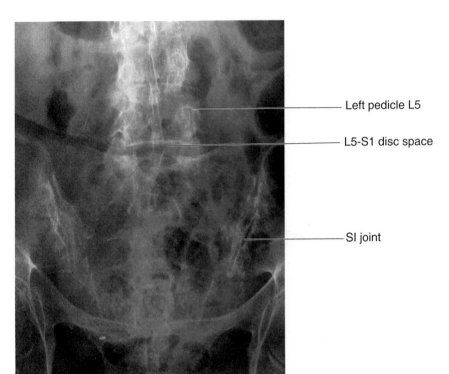

Left pedicle L5

L5-S1 disc space

SI joint

FIGURE 6-9. Lumbar spine angled view of lumbosacral junction. Note how the L5-S1 disc is now easily seen when compared to Fig. 6-8. The facets are prominent because of arthritis. The *small straight arrows* show the arcuate line of the right S1 anterior sacral foramen.

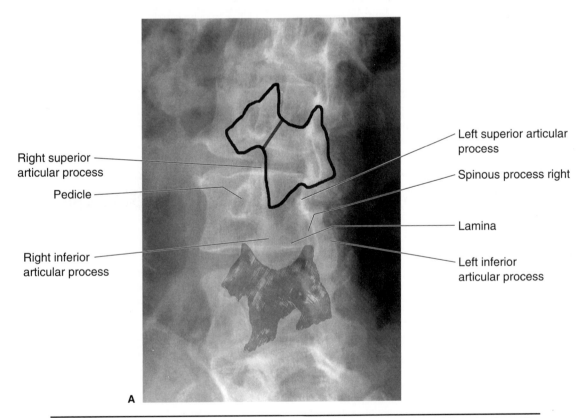

Right superior articular process

Pedicle

Right inferior articular process

Left superior articular process

Spinous process right

Lamina

Left inferior articular process

A

FIGURE 6-10. A: Visible "Scotty dog" and the anatomy that it represents on oblique lumbar spine radiographs. The neck of the Scotty dog represents the pars interarticularis. When the Scotty dog neck is absent, the condition is called spondylolysis.

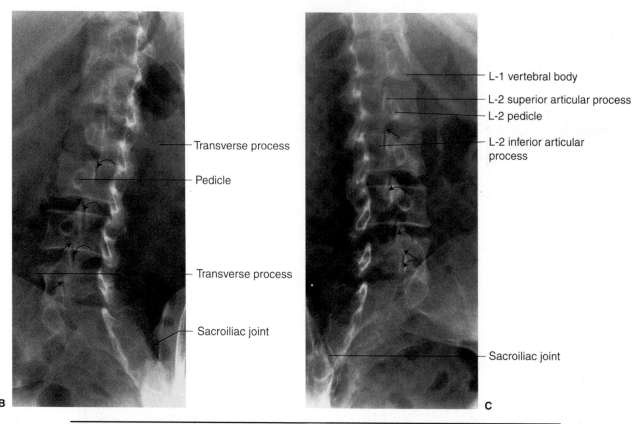

B

C

FIGURE 6-10. B, C: Lumbar spine right (B) and left (C) oblique radiographs. Normal. Note on these oblique views how well you visualize the normal pars interarticularis or the neck of the Scotty dog *(straight arrows)* and the normal apophyseal (facet) joints between the superior and inferior articular processes *(curved arrows)*.

observation checklist for spine radiographs is outlined in Table 6-3.

MRI of the lumbar spine is often requested to evaluate the vertebrae, intervertebral disc spaces, and the spinal cord (Fig. 6-11), which usually ends at the level of L1. As elsewhere in the spine, CT imaging may be requested to determine the presence and extent of fractures and the presence of intervertebral disc disease (Fig. 6-12).

In the past, the myelogram was the gold standard for the diagnosis of disease in and around the neural canal. The myelogram is an invasive procedure that is accompanied by discomfort. It is accomplished by injecting contrast material into the subarachnoid space via a lumbar or cervical puncture, and typical images are shown in Fig. 6-13. Fortunately, water-soluble myelographic contrast agents do not require physical removal as oil-based contrast once did.

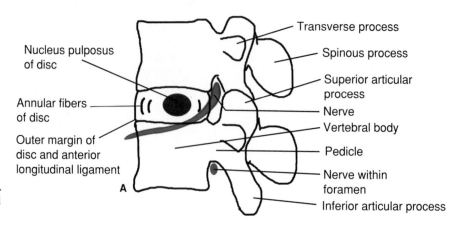

A

FIGURE 6-11. A: Lumbar spine lateral illustration. Normal.

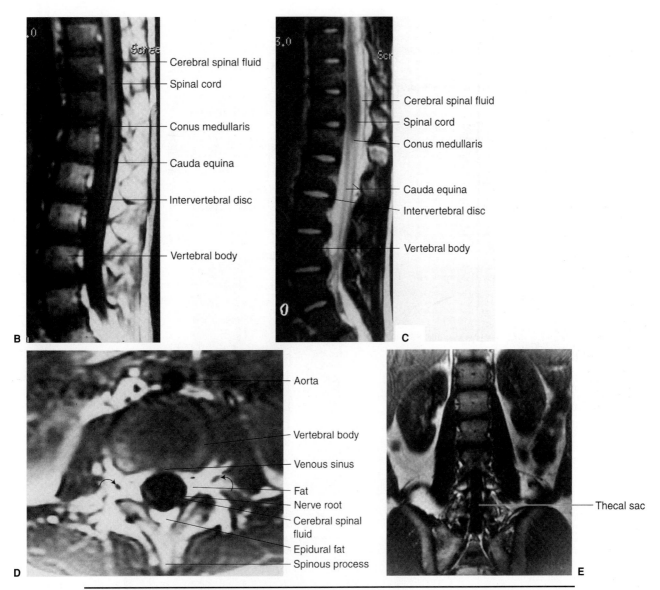

Cerebral spinal fluid
Spinal cord

Conus medullaris

Cauda equina

Intervertebral disc

Vertebral body

Cerebral spinal fluid
Spinal cord
Conus medullaris

Cauda equina
Intervertebral disc

Vertebral body

Aorta

Vertebral body

Venous sinus

Fat
Nerve root
Cerebral spinal
fluid
Epidural fat
Spinous process

Thecal sac

FIGURE 6-11. **B, C:** Lumbar spine T1 (A) and T2 (B) sagittal MR images. Normal. Notice again that the cerebral spinal fluid is black on a T1 image and white on a T2 image. Also, the bone marrow fat is whiter (high-intensity signal) on the T1 image. The intervertebral disc is whiter on the T2 image. **D:** Lumbar spine T1 axial image. Normal. Note that the nerve roots *(curved arrows)* are well visualized. **E:** Lumbar spine T1 coronal MR image. Normal. The coronal plane passes through the upper lumbar vertebral bodies and the lower lumbar neural sac.

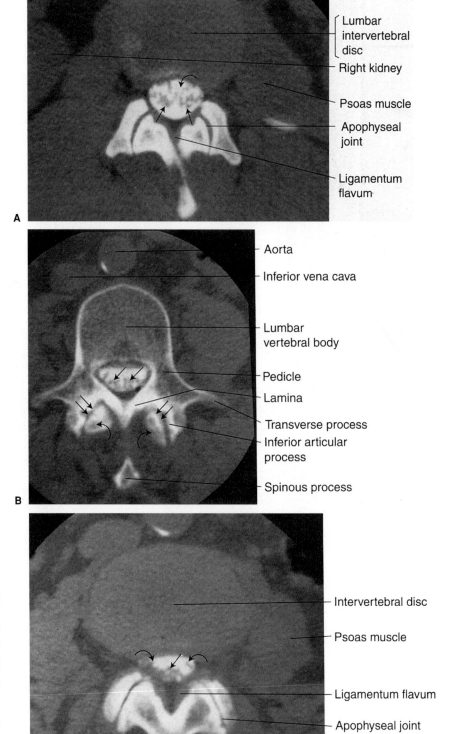

Lumbar
intervertebral
disc

Right kidney

Psoas muscle

Apophyseal
joint

Ligamentum
flavum

A

Aorta

Inferior vena cava

Lumbar
vertebral body

Pedicle

Lamina

Transverse process

Inferior articular
process

Spinous process

B

Intervertebral disc

Psoas muscle

Ligamentum flavum

Apophyseal joint

C

FIGURE 6-12. A: Lumbar spine axial CT image through the L1-2 intervertebral disc level. Normal. The *straight arrows* indicate the cauda equina surrounded by contrast media in the subarachnoid space cerebral spinal fluid *(curved arrow)*. **B:** Lumbar spine axial CT image through a lumbar vertebra. Normal. The *straight arrows* indicate multiple nerve roots. Notice how the inferior articular processes of the vertebra articulate with the superior articular processes *(curved arrows)* from the vertebra below to form the apophyseal joints *(double arrows)*. **C:** Lumbar spine axial CT image through a lumbar intervertebral disc. Normal. The *straight arrow* indicates nerve roots in the posterior aspect of the subarachnoid space whereas the *curved arrows* indicate nerve roots about to exit through the neural foramina.

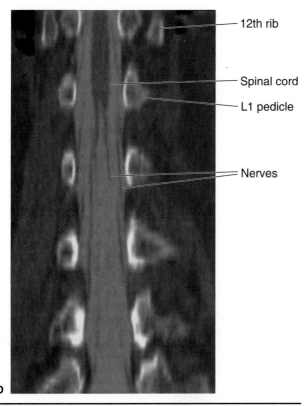

— 12th rib

— Spinal cord

— L1 pedicle

— Nerves

D

FIGURE 6-12. D: Lumbar spine coronal reformatted CT. The image was obtained following a myelogram and reformatted through the thecal space. This has a similar appearance to the conventional myelogram radiographs and shows the conus quite well.

CT routinely follows the injection to better define the disc and nerve pathology. Understandably, CT and MR examinations are more acceptable to the patient than the invasive spinal puncture associated with myelography.

The sacrum should be evaluated with both the spine and the pelvis, playing a role in both. Unfortunately, it may be difficult to evaluate, especially in an older patient with osteoporosis. The normal sacrum has an anterior concavity and is tilted posteriorly at the L5-S1 junction. The arcuate lines of the neural foramina should be evaluated closely on the AP view. They should be smoothly curved and symmetric (Fig. 6-14). Asymmetry may be the result of fracture or tumor involvement. The sacroiliac (SI) joints should be evaluated as they are important in the evaluation of several arthritides and may be widened as a result of trauma. Both CT and MRI can be useful in the evaluation of the sacrum and SI joints.

Pelvis

An AP pelvis radiograph is the standard view (Fig. 6-15). A lateral view is not obtained, but on occasion up- and down-tilt AP (outlet and inlet) views are indicated to assess fracture displacement. A modified outlet view is also useful for assessing the SI joints. As elsewhere, you must know the anatomy and have a system for looking at the pelvis radiograph. First look at the sacrum and coccyx followed by the iliac bones bilaterally. Compare the sacroiliac joints as they may be narrowed or even absent in diseases like ankylosing spondylitis (Fig. 6-45C). Then check out the ischial bones bilaterally as well as the pubic rami and the symphysis pubis. *Remember that the hamstring muscles arise from the ischial tuberosity*; this explains why someone with a hamstring injury runs off the athletic field clutching his or her buttock. As you know, all of the pelvic bones must be evaluated for fractures, density, anomalies, and metastatic lesions.

ANOMALIES

Anomalies of the spine and pelvis (Table 6-5) vary in severity from mild to severe. *As a general rule, most mild spinal anomalies are asymptomatic.* Small extra bones or supernumerary bones called *accessory ossicles* are usually asymptomatic, and they may be located near many different bones including the spine. Examples of accessory ossicles are shown in Fig. 6-16A and B. Accessory ossicles are simply normal variants and should not be confused with a fracture. The smoothly corticated, usually rounded margins help differentiate them from fractures.

Occasionally, extra ribs arise from the cervical spine, and they are called *cervical ribs* (Fig. 6-16C). Cervical ribs are generally asymptomatic, but have the potential to cause symptoms secondary to extrinsic pressure on the brachial plexus and the vessels of the upper extremities. A common anomaly at the lumbosacral junction is a *transitional vertebra* in which the L5 vertebra begins to have the appearance of the sacrum or the sacrum begins to look like a lumbar vertebra. *Partial sacralization* of L5 is the

TABLE 6-5 A Partial List of Spine and Pelvis Anomalies

Mild
Accessory ossicles
Cervical ribs
Hemivertebra
Osteitis condensans ilii
Scoliosis
Spina bifida
Transitional vertebrae

Severe
Absence of the sacrum
Meningocele and myelomeningocele
Scoliosis
Symphysis diastasis

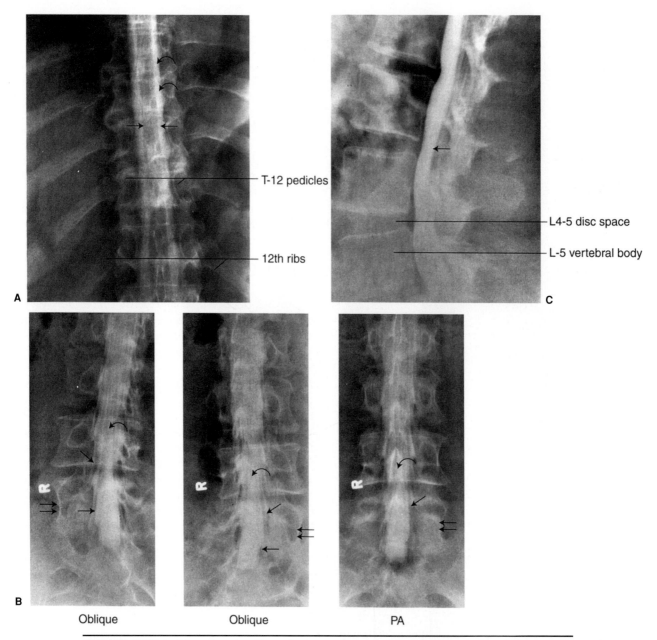

FIGURE 6-13. **A:** Thoracic spine PA myelogram radiograph. Normal. The spinal cord *(between the straight arrows)* is outlined by the injected subarachnoid contrast media *(curved arrows).* **B:** Lumbar spine oblique and PA myelogram radiographs. Normal. The *straight arrows* indicate the nerve roots surrounded by contrast media exiting the spinal canal. The *curved arrows* indicate nerve roots within the thecal sac. The *double arrows* indicate the L5 lumbar vertebra. **C:** Lumbar spine lateral myelogram radiograph. Normal. The thecal sac contains contrast media *(straight arrow).*

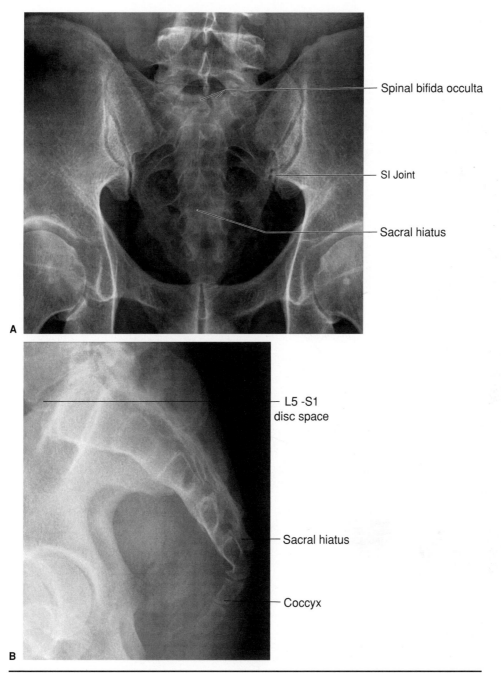

Spinal bifida occulta

SI Joint

Sacral hiatus

L5 -S1
disc space

Sacral hiatus

Coccyx

FIGURE 6-14. Sacrum AP with cephalad angulation **(A)** and lateral **(B)** radiographs. Normal. The *short arrows* demonstrate the normal arcuate lines of the anterior openings of the sacral neural foramina. The *arrowheads* demarcate the posterior margin of the left S1 foramen. There is a spina bifida occulta. The sacral hiatus represents the termination of the posterior elements at the midline.

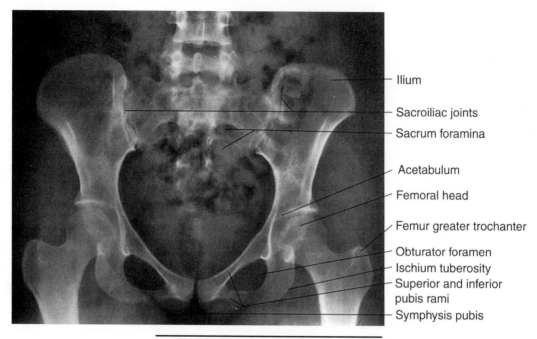

Ilium

Sacroiliac joints

Sacrum foramina

Acetabulum

Femoral head

Femur greater trochanter

Obturator foramen

Ischium tuberosity

Superior and inferior
pubis rami

Symphysis pubis

FIGURE 6-15. Pelvis AP radiograph. Normal.

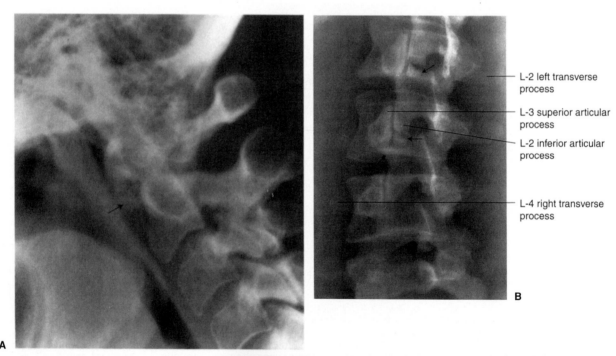

L-2 left transverse
process

L-3 superior articular
process

L-2 inferior articular
process

L-4 right transverse
process

A

B

FIGURE 6-16. A: Cervical spine lateral radiograph. This accessory ossicle is located inferior to the anterior arch of the atlas or C-1. This supernumerary bone or os *(straight arrow)* is a normal variant. **B:** Lumbar spine right oblique radiograph. Lumbar spine accessory ossicles *(straight arrows)*. This 22-year-old gymnast experienced a sudden onset of back pain. The accessory ossicles are variants of normal and had nothing to do with the patient's back pain. They are usually found around the L-2 and L-3 levels. **C:** Lower cervical and upper thoracic spine AP radiograph. Bilateral cervical ribs. The small bilateral ribs *(arrows)* arise from the C-7 vertebra; hence the name cervical ribs.

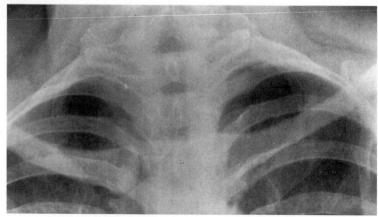

C

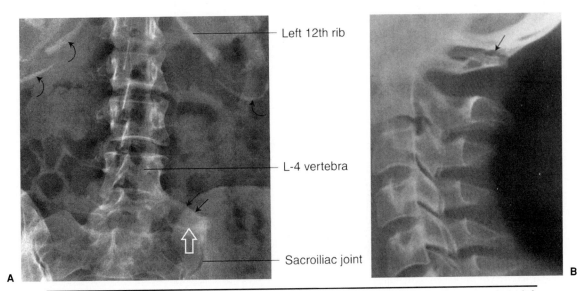

FIGURE 6-17. **A:** Lumbar spine AP radiograph. Partial sacralization of L-5. L-5 articulates with the left sacrum in an anomalous fashion *(straight arrows)*. There is a pseudarthrosis *(open arrow)*. Transitional vertebrae describe a situation in which L-5 begins to look like a part of the sacrum or the sacrum begins to look like a part of the lumbar spine. The *curved arrows* indicate calcifications within the cartilaginous portion of the ribs. **B:** Cervical spine lateral radiograph. Partial occipitalization of C1. The spinous process of C1 articulates with the occiput *(arrow)*. Normally the spinous process of C1 does not articulate with the occiput.

term used when fusion exists between a portion of the L5 vertebra and the sacrum (Fig. 6-17A). Usually one of the L5 transverse processes is enlarged and fused with the sacrum, but there are many variations. Occasionally, the anatomic L5 is completely sacralized, having the appearance of the first portion of the sacrum. Transitional vertebra may become symptomatic, especially after excessive back strain or when there is a *pseudarthrosis* (two bones articulating without a joint between them) as seen in Fig. 6-17. A less common anomaly is an abnormal articulation between the C1 spinous process and the occiput (Fig. 6-17B). A more severe anomaly of the spine is total absence of the posterior vertebral arch as in a meningomyelocele.

An important anomaly is spina bifida (Fig. 6-18), which occurs in approximately 5% of the population. Spina bifida occulta is a midline defect of the vertebral arch (usually posterior), and it is generally asymptomatic. When spina bifida has an associated soft tissue mass associated, it is called a meningocele. Meningoceles contain cerebral spinal fluid, and the sac envelope consists of the meninges. When the sac contains spinal cord and/or nerve roots, it is called a *myelomeningocele* ("myelo-" refers to the cord). A *meningocele* (Fig. 6-19) is a herniation of neural tissue through a bone defect. The size of these herniations is variable, and the herniation direction most commonly is posterior, but can be anterior or lateral. The symptoms vary from nonexistent to extensive and disabling. Visceral innervation of the bladder and/or rectum may be affected, as well as sensory and motor nerves. Another unfortunate

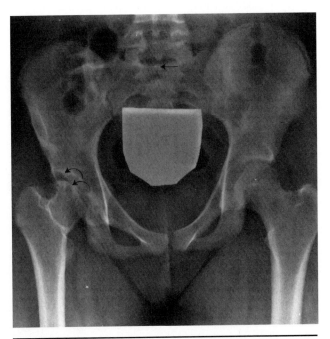

FIGURE 6-18. Pelvis AP radiograph. Spina bifida occulta and developmental dysplasia of the hip. Spina bifida occulta is indicated by the *straight arrow* and represents incomplete fusion of the posterior sacral segments. Right hip developmental dysplasia *(curved arrows)* is characterized by the steep slant of the acetabulum compared to the left. The femoral head remodels as it grows in the shallow socket. Note the presence of a gonadal shield.

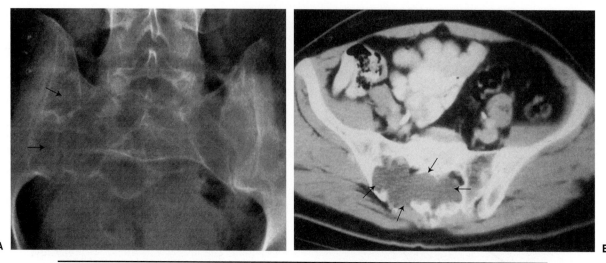

FIGURE 6-19. A: Pelvis AP radiograph. Sacral meningocele. This 54-year-old patient consulted a physician because of urinary retention. The lucent areas in the sacrum *(straight arrows)* indicate the bone defect secondary to the meningocele mass. **B:** Pelvis axial CT image. The full extent of the meningocele mass within the sacrum is indicated by the *straight arrows.*

anomaly in this category is complete absence of the sacrum (sacral agenesis), and it is often associated with a variety of other anomalies. Another severe anomaly is exstrophy of the urinary bladder, which is associated with abnormal widening of the symphysis pubis. This widening of the symphysis pubis, or diastasis, is most often the result of trauma (Fig. 6-20), but can occasionally be associated with a difficult or large baby birth, some

bone dysplasias, epispadias, hypospadias, and the prune belly syndrome (loss or absence of abdominal wall muscles).

One of the most clinically important anomalies of the spine is scoliosis. Some of the many etiologies of scoliosis include idiopathic, disc degeneration and osteoarthritis, neuromuscular diseases, trauma, infections, tumors, radiation therapy, acromegaly, and underlying congenital

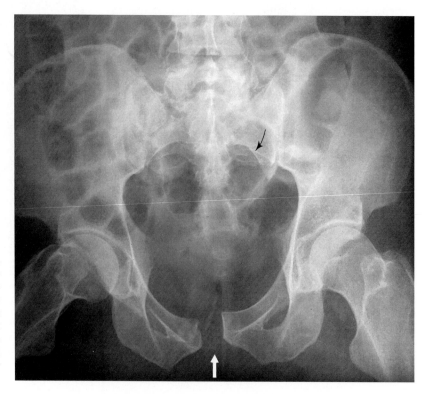

FIGURE 6-20. AP pelvis. Symphysis pubis diastasis. Widening of the normal close relationship of the left and right pubic bones *(white arrow)* is due to trauma in this patient. Note the irregular margin from fracture of the right side of the symphysis. The disrupted arcuate line of the left sacral foramen *(arrow)* should be searched for since the pelvic "ring" typically breaks in at least two places.

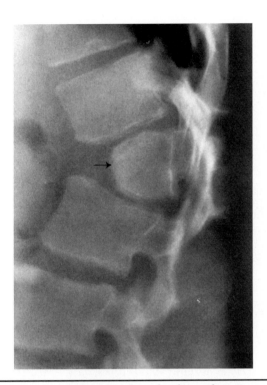

FIGURE 6-21. Lumbar spine lateral radiograph. L-1 posterior hemivertebra *(arrow)*. This is usually asymptomatic.

problems such as hemivertebrae (Fig. 6-21) and pedicle bars. A *hemivertebra* is a vertebra with formation of only one side secondary to absence of a lateral ossification center. Typically, there is a body, pedicle, lamina, and corresponding rib on only one side (Fig. 6-22). Pedicle bars occur when two or more pedicles on the same side are joined by a bony bridge. While the normal side grows, the absent side of a hemivertebra or side with a pedicle bar cannot grow as much, and a curvature develops. Approximately 10% of scoliosis cases are congenital with associated vertebral and rib abnormalities as shown in Fig. 6-22, but, by far, most cases are idiopathic (Fig. 6-23). Scoliosis may be associated with abnormalities of the spinal cord, such as a syrinx. When scoliosis is severe or rapidly progressive, it may be treated by fusion of a long segment of the spine (Fig. 6-24). Degenerative lumbar scoliosis (Fig. 6-25) is an increasing problem in the older population. It is likely multifactoral and may be related to altered load due to compression deformities, degenerative disc changes, leg length discrepancies, and lumbosacral anomalies. This deformity may be slow or rapidly progressive and can lead to back pain, radiculopathy, and spinal

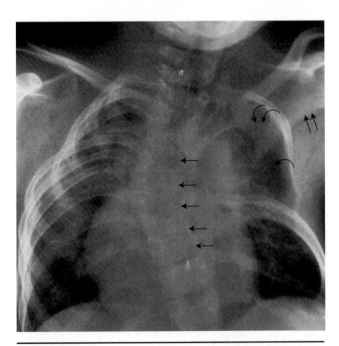

FIGURE 6-22. Thoracic spine AP radiograph. Congenital scoliosis. The thoracic spine is convex to the right, and the thorax is markedly asymmetric. Underlying the scoliosis are multiple hemivertebrae or incompletely formed thoracic vertebrae *(straight arrows)*. There are multiple absent left ribs *(curved arrows)*, and several left upper ribs are fused *(double curved arrows)*. The left scapula is abnormally elevated *(double straight arrows)*.

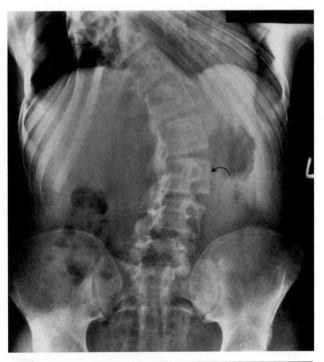

FIGURE 6-23. Thoracolumbar spine AP radiograph. Idiopathic scoliosis of the thoracic and lumbar spine. The lumbar spine is convex to the left *(curved arrow)*, and the lumbar vertebrae are markedly rotated. This rotation component causes the lumbar vertebra to appear oblique on the radiograph. The lower thoracic spine is convex to the right *(straight arrow)*, resulting in asymmetry of the ribs and thorax. Interestingly, the foramen magnum and sacrum usually form a vertical line when a line connects the two.

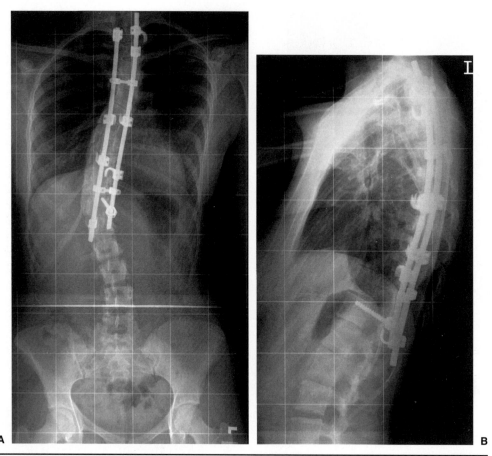

A   B

FIGURE 6-24. AP (**A**) and lateral (**B**) thoracolumbar radiographs. Posterior spinal fusion for idiopathic scoliosis. Fusion rods, screws, and hooks are used to decrease the curvature. Bone graft is usually placed as well to prevent progression of the curves.

stenosis. It is occasionally treated by decompression of the stenosis and fusion.

Osteitis condensans ilii (Fig. 6-26) is a well-marginated, triangular-shaped area of increased bone density found predominately in women of childbearing years. It is located in the iliac bone just lateral to the sacroiliac joint, but the sacrum and sacroiliac joints are not involved. This abnormality may or may not be symptomatic. The differential diagnosis should include osteoblastic metastatic disease, ankylosing spondylitis, and other inflammatory arthritides such as rheumatoid arthritis. It usually can be differentiated from metastatic disease that commonly involves multiple widespread sites. The sacroiliac joints are usually narrowed or absent in ankylosing spondylitis and often appear irregular in the other inflammatory arthritides such as rheumatoid arthritis.

A sometimes confusing variant in the pelvis is *os acetabulare*. This is an accessory center of ossification at the superolateral margin of the acetabulum (Fig. 6-27). It is typically triangular in shape. The margins are smooth and corticated, which should allow differentiation from a fracture.

TRAUMA

Fractures

Fractures of the spine and pelvis are common and result from a wide variety of traumas including motor vehicle accidents, sports, falls, and normal activity in those who have osteoporosis or bone loss due to tumor. Fractures of the spine are obviously important as the spinal cord and cauda equina are vulnerable to injury because of their close proximity to the vertebrae. Roughly 40% of cervical spine fractures have neurologic complications, 10% in the thoracic spine and 4% at the thoracolumbar junction.

Cervical Spine Injuries

Most cervical spine fractures occur between C5 and C7, with another peak at C1 and 2. A variety of injuries occur when the cervical spine undergoes acute hyperflexion and hyperextension (Table 6-6). The flexion teardrop fracture (Fig. 6-28) is one type of injury that results from acute cervical spine hyperflexion. The teardrop-shaped fracture

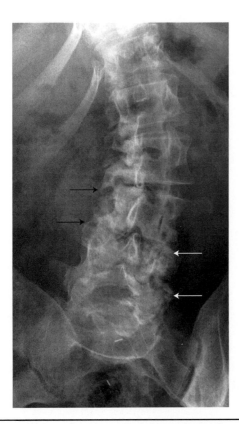

FIGURE 6-25. Lumbar spine AP radiograph. Senile scoliosis. The lumbar spine is convex to the left. The discs are asymmetrically narrowed and there is prominent osteoarthritis of facets *(arrows)*, which is worse on the concave sides.

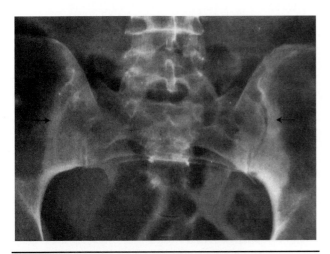

FIGURE 6-26. Pelvis AP radiograph. Osteitis condensans ilii. The sharply marginated, bilateral increased densities (sclerosis) involve the iliac sides of the sacroiliac joints and spare the sacrum. This is a benign condition that is usually found in women in their childbearing years and seldom found in older women. This can be an incidental finding on a radiograph, or the patient may present with acute or chronic back pain.

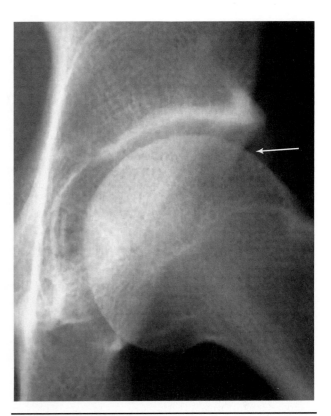

FIGURE 6-27. Hip AP radiograph. Os acetabulare. The smoothly marginated, oval density near the superolateral margin of the acetabulum *(arrow)* is a normal variant and should not be confused with a fracture.

fragment is the result of compression at the anterior inferior aspect of the vertebral body. This fracture is usually accompanied by disruption of the interspinal ligaments between the spinous processes, thus making the spine very unstable. Other ligaments that may be involved are the supraspinous ligament and the ligamentum flavum. The involved vertebral body may be displaced posteriorly, and this situation is a good indication for CT imaging to determine the extent of the fracture lines and to determine the precise location of the fracture fragments, especially their relationship to the cervical spinal cord. Particularly

▶ **TABLE 6-6 Cervical Spine Injuries**

Flexion
Anterior wedge fracture
Facet locking
Ligament disruption
Odontoid process fracture
Teardrop fracture (C5)

Extension
Hangman fracture (C2)
Ligament disruption
Odontoid process fracture
Spinous process fracture
Teardrop fracture (C2)

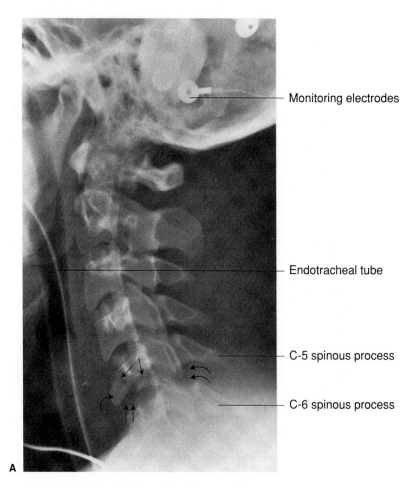

Monitoring electrodes

Endotracheal tube

C-5 spinous process

C-6 spinous process

FIGURE 6-28. A: Lateral cervical spine radiograph. C-5 flexion teardrop fracture. This 21-year-old man was involved in a motor vehicle accident. There is mild compression anteriorly of the C-5 vertebral body secondary to the comminuted fracture *(straight arrows)*, and there is mild separation of the fracture fragments. The major fracture fragment has a teardrop shape *(curved arrow)* due to avulsion at the site of the anterior longitudinal ligament. The hyperflexion injury has resulted in a mild separation or fanning of the space between the C-5 and C-6 spinous processes secondary to ligamentous disruption *(double curved arrows)*. The disrupted ligaments are the interspinal and supraspinal ligaments and possibly the ligamentum flavum. Also, the hyperflexion injury created minimal widening of the C5-C6 disc space *(double straight arrows)* and mild angulation of the spine at this level with minimal retrolisthesis of C-5 on C-6. This type of cervical fracture usually is associated with severe cord injury as the vertebral body is often displaced posteriorly into the spinal canal.

FIGURE 6-28. *Continued* **B:** Cervical spine axial CT image of the C-5 vertebra. The comminuted fracture lines in the vertebral body are separated or distracted *(straight arrows)*, and the anterior fracture fragments are displaced anteriorly approximately 3 mm *(curved arrow)*. **C:** Lateral cervical spine radiograph. Posterior wire stabilization of the cervical spine between the spinous processes of C5 and C6 vertebrae *(curved arrow)*. The major fracture fragment *(straight arrow)* is in fairly good alignment with mild offset of the fragments *(double straight arrows)*, but no attempt is made to reduce this fragment.

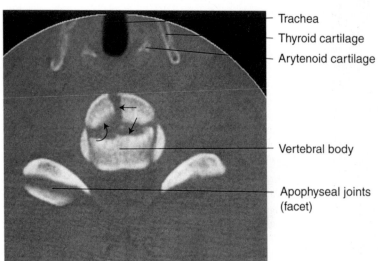

Trachea
Thyroid cartilage
Arytenoid cartilage

Vertebral body

Apophyseal joints
(facet)

B

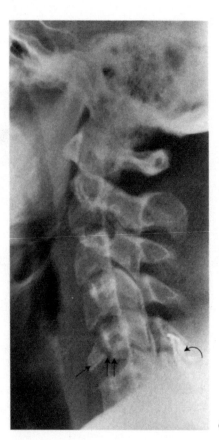

C

with neurologic deficit, MRI may be used to evaluate the spinal cord for injury and the soft tissue structures such as the ligamentum flavum and interspinous ligaments.

Facet locking (Fig. 6-29) is another hyperflexion injury. Locking will occur when the inferior articular process of the upper vertebra moves forward or anteriorly over the superior articular process of the lower vertebra, which results in an anterior dislocation of the upper vertebra. Once

again, the spine is unstable as there usually is posterior and sometimes anterior ligamentous disruption, and cervical spinal cord injury is common. The lateral radiograph is usually sufficient to make the diagnosis (see Fig. 6-29A), but occasionally a reconstructed sagittal CT image (Fig. 6-29B, C) is necessary to confirm the diagnosis. Unilateral locked facet (Fig. 6-29C) has a rotational component and does not have the extensive ligamentous disruption as the bilateral form does.

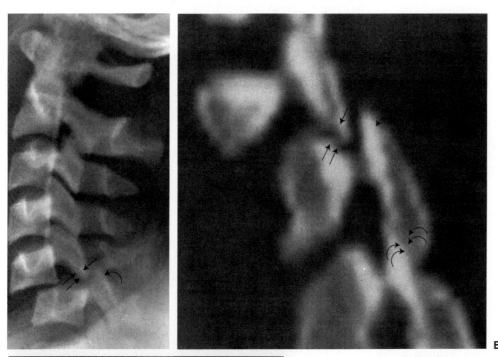

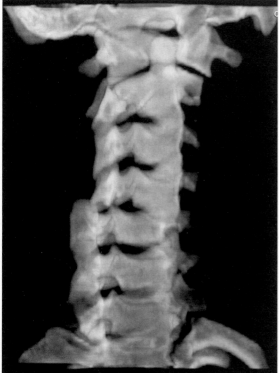

FIGURE 6-29. A: Cervical spine lateral radiograph. Bilateral facet locking at the C5-6 level. The inferior articular process of C-5 *(straight arrow)* is anterior to the superior articular process of C-6 *(curved arrow)*. The *double straight arrows* indicate the expected normal position for the superior articular process of the C-6 vertebra. There is obvious anterior dislocation of the C-5 vertebral body referable to the C-6 vertebral body. No fractures are apparent. **B:** Cervical spine sagittal reconstructed CT image on a different patient. Bilateral facet lock. The inferior articular processes of the upper vertebra *(straight arrow)* is in an abnormal relationship with the superior articular process of the lower vertebra *(curved arrow)*. The *double straight arrows* indicate the expected normal location of the displaced superior articular process. A normal apophyseal articulation is visible at the level below *(double curved arrows)*. **C:** Reformatted CT image in another patient with unilateral locked facets at C4-5 on the right. Note how the upper cervical spine appears rotated while the lower cervical spine is straight. The left facets are not shown on this 3D reformat, but had a normal relationship.

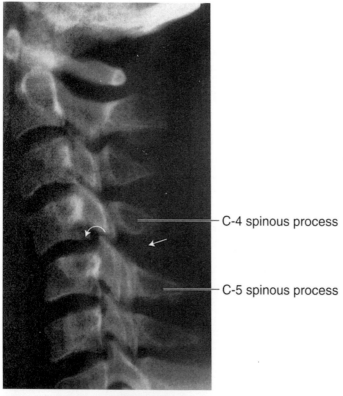

A

C-4 spinous process

C-5 spinous process

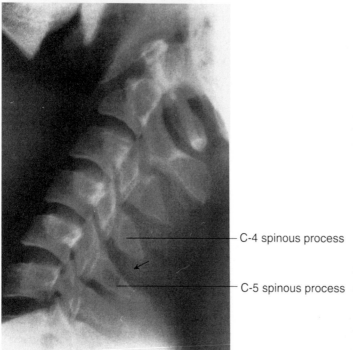

B

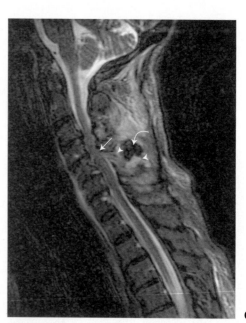

C

C-4 spinous process

C-5 spinous process

FIGURE 6-30. A: Cervical spine cross-table lateral radiograph with the patient supine. Posterior liga-ment disruption at C4-5. There is an increase in the height of the interspinous space between the C4-5 spinous processes *(straight arrow)* secondary to disruption of the C4-5 interspinal ligament, supraspinal ligament, and possibly the ligamentum flavum. Compare the height of the C4-5 interspinous space to those above and below. The mild anterior spondylolisthesis of C-4 referable to C-5 *(curved arrow)* has resulted in mild kyphotic angulation and reverse of the normal cervical curvature at the C-4 level. **B:** Cer-vical spine extension lateral radiograph in the same patient. When the cervical spine is in full extension, the C4-5 interspinous space *(straight arrow)* is now normal in height and the anterolisthesis of C-4 on C-5 has been reduced. **C:** Sagittal T2-weighted MRI cervical spine in a different patient. Ligament disruption without fracture. There is widening between the spinous processes at C5-6 and increased signal (white) *(arrowheads)*. Disruption of the ligamentum flavum *(arrow)* is also seen. A hematoma *(curved arrow)* can be seen, which would explain persistent widening of spinous processes on radiographs. There is a small amount of high signal within the posterior aspect of the C5-6 disc, which may suggest a disc injury as well.

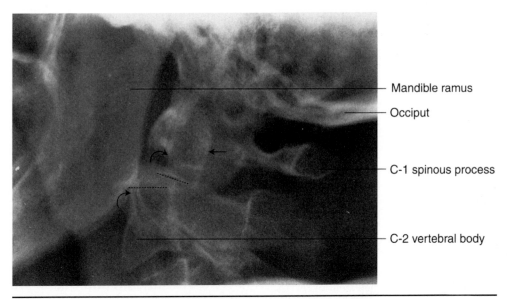

— Mandible ramus

— Occiput

— C-1 spinous process

— C-2 vertebral body

FIGURE 6-31. Cervical spine lateral radiograph. Displaced fracture through the caudad or inferior aspect of the dens or odontoid process of C2. The actual fracture edges are indicated by the *dotted lines*, and the dens *(arrow)* is displaced posteriorly approximately 8 mm. The *curved arrows* indicate the amount of displacement of the dens.

Occasionally hyperflexion injury results in ligamentous injury without fracture (Fig. 6-30). As with other hyperflexion injuries, this has the potential for spinal instability and cord injury.

Dens or odontoid process fractures are relatively common in the older population, and they may result from hyperflexion or hyperextension injuries. The fractures are often not displaced initially and may be difficult to detect. The best methods for the diagnosis of odontoid process fracture are AP open mouth and lateral cervical radio-graphs, and, of course, CT imaging. The odontoid fracture in Fig. 6-31 is probably a hyperextension injury as the odontoid is displaced posteriorly.

Thoracic Spine Fractures

Most fractures of the thoracic (dorsal) spine occur in the lower thoracic region. Fractures of the thoracic spine may result from significant trauma; however, underlying bone diseases can weaken the vertebrae and pathologic

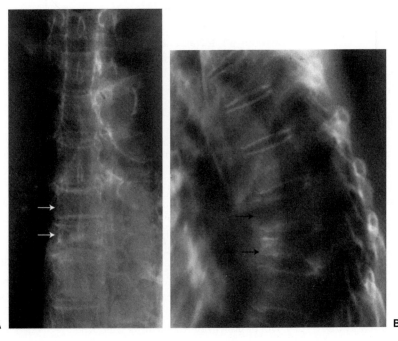

A
B

FIGURE 6-32. Thoracic spine AP **(A)** and lateral **(B)** radiographs. Osteopenia due to senile osteoporosis with secondary pathologic compression fractures of the T-7 and T-8 vertebral bodies. The compression fractures *(straight arrows)* are manifest by a decrease in the vertical height of the T-7 and T-8 vertebral bodies when compared to the other dorsal vertebral bodies. Notice the overall decreased density (osteopenia) of all the osseous structures due to osteoporosis.

fractures may occur with little or no trauma. These fractures are usually wedged-shaped compression fractures, often with no canal compromise and are, by far, the most common thoracic spine fracture. A few of the underlying diseases that may cause pathologic fractures are osteoporosis, primary and secondary bone tumors, Paget's disease, osteopetrosis, and osteomalacia (Fig. 6-32). If there are neurologic symptoms, imaging with MR or CT is usually warranted.

Lumbar Spine Fractures

Fractures commonly occur in the lumbar spine and are usually diagnosed by radiography (Fig. 6-33A, B). MRI may be helpful in assessing the effect of the fracture fragments on the thecal sac (Fig. 6-33C). As in other areas of the spine, CT imaging is helpful in evaluating the extent of the fractures and precisely locating the fracture fragments within the neural canal and their relationship relative to the thecal sac (Fig. 6-33D, E).

Spondylolysis and Spondylolisthesis

Spondylolysis and spondylolisthesis are difficult and confusing terms for the beginner. To add to the confusion, many will use the term "spondylosis" to describe degenerative changes in the spine. However, an understanding of these conditions and their clinical significance is necessary as they will commonly be encountered in clinical practice.

Spondylolysis refers to a defect in the pars interarticularis that lies between the superior and inferior articular processes of a vertebra. In other words, the neck of the Scotty dog is missing or some say that a collar has been placed (Fig. 6-10A). The defect occurs in about 5% of the population and, in most cases, is thought to be a stress fracture. It is seen on lateral radiographs, but seen particularly well seen on oblique views (Fig. 6-34). It is seen more often in athletes whose activities require prolonged or forced extension of the lower back.

Spondylolisthesis is the forward movement of a vertebra relative to the more stable vertebra below. The forward movement may be made possible by a bilateral spondylolysis defect in the vertebra (Figs. 6-34 and 6-35). Actually, with a pars defect, it is the vertebral body, pedicles, and superior articular processes that move forward or ventrally, whereas the laminae, inferior articular processes, and the spinous process remain in their normal positions (Fig. 6-35). This actually increases the size of the canal at this level. The majority of the spondylolysis with spondylolisthesis cases occur in the lumbar spine, especially at L5-S1 levels, and it is uncommon in the thoracic and cervical spine. Spondylolisthesis may be asymptomatic, and the most frequent symptom is low back pain probably due

to muscle spasm and instability. Symptoms, when they occur, are not necessarily related to the severity of the disease.

Spondylolisthesis secondary to spondylolysis must be differentiated from the spondylolisthesis secondary to disc and facet degeneration without spondylolysis. Degenerative spondylolisthesis is best imaged on a lateral radiograph of the lumbar spine (Fig. 6-36), and it most commonly occurs at the L4-5 level. There are degenerative changes in the disc space and the apophyseal (facet) joints *without a defect in the pars interarticularis.* Because there is no defect in the region of the pars interarticularis, however, there is more likely to be encroachment of bony structures into the neural foramina, which may lead to nerve compression.

Pelvic, Acetabular, and Sacral Fractures

Fractures of the pelvis are common and result from a variety of injuries (Fig. 6-37). Stable pelvic fractures break the "ring" of the pelvis in only one place. These include fractures of unilateral pubic rami, acetabulum, or sacrum. Typically both superior and inferior pubic rami are broken on one side since the rami form a ring. However, it is virtually impossible to break a ring in only one place and most pelvic fractures are unstable, disrupting the pelvic bones, symphysis, and/or sacroiliac joints. These fractures may be better evaluated by CT, which also allows evaluation of many of the soft tissue structures such as the bladder, urethra, and other pelvis soft tissues that may be damaged by fracture fragments. CT reformatted images are often useful for better evaluating the pelvic fractures.

Acetabular fractures result most commonly from motor vehicle accidents as the femoral head is driven into the acetabulum. Depending on the direction of force, the femoral head may dislocate, typically posteriorly, with or without an acetabular fracture. Avascular necrosis is a complication of hip dislocation as the vascular supply to the femoral head is stretched or disrupted during the dislocation. Pelvic oblique, or Judet, views and CT are useful in the evaluation of acetabular fractures (Fig. 6-38).

Sacral fractures may occur with major pelvic trauma, but may be an isolated insufficiency-type fracture in the elderly, osteoporotic population. When the fracture enters the sacral foramina, the arcuate lines are disrupted (Fig. 6-20). Sacral insufficiency fractures, which occur in weakened (usually osteoporotic) bone, may occur with little or no trauma. An older patient may present with lower back, buttock, or hip pain. Radiographs frequently will not demonstrate the fracture. Bone scan or MRI may be the next study to evaluate for an occult or developing hip fracture and the sacral fracture discovered (Fig. 6-39). Occasionally, these studies have an atypical appearance, but CT will demonstrate the healing fracture.

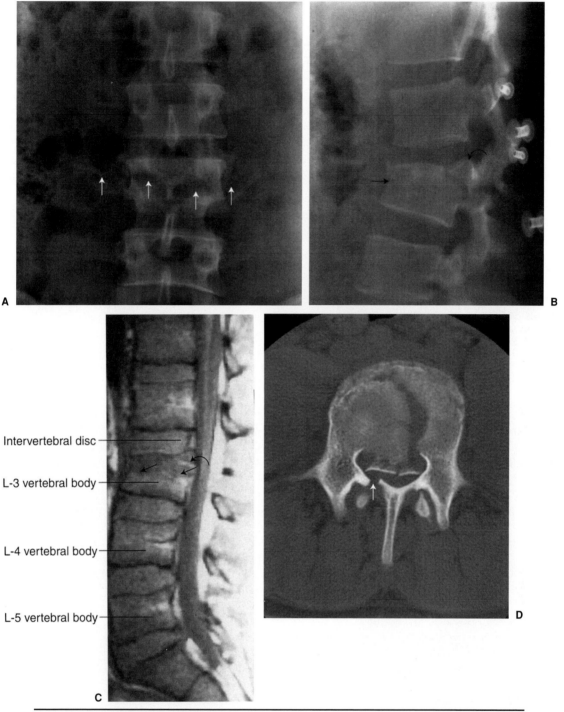

Intervertebral disc —

L-3 vertebral body —

L-4 vertebral body —

L-5 vertebral body —

A

B

C

D

FIGURE 6-33. Lumbar spine AP **(A)** and lateral **(B)** radiographs. Seat belt fracture of the L-3 vertebrae. This 30-year-old was wearing a lap seat belt when involved in a motor vehicle accident, and this is a flexion injury caused by the mobile upper body flexing on the lower body that is fixed by the lap seat belt. There is a transverse fracture through the L-3 vertebra involving the vertebral body and the transverse processes *(straight arrows in A and B)*. A large fracture fragment arising posteriorly from the vertebral body is displaced into the neural canal *(curved arrow in B)*. The L-3 vertebral body height is less than normal secondary to compression or collapse caused by the fracture. There is mild dorsal angulation of the spine at the level of the L-3 fracture. These fractures may be either stable or unstable. The remainder of the lumbar spine is normal. Note the clothing snaps. **C:** Lumbar spine sagittal proton-density MR image. A lap seat belt L3 displaced fracture in another 30-year-old patient. The L-3 vertebral body is mildly compressed secondary to a fracture *(straight arrows)*, and a posterior fracture fragment resides in the neural canal compressing the neural canal *(curved arrow)*. **D:** Lumbar spine axial CT image. L-4 vertebra displaced burst-type fracture in a 28-year-old involved in a motor vehicle accident. The mechanism of injury is axial compression with or without flexion and/or rotation. There is severe compromise of the neural canal *(asterisk)* with resultant neurologic injury. The *straight arrow* demonstrates a fracture of the right lamina in this unstable fracture.

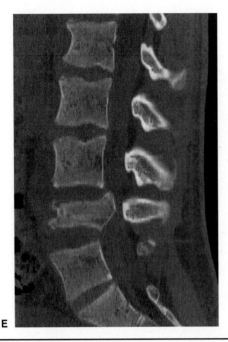

E

FIGURE 6-33. E: Sagittal reformatted CT image on the same patient shows the severity of the canal compromise compared to the other levels.

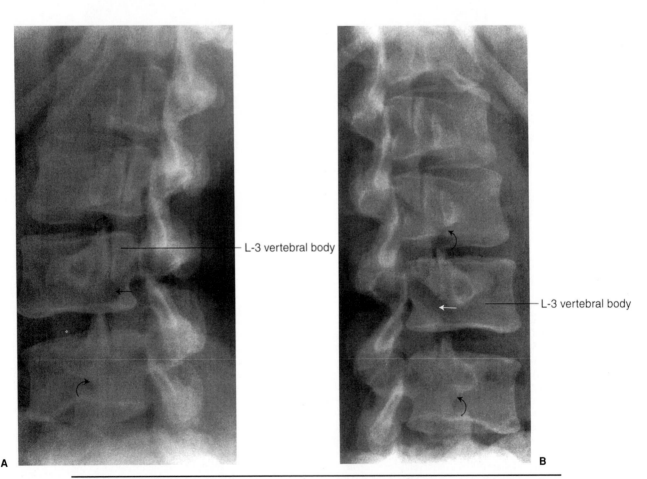

— L-3 vertebral body

— L-3 vertebral body

A

B

FIGURE 6-34. Lumbar spine right **(A)** and left oblique **(B)** radiographs. Bilateral spondylolysis of L-3 *(straight arrows)*. The pars interarticularis or the Scotty-dog neck is absent bilaterally in the L-3 vertebra. Normal Scotty-dog necks or pars interarticulares are present in the L-2 and L-4 vertebrae bilaterally *(curved arrows)*. (*continued*)

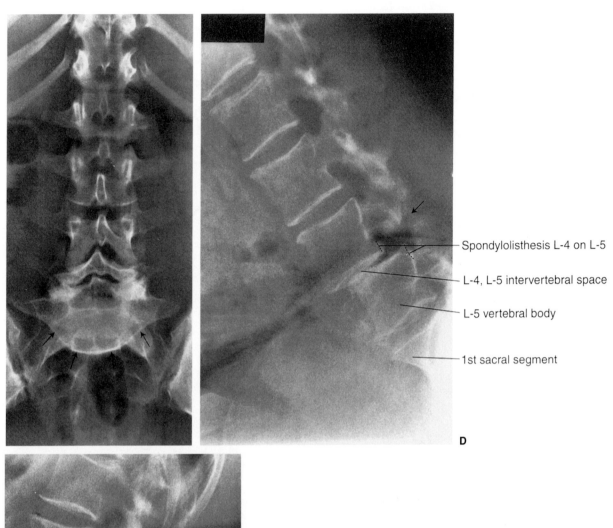

C

Spondylolisthesis L-4 on L-5

L-4, L-5 intervertebral space

L-5 vertebral body

1st sacral segment

D

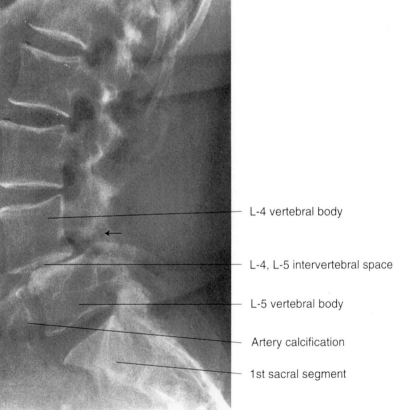

L-4 vertebral body

L-4, L-5 intervertebral space

L-5 vertebral body

Artery calcification

1st sacral segment

E

FIGURE 6-34. C: Lumbar spine AP radiograph. The classical appearance of the Napoleon hat sign *(straight arrows)* on an AP radiograph is secondary to severe (grade 4) spondylolisthesis of L-5 referable to S1. The Napoleon hat is inverted or upside-down. Lumbar spine lateral flexion **(D)** and extension **(E)** radiographs. This is a different patient with L-4 spondylolysis and grade 2 anterior spondylolisthesis of the L-4 vertebral body referable to the L-5 vertebral body. The spondylolysis defect in the pars interarticularis *(straight arrows)* can be visualized on both views, but the flexion radiograph opens the defect for easier visibility. The degree of spondylolisthesis is slightly less on the lateral extension radiograph as extension would counteract the forward slip. Notice the marked narrowing of the L4-5 intervertebral disc space.

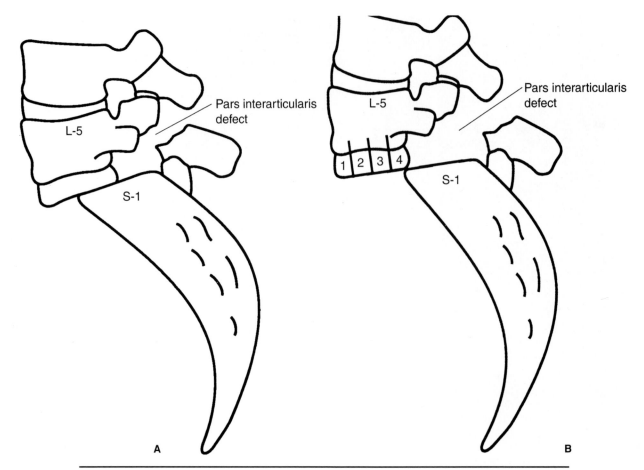

FIGURE 6-35. A: Illustration of spondylolysis and spondylolisthesis on a lateral radiograph. The L-5 vertebral body, pedicles, and superior articular processes have moved forward or ventral relative to the sacrum. However, the L-5 inferior articular processes, laminae, and the spinous process remain in their normal position. **B:** Illustration of spondylolisthesis classification or grading system. The sacrum is divided into fourths and the forward movement of L-5 is simply given a grade of 1-4.

Herniated Intervertebral Disc Disease

Intervertebral disc herniations may occur at any level in the spine. Although intervertebral discs cannot be visualized on radiographs, disc disease should be suspected whenever there is intervertebral disc space narrowing on radiographs. However, a narrowed disc level identified on radiographs cannot predict whether or not that level is symptomatic. Often the disc spaces are narrowed because of chronic disc degeneration and not an acute herniation. Noninvasive CT and MRI are increasingly being used in conjunction with, or in place of, the myelogram as they are more accurate and have a lower complication rate than myelography.

The normal disc structures are shown in Fig. 6-11. Some confusing terms have developed in the classification of herniated intervertebral discs, but the following is the current most accepted approach to this terminology problem. There is some "normal" drying out of discs with aging, which may lead to decreased disc space height. Disc *degen-eration* usually refers to this drying out, narrowing, and/or numerous small tears of the annulus fibrosis in all directions, which allows the nucleus of the disc to spread out. *Annular fissure (tear)* usually refers to a focal tear in the annulus allowing nuclear material to extend toward the outer margin of the disc without extending beyond the margin. A *bulging disc* means that 50% or more of the circumference of the disc is mildly displaced outward relative to the margin of the vertebral body. Scoliosis often leads to multiple asymmetric bulging discs due to the change in bony alignment. In this instance, the appearance is not due to structural problems within the discs.

Herniation is a general umbrella term, and it can be divided into three main categories, that is, protruded, extruded, and sequestered discs (Table 6-7). A *protrusion* implies the depth of disc extension is less than the width of its base at the disc margin. A *broad-based protrusion* involves over 25% of the circumference of the disc whereas *focal protrusion* involves less than 25% of the disc margin.

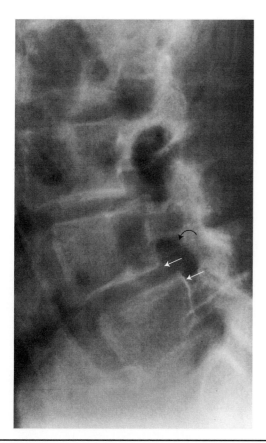

FIGURE 6-36. Lumbar spine lateral radiograph. Degenerative grade 1 spondylolisthesis of L-4 on L-5 *(straight arrows)*. This is a common complication of degenerative spine changes. The pars interarticularis is intact *(curved arrow)*. The spondylolisthesis is secondary to the degenerative changes in the intervertebral space and the apophyseal joints that allow L-4 to move forward relative to L-5.

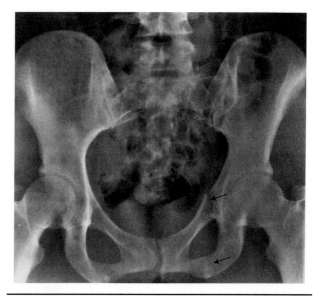

FIGURE 6-37. Pelvis AP radiograph. Fractures of the left superior and inferior pubis rami *(straight arrows)*. Sacral fractures are present but are partly obscured by the overlying intestinal gas. Note how the sacral arcuate lines are poorly seen on the left compared with those on the right.

complain of back pain. The diagnosis of Scheuermann's disease usually can be made on lateral spine radiographs. The radiographic features include fragmented and sclerotic epiphyseal plates of the vertebrae, wedge-shaped vertebral bodies with increased AP diameter, and narrowed disc spaces. Limbus vertebrae and Schmorl's nodes may be present.

ARTHRITIDES

Because the spine has multiple joints, it is not surprising that most of the arthritides involve the spine in some fashion (Table 6-8).

If the extension of disc material is greater than the width of its base or extends superior or inferior to the endplate, it is termed *extrusion*. If the fragment becomes detached, it is termed a *sequestered fragment*. Herniated lumbar intervertebral disc disease is common, especially at the L4-5 and L5-S1 levels (Fig. 6-40). MRI with the use of intravenous contrast has proved useful in determining whether or not there has been a recurrent disc herniation (Fig. 6-41).

Usually, disc herniations are lateral and/or posterior. However, when the disc herniates anteriorly into the vertebral body, this results in a vertebral defect with a classical appearance called a *limbus vertebra* (Fig. 6-42). When the disc herniates into the vertebral endplate, the resulting defect is called a *Schmorl's node* (Fig. 6-42). There are some people who feel that these are congenital or developmental variants. *Scheuermann's disease* (Fig. 6-42) is osteochondrosis of the epiphyseal plates in teenagers who often

> **TABLE 6-7   Intervertebral Disc Herniation Nomenclature**

Annular fissure (tear)—focal disruption in the outer fibrous layers of disc
Bulge—> or = 50% width of disc displaced beyond vertebral body margin

Herniation
Protrusion—depth of extent of disc < width of base at disc margin
Extrusion—depth of extent of disc > width of base at disc margin
Sequestration—detached disc fragment
Limbus vertebra
Schmorl's node
Scheuermann's disease

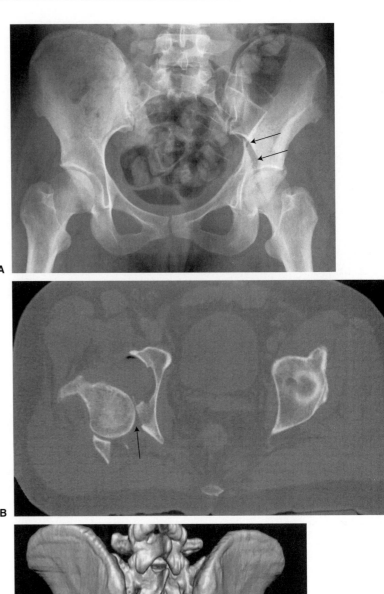

A

B

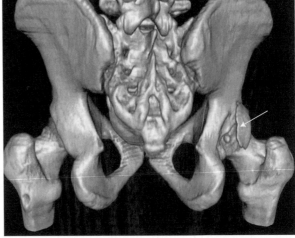

C

FIGURE 6-38. **A:** Pelvis AP radiograph. Acetabular fracture. There is a left acetabular fracture *(arrows)*. The fracture that involves the iliac wing is considered part of the acetabular fracture. **B:** Axial CT at level of the acetabulum. This 23-year-old was involved in a motor vehicle accident. The right femoral head is dislocated posteriorly, nicely demonstrating the mechanism for a fracture of the posterior wall of the acetabulum. The *arrow* shows the fracture site from which the posterior wall fragment came. **C:** Posterior view of a 3D CT reformatted image in a different patient with a posterior wall acetabular fracture *(arrow)*. These images can sometimes allow better demonstration of the location of fracture fragments.

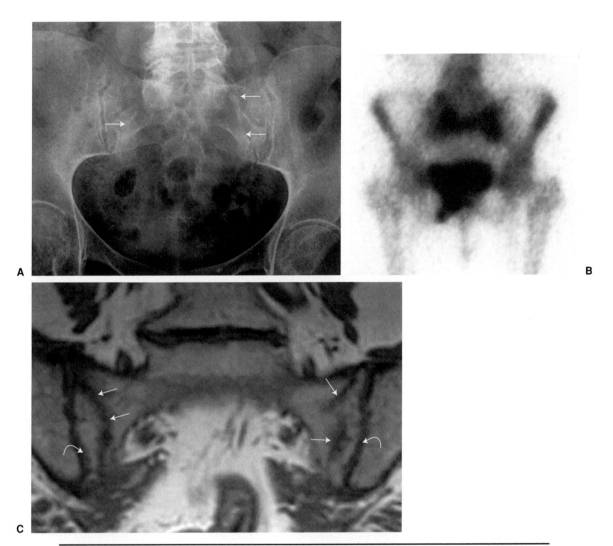

FIGURE 6-39. A: Sacrum AP radiograph. Insufficiency fractures of the sacrum. There is subtle sclerosis in a vertical orientation involving each sacral ala *(arrows)*. Compare this to the normal sacrum in Fig. 6-14A. **B:** Radionuclide bone scan posterior view of the pelvis in this same patient reveals increased activity (black) due to the healing fractures. The vertical orientation of each side with a horizontal connecting fracture line has been termed the "Honda sign." **C:** Coronal T1-weighted MR pelvis in a different patient. The characteristic sacral insufficiency fracture lines are easily seen *(arrows)*, but should not be confused with the normal sacroiliac joints *(curved arrows)*.

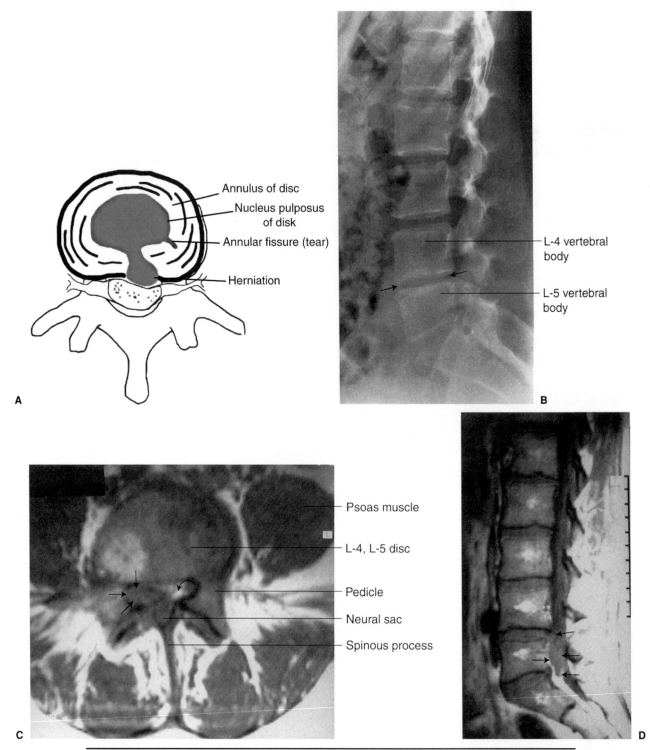

FIGURE 6-40. A: Lumbar intervertebral disc illustration. A disc herniation is a tear extending from the nucleus pulposis through all the layers of the annulus fibrosis. There may be compression of the thecal sac and possibly nerve roots. Smaller annular fissures may or may not cause pain. **B:** Lumbar spine lateral radiographs. Herniated L4-5 intervertebral disc. The patient is a 30-year-old woman with bilateral leg weakness greater on the right than the left. There is significant narrowing of the L4-5 intervertebral disc space *(straight arrows),* suggesting disc disease at this level. Again, the disc is not visible on the radiograph. The disc space narrowing is more apparent when you compare the L4-5 disc space to the other lumbar disc spaces. Normally the L4-5 disc space height is greater than the other lumbar spine disc spaces. *(continued)*

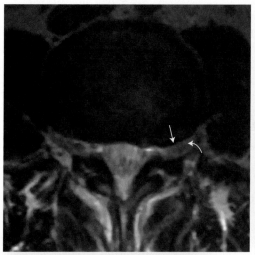

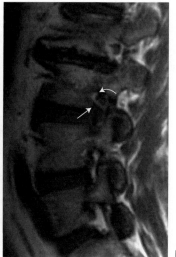

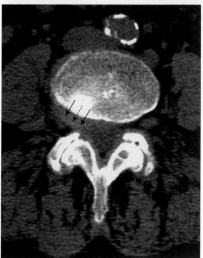

E

F

G

FIGURE 6-40. C: Lumbar spine axial T1 MR image in the same patient. Large extruded L4-5 intervertebral disc. The disc is extruded posterolaterally to the right *(straight arrows),* and it is creating extrinsic pressure on the neural sac and obliterating the epidural fat on the right side. Normal epidural fat is present on the left *(curved arrow).* **D:** Lumbar spine sagittal T1 MR image in the same patient. Caudally extruded L4-5 intervertebral disc and a protruding L5-S1 intervertebral disc. Notice that the extruded L4-5 disc *(arrows)* has migrated inferiorly to the level of the L5-S1 disc space posteriorly and is severely compressing the neural sac. A bulging disc at L5-S1 does not touch the thecal sac at this level. **E:** Axial T2 MR image at L3-4 in a 43-year-old man. Foraminal disc protrusion. The disc protrusion *(arrow)* narrows the left foramen and displaces the L-3 nerve *(curved arrow).* **F:** Sagittal PD (proton density) MR on the same patient. This view shows the disc extension into the neural foramen *(arrow)* and relationship to the nerve *(curved arrow).* There are degenerative disc changes at L2-3 as well with some foraminal narrowing seen at that level. **G:** Lumbar spine axial CT image. Protruded L4-5 intervertebral disc. The *straight arrows* mark the protruded disc with narrowing of the right foramen by the disc and facet arthritis.

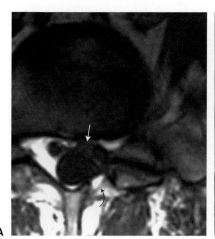

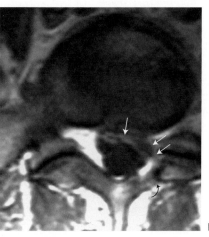

A

B

FIGURE 6-41. Axial T1 weighted MR image at L5-S1 without **(A)** and with **(B)** intravenous contrast. Scar tissue in a person with recurrent back pain. The *curved arrow* demonstrates an absent portion of lamina from this patient's prior surgery. The *arrow* in A shows abnormal signal, which could be a new disc herniation or scar tissue. B demonstrates that this area *(arrow)* enhances completely. Disc material does not enhance. The left S-1 nerve root *(double arrow)* is displaced and enhances suggesting, that it is affected by the scar tissue.

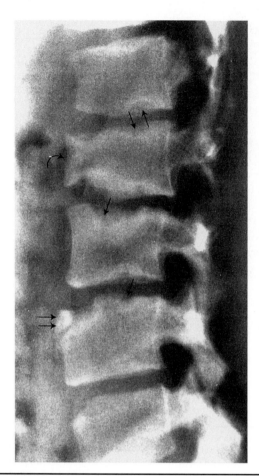

FIGURE 6-42. Lumbar spine lateral radiograph. Scheuermann's disease. The involvement of three or more vertebrae by Schmorl's nodes *(straight arrows)* defines Scheuermann's disease. Anterior wedging and increased AP diameter of the vertebral bodies *(curved arrow)* may result from this process. There is a limbus vertebra *(double straight arrows)*. Note the wavy appearance of the endplates.

Osteoarthritis

Osteoarthritis or degenerative arthritis (Fig. 6-43) is the most common arthritis, and the facet joints of the spine are frequently involved. Patients with osteoarthritis will usually complain of pain and/or limited motion in the involved spine. As in the extremities, the typical radiologic features include irregular joint narrowing, sclerosis, and osteophyte formation. The differential diagnosis of degenerative or osteoarthritis must include neuropathic joints and diffuse idiopathic skeletal hyperplasia. Common com-

▶ **TABLE 6-8 Arthritides**

Osteoarthritis
Inflammatory arthritis (rheumatoid arthritis and ankylosing spondylitis, psoriasis, Reiter's disease)
Neuropathic joint (Charcot's joint)
Infectious arthritis

plications of osteoarthritis are spinal stenosis (Fig. 6-44) and spondylolisthesis.

Spinal stenosis describes a vertebral or neural canal that is too narrow, and the multiple etiologies can be classified as congenital, developmental, and idiopathic. Although myelography dramatically demonstrates this abnormality, CT enjoys excellent patient acceptance and determines the causes and precise location (foraminal, lateral recess, or central) of the stenosis. Often, the stenosis is due to a combination of bulging disc, facet arthritis with osteophytes, and thickened ligamentum flavum (Fig. 6-44B).

Ankylosing Spondylitis, Psoriasis, and Reiter's Disease

A group of arthritides that have prominent axial skeleton involvement are collectively known as *spondyloarthropathies*. The three most frequently discussed are ankylosing spondylitis, psoriasis and Reiter's disease.

Ankylosing spondylitis, or Marie-Strumpell disease, is a chronic inflammatory arthritis. It is most common in young men and most frequently involves the spine and sacroiliac (SI) joints (Fig. 6-45). The SI joints become symmetrically narrowed or completely obliterated. Ankylosing spondylitis in the spine often results in squaring of the vertebral bodies and syndesmophytes, ossification between the outer margin of the vertebral bodies and the disc annulus. These changes radiographically simulate a piece of bamboo and have been termed the "bamboo spine" (Fig. 6-45B, C). Because of the rigidity of the spine and relatively weak fusion across discs, even mild trauma may lead to fractures at the disc levels (Fig. 6-45D). Ankylosing spondylitis may involve other joints, and these joints will have an appearance similar to rheumatoid arthritis.

Psoriasis is probably most known for its characteristic dermatologic manifestations, but its arthritis may coincide or even predate the skin changes. Psoriatic arthritis features both erosions and bony proliferation. When the SI joints are involved, they are asymmetrically involved (Fig. 6-46). Sporadic paravertebral ossification will connect adjacent vertebral bodies.

Reiter's disease consists of a constellation of conjunctivitis, urethritis, and arthritis. The radiographic features are quite similar to psoriasis but more likely to involve the lower extremity rather than upper extremity joints. The spine and SI joint changes are indistinguishable from psoriasis.

Rheumatoid Arthritis

There are many synovial joints in the spine; thus rheumatoid arthritis often involves the spine. The severity of rheumatoid arthritis of the spine ranges from mild to severe. There may be only mild narrowing of cervical disc spaces. However, when rheumatoid arthritis involves the

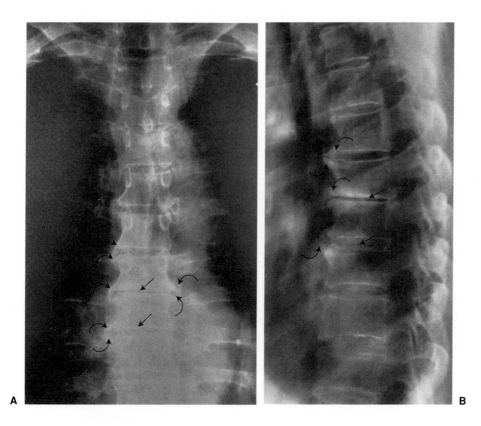

FIGURE 6-43. Thoracic spine AP **(A)** and lateral **(B)** radiographs. Osteoarthritis or degenerative arthritis. Multiple osteophytes *(curved arrows)* are present and multiple disc spaces are narrowed *(straight arrows)* secondary to degenerative disc disease.

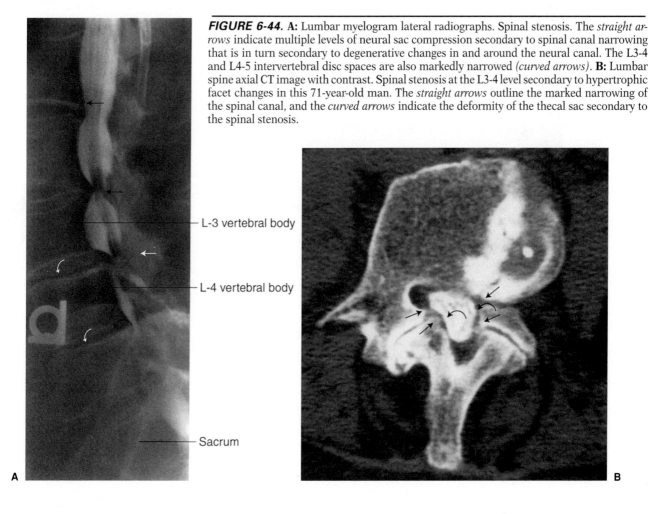

FIGURE 6-44. A: Lumbar myelogram lateral radiographs. Spinal stenosis. The *straight arrows* indicate multiple levels of neural sac compression secondary to spinal canal narrowing that is in turn secondary to degenerative changes in and around the neural canal. The L3-4 and L4-5 intervertebral disc spaces are also markedly narrowed *(curved arrows)*. **B:** Lumbar spine axial CT image with contrast. Spinal stenosis at the L3-4 level secondary to hypertrophic facet changes in this 71-year-old man. The *straight arrows* outline the marked narrowing of the spinal canal, and the *curved arrows* indicate the deformity of the thecal sac secondary to the spinal stenosis.

L-3 vertebral body

L-4 vertebral body

Sacrum

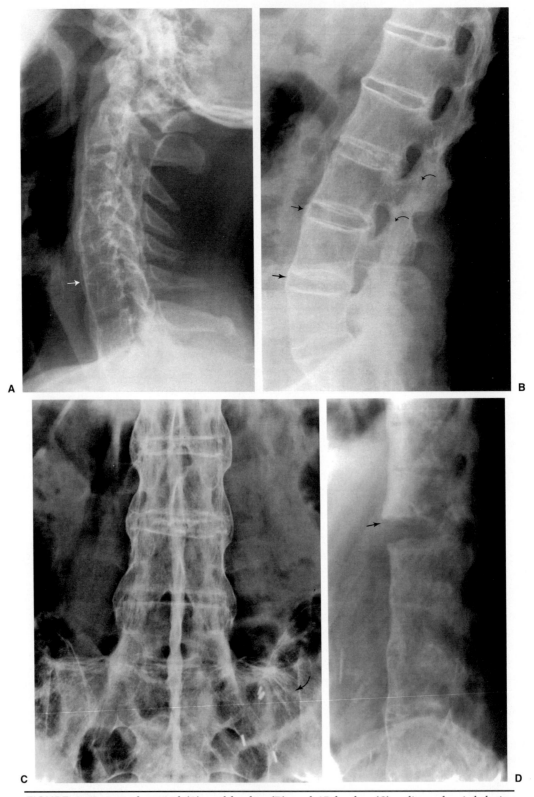

FIGURE 6-45. Lateral cervical **(A)**, and lumbar **(B)**, and AP lumbar **(C)** radiographs. Ankylosing spondylitis. *Straight arrows* demonstrate the syndesmophytes that bridge across disc levels forming a solid "bamboo" spine. The *curved arrows* in B marks the fused apophyseal joints while the *curved arrow* in C is in the expected location of the sacroiliac joint, which has fused. **D:** Lateral radiograph in man with ankylosis spondylitis following a relatively minor fall. There is anterolisthesis of L-1 on L-2 and a widened L1-2 disc *(arrow)* due to a fracture through this disc level.

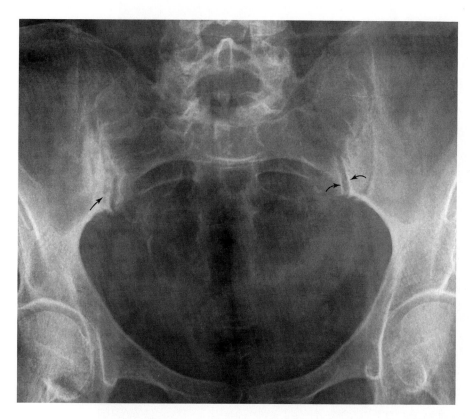

FIGURE 6-46. Pelvis AP radiograph. Psoriasis. There is sclerosis and irregularity of the right sacroiliac (SI) joint *(arrow)* due to sacroiliitis associated with psoriatic arthritis. Compare the appearance to the sharply defined margins of the left (SI) joint *(curved arrows)*.

odontoid and the atlantoaxial joint, the result can be weakening of the transverse atlantal ligament that holds the odontoid close to the anterior arch of C1. When this ligament becomes involved, subluxation or even dislocation of the atlantoaxial joint may occur (Fig. 6-47). These patients can experience cervical pain either at rest or with head movement. On a lateral radiograph, the normal distance between the anterior border of the odontoid and posterior aspect of the C1 anterior arch is usually less than 2.5 mm in adults. When there is subluxation or dislocation of this joint, the distance becomes greater than 2.5 mm, especially when the cervical spine is flexed.

Flexion and extension lateral cervical spine radiographs are indicated in rheumatoid arthritis patients when they experience pain with head movement, and before undergoing general anesthesia or any other procedure in which their head might be hyperflexed or hyperextended. These precautions help to prevent spinal cord injury. As elsewhere, rheumatoid arthritis often is associated with osteopenia and secondary pathologic fractures. The differential diagnosis for osteopenia and vertebral fracture includes osteoporosis, metastatic disease, multiple myeloma, infection, and trauma.

Neuropathic Joints

Charcot joints or neuropathic or neurotrophic joints can occur in the spine as well as the extremities (Fig. 6-48).

The joint changes are secondary to lost pain sensation and/or unstable joints found in a variety of neurologic conditions including diabetes mellitus, syringomyelia, and spina bifida with meningocele. The radiographic findings are disc space narrowing, bone destruction and fragmentation, sclerotic subchondral bone, subluxation and dislocation, and marginal bone mass formation. Many of these findings can be found in osteoarthritis, and the appearance is that of severe osteoarthritis of the spine.

INFECTION

Osteomyelitis or bone infection is common and has been discussed in Chapter 5. Spine infections are caused by a wide range of organisms, but staphylococcal infections are the most common. As with osteomyelitis elsewhere, patients with spinal osteomyelitis usually have fever and localized pain. The radiographic findings are subtle, and often poor definition of a vertebral endplate is the only finding (Fig. 6-49). With progression, frank bony destruction may be found. Osteomyelitis is in the differential diagnosis of lytic bone lesions. Radionuclide bone scans are often helpful for detecting osteomyelitis, especially when the radiographs are negative. MRI is sensitive in detecting osteomyelitis (Fig. 6-50). On T1 MR images, the infections have a decreased signal intensity (they appear dark gray), whereas on T2 images the infections have an increased

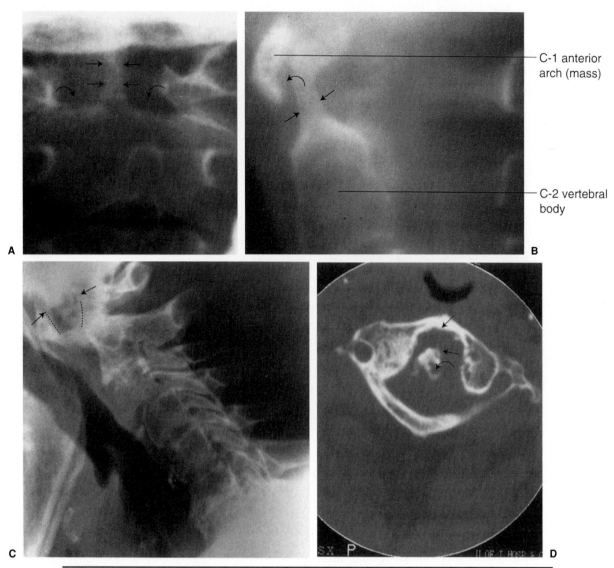

FIGURE 6-47. **A:** Cervical spine AP open-mouth radiograph. Rheumatoid arthritis. The odontoid process *(straight arrows)* is narrowed, osteopenic, and poorly marginated. Note the increased distances between the odontoid process of C-2 and the inferior articular processes of C-1 *(curved arrows)* due to partial loss of odontoid bone. **B:** Cervical spine lateral tomograph in the same patient. Rheumatoid arthritis. The odontoid *(straight arrows)* is markedly narrowed. The space between the anterior odontoid and the anterior arch of C-1 *(curved arrow)* is greater than the normal-2.5 mm or less. This can also occur in ankylosing spondylitis. **C:** Cervical spine lateral flexion radiograph in a different patient than shown in B. Rheumatoid arthritis. When the cervical spine is flexed, the space *(straight arrows)* between the anterior surface of the odontoid and the posterior aspect of the anterior arch of C-1 *(dotted lines)* is dramatically widened. This widening represents an unstable dislocation of C-1 relative to C-2. There is grade 1 anterior spondylolisthesis of C-3 relative to C-4. Note the narrowing of all the cervical disc spaces and the generalized osteopenia. **D:** Cervical spine axial CT image. Rheumatoid arthritis with spinal stenosis in a 55-year-old man. The C1-2 joint is abnormal with 8 mm distance between the anterior arch of C-1 and the odontoid *(between the straight arrows)*. There are advanced erosive changes in the odontoid *(curved arrow)*. Cervical spine CT sagittal reconstruction **(E)** and sagittal CT three-dimensional reconstruction **(F)** in the same patient as shown in D. The odontoid is involved with erosive changes and has a distal penciled appearance *(curved arrows)*. There is redemonstration of the abnormal C1-2 joint *(between the straight arrows)*. **G:** Cervical spine sagittal T2 MR image in the same patient as shown in D–F. The odontoid *(double arrows)* is displaced posterior, resulting in spinal stenosis and cervical cord compression *(curved arrow)*. The increased signal in the compressed cord *(arrowhead)* probably represents edema and/or chronic reaction to the compression. The *single straight arrows* indicate multiple levels of mild spinal stenosis. **G:** Cervical spine sagittal T2 MR image in the same patient as shown in D–F. The odontoid *(double arrows)* is displaced posterior, resulting in spinal stenosis and cervical cord compression *(curved arrow)*. The increased signal in the compressed cord *(arrowhead)* probably represents edema and/or chronic reaction to the compression. The *single straight arrows* indicate multiple levels of mild spinal stenosis.

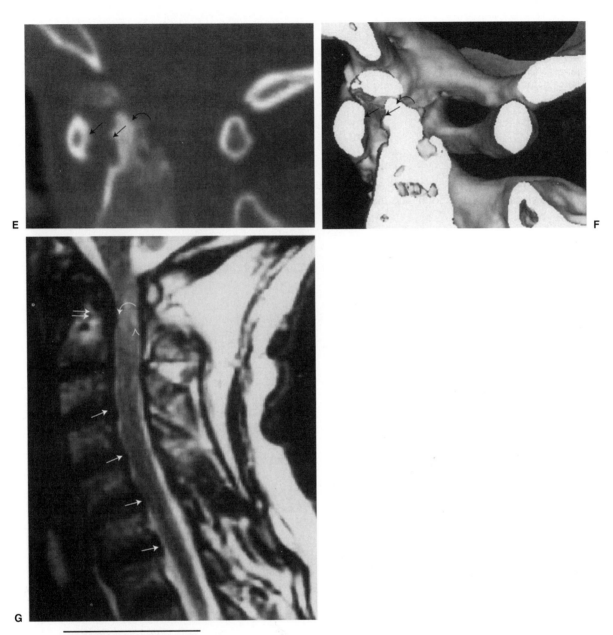

FIGURE 6-47. (*Continued*)

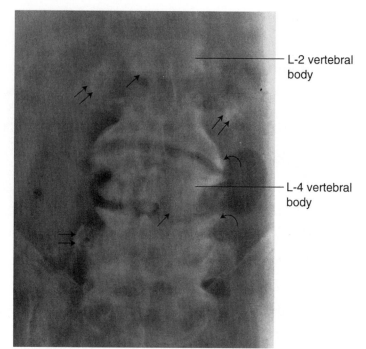

L-2 vertebral body

L-4 vertebral body

FIGURE 6-48. Lumbar spine AP radiograph. Diabetic neuropathic arthropathy. The characteristic changes of neuropathic arthropathy are present including sclerotic and destructive changes *(single straight arrows)*, fragmentation and marginal bone mass formation *(double straight arrows)*, and osteophyte formation *(curved arrow)*.

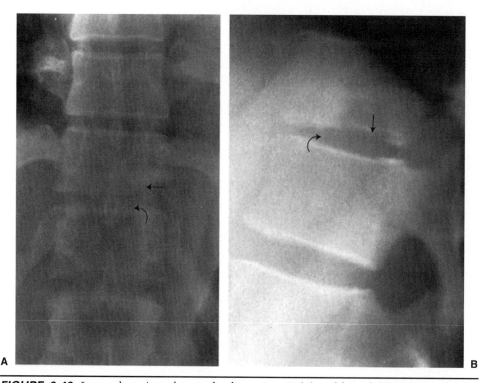

A

B

FIGURE 6-49. Lower thoracic and upper lumbar spine AP **(A)** and lateral **(B)** radiographs. Osteomyelitis of T-11 vertebral body. This 41-year-old patient had back pain and a low-grade fever. There is destruction of the posterior portion of the T-11 inferior endplate *(straight arrows)*, and the marked narrowing of the T11-12 intervertebral disc space *(curved arrows)* suggests disc and joint destruction.

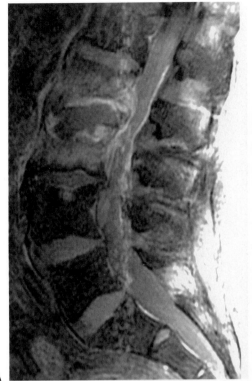

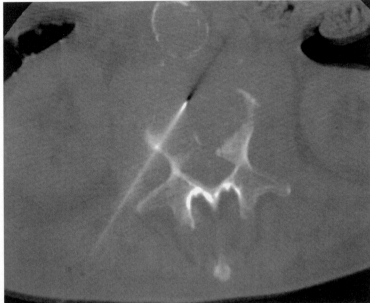

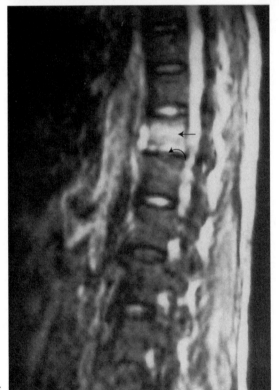

A

B

C

FIGURE 6-50. A: Sagittal T1 MR with intravenous contrast. Discitis. The L2-3 disc appears enlarged because the adjacent endplates have been destroyed by the infection. There is contrast enhancement (white) surrounding the infected disc and of the involved vertebral bodies. **B:** Axial CT during biopsy in the same patient. The tip of the biopsy needle *(arrow)* is in the infected disc. In only about half of biopsies performed for discitis will an organism be identified. **C:** Thoracic and lumbar spine T2 sagittal MR image. Osteomyelitis of the T-11 vertebral body and infectious destruction of the T11-12 intervertebral disc space. The white appearance of the T-11 vertebral body confirms the clinical impression of osteomyelitis *(straight arrow)*. Compare the abnormal density of T-11 vertebral body to the normal density of the uninvolved vertebral bodies above and below the T-11 vertebra. Notice that a large portion of the T11-12 intervertebral disc is missing *(curved arrow)*, compatible with probable disc destruction. Compare the involved abnormal disc space at T11-12 to the normal-appearing discs above and below.

signal intensity (they appear white). Contrast enhancement is fairly intense. The disc is invariably involved, which often helps to differentiate infection from fractures and metastases. CT scans may detect bone and joint destruction that is not visible on radiographs (Fig. 6-50B).

MISCELLANEOUS DISEASES

Diffuse Idiopathic Skeletal Hyperostosis

Diffuse idiopathic skeletal hyperostosis (DISH) or Forestier's disease is best demonstrated on a lateral spine radiograph (Fig. 6-51) and is characterized by ossification involving the anterior longitudinal ligament. It is characteristically accompanied by exuberant osteophytes. The overall appearance is similar to the bamboo spine of ankylosing spondylitis; however, ankylosing spondylitis is usually accompanied by obliteration of the sacroiliac joints. Spinal stenosis is a significant complication of DISH (Fig. 6-52). As in ankylosing spondylitis, fractures may occur from a relatively minor trauma. Elsewhere

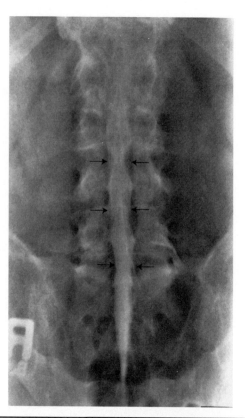

FIGURE 6-52. Lumbar myelogram PA radiograph in a different patient. Spinal stenosis secondary to diffuse idiopathic skeletal hyperostosis (DISH). The *straight arrows* indicate multiple levels of spinal stenosis and neural sac compression due to DISH changes in the spinal canal. The overall appearance of the spine is somewhat similar to the bamboo spine of ankylosing spondylitis.

in the body, DISH is manifested by prominent bony projections at ligament attachment sites.

Paget's Disease

Paget's disease is due to an imbalance of osteoclastic and osteoblastic activity that may be metabolic in origin, and this has been discussed in Chapter 5. It often involves the spine and, more frequently, the pelvis (Fig. 6-53). The classic spine appearance is the picture frame vertebra caused by increased peripheral vertebra density and central lucency.

Tumors

Benign tumors may involve the spine (Table 6-9). One such tumor is the hemangioma. These are usually asymptomatic and an incidental finding in the spine. Hemangiomas in the spine require no therapy unless they become symptomatic. Symptoms may develop when the tumor causes a pathologic fracture or the lesion extends

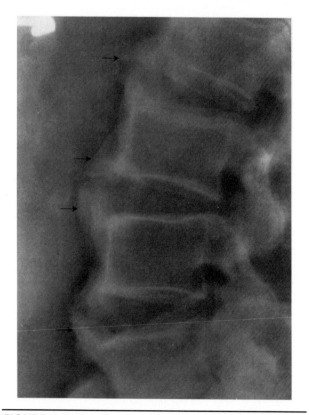

FIGURE 6-51. Lumbar spine lateral radiograph. Diffuse idiopathic skeletal hyperostosis, or DISH. Note the large osteophytes (*straight arrows*) along the anterior vertebral bodies that extend anteriorly across the disc spaces and ossification of the anterior longitudinal ligament. The intervertebral disc spaces are normal in height.

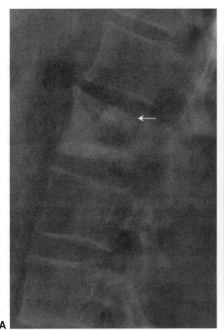
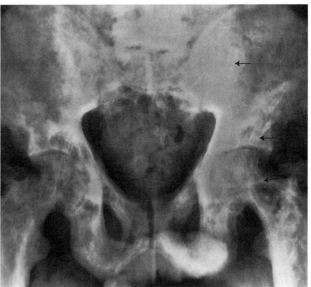

A

B

FIGURE 6-53. **A:** Lumbar spine lateral radiograph. Paget's disease L-2 vertebra *(straight arrow)*. The L-2 vertebra has the classic picture frame appearance secondary to the increased trabecular density in the periphery of the vertebral body. There is mild loss of the L-2 vertebral body height compared to the vertical heights of L-1 and L-3, and this is compatible with a mild compression fracture. The remainder of the lumbar spine is not involved by the Paget's disease. **B:** Pelvis AP radiograph. Paget's disease. The bone trabeculae are coarse *(straight arrows)* with an overall increased density and widening or expansion of the bones.

outside the vertebrae and compresses the spinal cord. Hemangiomas can develop in other bones, but in the spine they have a classic appearance with prominent or thickened vertical trabeculae that simulate jail bars or corduroy fabric (Fig. 6-54). The MRI and CT appearances are also quite characteristic and do not pose a diagnostic dilemma.

As previously discussed in Chapter 5, *metastatic disease is the most common neoplasm in bone and this includes the spine.* As in other bones, metastatic disease involving the spine can be osteolytic (Fig. 6-55) with or without de-

struction and/or osteoblastic activity (Fig. 6-56). The primary neoplasms causing osteolytic and osteoblastic bone lesions are listed in Table 6-10.

The importance of visualizing the vertebral pedicles is emphasized in Fig. 6-57. When one or both pedicles are missing in patients with known or suspected cancer, the first diagnosis that must come to mind is metastatic disease. MRI is very useful for confirming the presence of metastatic disease in a vertebra with a missing pedicle (see Fig. 6-57B) and for assessing the extent and location of the metastases (Fig. 6-58).

▶ **TABLE 6-9 Some Primary Spine Bone Tumors**

Benign
Hemangioma
Osteoid osteoma
Osteoblastoma
Aneurysmal bone cyst
Osteochondroma

Malignant
Multiple myeloma (most common)
Chondrosarcoma
Osteosarcoma
Ewing's sarcoma

▶ **TABLE 6-10 Characteristics of Metastases**

Osteoblastic
Prostate
Breast
Lymphoma
Carcinoid
Neuroblastoma (occasional)

Osteolytic
Breast
Lung
Almost all other metastatic tumors

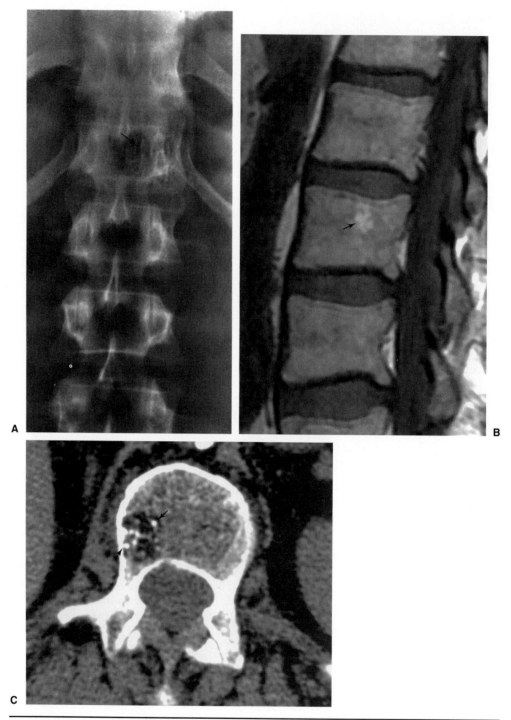

FIGURE 6-54. A: Thoracolumbar spine AP radiograph. T-12 vertebral body hemangioma. The prominent vertical trabecular pattern is characteristic of bone hemangioma *(straight arrow)*. Compare the appearance of the T-12 vertebral body to those above and below that level. **B:** Sagittal T1 MR of the lumbar spine. The round focal area of higher signal *(arrow)* is quite characteristic of hemangioma in the spine since it contains a moderate amount of fat. **C:** Axial CT of a thoracic vertebral body demonstrates the punctate appearance of the cross section of coarse trabeculae *(arrows)*, similar to that seen in A. Note the very low density of the fat within the hemangioma (black).

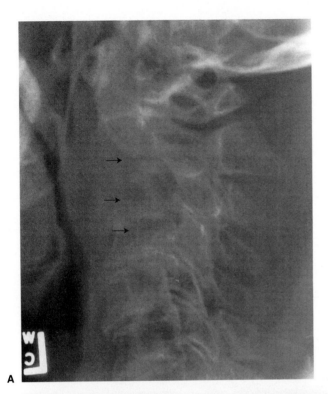

A

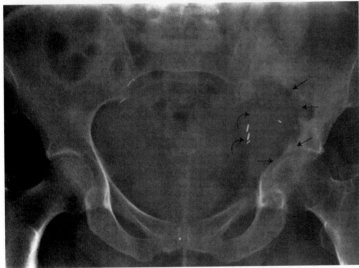

B

FIGURE 6-55. A: Cervical spine lateral radiograph. Osteolytic metastatic disease of multiple cervical vertebrae. The C-2, C-3, and C-4 vertebral bodies are involved by destructive (lytic) metastatic disease from the lung *(straight arrows)*. **B:** Pelvis AP radiograph. Osteolytic metastatic carcinoma of the cervix involving the left ilium and ischium *(straight arrows)*. The extensive involvement of the left ischium has resulted in left acetabular protrusio. There is a large soft tissue metastatic mass in the left pelvis *(curved arrows)*.

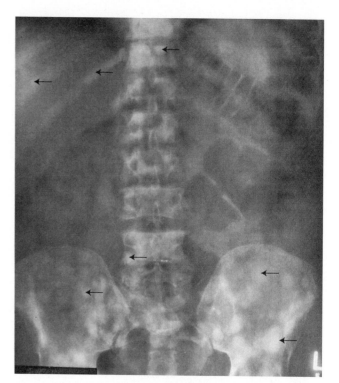

FIGURE 6-56. Abdomen AP radiograph. Osteoblastic metastatic carcinoma of the prostate. The multiple areas of increased density *(straight arrows)* represent the metastases that involve the pelvis, lumbar spine, dorsal spine, and ribs.

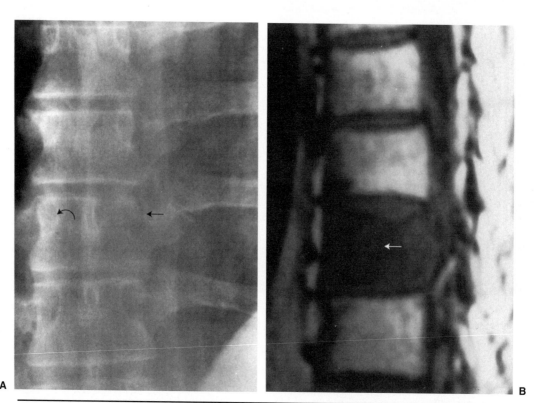

A

B

FIGURE 6-57. A: Thoracic spine AP radiograph. Osteolytic metastatic lesion of the left T-9 vertebral pedicle. The missing left T-9 pedicle *(straight arrow)* was destroyed by metastatic disease while the uninvolved normal right T-9 pedicle *(curved arrow)* remains clearly visible. This finding prompted further investigation by MRI that proved the missing pedicle was destroyed by a metastatic lesion. **B:** Thoracic spine sagittal T1 MR image in the same patient. Metastatic disease of the T-9 vertebra. The metastatic disease involving the T-9 vertebral body *(straight arrow)* has replaced almost all of the bone marrow fat, resulting in a low-intensity signal. This abnormality of T-9 is quite obvious when compared to the high-intensity signals from the normal bone marrow of the uninvolved vertebral bodies above and below T-9.

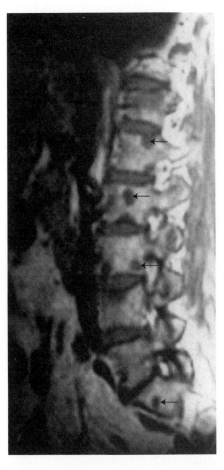

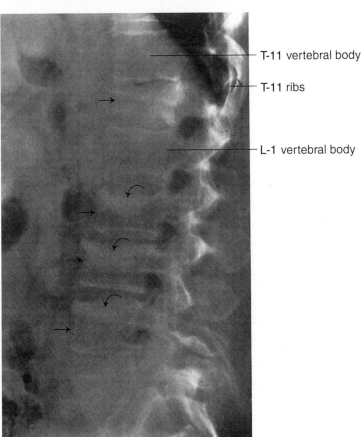

FIGURE 6-58. Lumbosacral spine sagittal T1 MR image. Metastatic carcinoma of the breast. The patient complained of severe back pain, but the radiographs were negative. The straight arrows indicate some of the many metastatic lesions present in the lumbar and sacral spine. The metastatic lesions appear black on the T1 MR image but white or gray on T2 images.

T-11 vertebral body

T-11 ribs

L-1 vertebral body

FIGURE 6-59. Lumbar spine lateral radiograph. Senile osteoporosis. Note the overall decreased density or osteopenia of the spine. There are multiple compression pathologic fractures secondary to osteoporosis *(straight arrows)*. The fractures of T-12, L2, -3, and -4 are manifest by a loss of the vertical heights of the involved vertebral bodies. Compare the fractured vertebrae to the normal vertical heights of the T-11 and L-1 vertebral bodies. Note the multiple fish-mouth deformities *(curved arrows)*.

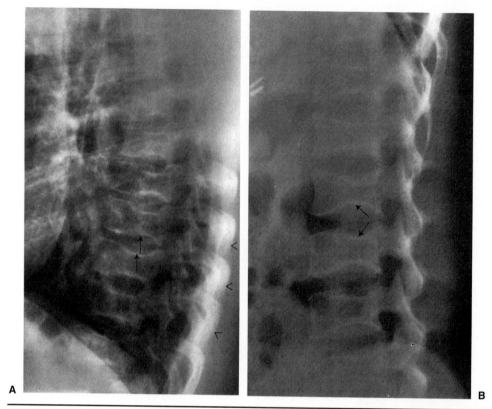

FIGURE 6-60. Thoracic spine **(A)** and lumbar **(B)** spine lateral radiographs. Sickle cell anemia. There is overall osteopenia, and the fish-mouth deformities of the vertebral bodies *(straight arrows)* are similar to those in senile osteoporosis (Fig. 12-59). Note the ribs in A *(arrowheads)*.

Primary tumors of the thecal sac and the spinal cord can mimic bone tumors of the spine. Thus tumors arising from these structures should be considered in the differential diagnosis when dealing with back pain and abnormal radiographs and myelograms.

Others

Osteoporosis and osteomalacia have been discussed in the metabolic disease section of Chapter 5. The typical patient with osteoporosis (Fig. 6-59) is elderly and complains of back pain, especially if secondary compression fractures are present. Vertebral fractures not only cause back pain, but often result in loss of height and kyphosis. The typical radiographic appearance of osteoporosis in the spine is decreased overall density of the vertebral bodies, and as a result the vertebral endplates appear prominent. As the vertebrae become softer than the discs, the endplates can sag, resulting in fish-mouth deformities of the vertebrae.

Sickle cell anemia is a Mendelian dominant hereditary trait. The disease is variable in severity and characterized by crises that include anemia, fever, severe abdominal and bone pain, and bone infarction. Radiographs may show

osteoporosis, bone infarcts, aseptic necrosis, and fish-mouth vertebrae (Fig. 6-60).

Dwarfism and several congenital anomalies have classic or typical appearances of the spine and pelvis, but a discussion is beyond the scope of this introductory text.

APPROACH TO CLINICAL PROBLEMS

Initial evaluation of a patient with back pain requires a thorough history and physical examination. If the patient experienced pain two or three days after playing in the father–son football game, he is more likely to have a muscle strain or delayed-onset muscle soreness. Acute pain after lifting a heavy object is more likely a herniated nucleus pulposis. Insidious onset of pain may be related to arthritis, developing osteoporotic compressions, or metastatic disease. The level of clinical suspicion will determine what steps to take next. Most patients will undergo a trial of conservative treatment of rest, physical therapy, and pain medications. If there is no improvement, imaging studies may then be considered. However, if the patient has a known primary neoplasm, MRI or radionuclide bone scan may be the initial study because of a higher clinical suspicion of metastases and the importance of the diagnosis.

KEY POINTS

- Basic observations on spine radiographs should include spinal alignment, the heights of the vertebral bodies and the intervertebral disc spaces, osseous density, presence of the pars interarticularis in the lumbar spine, and presence of the pedicles of each vertebra.
- An absent pedicle is abnormal and should make you suspicious of a destructive process such as primary and secondary bone neoplasms.
- Spine CT is good for bone detail, localization of fracture fragments and their relationship to the spinal canal and cord, and diagnosis of herniated intervertebral disc disease.
- Spine MRI is good for imaging disease processes that involve the bone marrow fat such as tumor and infection. MRI is also valuable for diagnosis and staging of herniated intervertebral disc disease and evaluating the spinal cord.
- Most congenital anomalies of the spine are asymptomatic.

- Hyperflexion injuries include teardrop fractures, posterior ligament injury, and facet locking. Locked facets commonly have associated spinal cord injury.
- Odontoid process fractures are frequent in the elderly and result from both hyperflexion and hyperextension injuries.
- Open-mouth AP radiographs and CT are useful tools for diagnosing odontoid fractures.
- A ring is rarely broken in only one location. At least two fractures are usually present in the pelvis.
- Acetabular fractures are evaluated by AP and oblique (Judet) views of the pelvis.
- Following an acetabular fracture, subsequent studies should closely evaluate for the presence of avascular necrosis in the femoral head.

FURTHER READING

Rogers LF. *Radiology of skeletal trauma*, 3rd ed. New York: Churchhill Livingstone, 2002.

El-Khoury GY. *Essentials of musculoskeletal imaging*. New York: Churchill Livingstone, 2003.

Renfrew DL. *Atlas of spine imaging*. Philadelphia: WB Saunders, 2003.

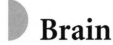

Brain

Wilbur L. Smith

BRAIN IMAGING

Neuroradiology was a relatively unsophisticated branch of imaging prior to 1970. Plain radiographs of the skull were insensitive for predicting neurologic disorders, and obtaining more useful diagnostic imaging information about the brain and spinal cord was cumbersome and painful, and yielded images that were difficult to interpret without advanced knowledge of neuroanatomy. The early brain imaging techniques were all at best minimally invasive and many involved such gruesome activities as injecting air into the spinal canal and rolling the patient about in a specially devised torture chair. Few patients willingly returned for another one of those exams! The highest level of comfort that the poor patient who needed brain imaging could anticipate was a direct puncture carotid arteriogram or a spinal tap.

The invention and widespread use of the technique of computerized axial tomography (CAT), or computed tomography (CT), allowed relatively painless access to the processes inside the skull and allowed the field of neuroradiology to become a premier subspecialty within radiology. The early CT scanners were slow, lacking in detail, and hard to manage (Fig. 7-1), but they were such a marvelous advance that they were embraced as a revolution in medical imaging. Indeed, Sir Godfrey Hounsfield, the pioneer of CT imaging, won many international awards and was knighted for his work. Despite the development of many other imaging modalities to date, CT still forms the basis for a majority of the diagnostic studies of the

brain and spine and is the most common neuroimaging study performed in the United States. The CT scanners of today are capable of obtaining simultaneous multiple slices and with new image processing techniques can produce reconstructed anatomical images in any plane. CT scans are routinely performed either with or without intravenous contrast enhancement, and the enhancement produced coupled with the speed of the new scanners makes real-time vascular mapping of the brain a practical clinical tool (Fig. 7-2). Certain clinical indications are generally predictive of the need for contrast, although there are many variations. Table 7-1 gives the usual indications for contrast use; however, if in doubt, radiologists are always available for consultation on individual cases.

In CT scanning, images of the brain are usually acquired in axial (horizontal) planes and then viewed at different digital levels, so that one can see the bones of the face and skull as well as the tissues of the brain itself. Two image acquisitions are not required to get these data, but rather, two different levels of viewing the same digital data. The sections that result from the CT scans depict the anatomy at predetermined intervals depending on the parameters of reconstruction of the slices (thickness) and timing of acquisition of the data. Generally, the thicker the slices the fewer the sections needed to get through the brain, but as the slices are thickened, anatomy is depicted in less detail. In the standard brain CT scan, there are several key landmarks to observe for proper orientation. Figure 7-3 illustrates some of the highlights for which you should

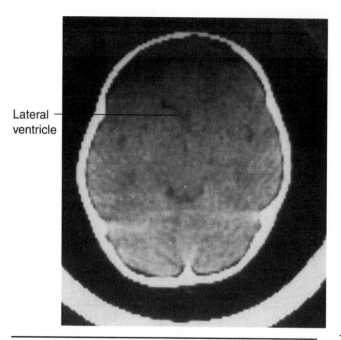

Lateral ventricle

FIGURE 7-1. A scan of the brain performed in 1976 on an EMI device. This single section took about 1 minute to acquire. The coarse pixels make anything but the larger brain structures such as the ventricles difficult to appreciate. This was, however, a huge improvement over the pneumoencephalogram.

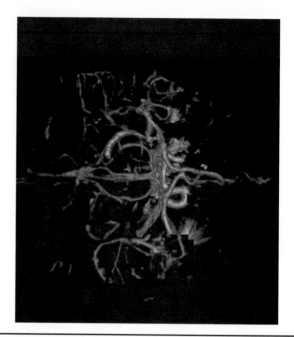

FIGURE 7-2. CT arteriogram of the brain obtained after intravenous contrast shows detail of the intracerebral vessels of the circle of Willis.

look in orienting yourself to the anatomy depicted by the slices.

Let's begin with the caudal sections and work cephalad. The fourth ventricle, a cerebrospinal fluid space located dorsal to the brain stem and in the midline of the posterior fossa, is a good marker for identifying the level of the pons, cerebellar vermis, and the base of the anterior cranial fossa (Fig. 7-3A). On the same section lying ventral to the brain stem is the suprasellar cistern and the dorsum sellae. Note that the figures depict the anatomy of the posterior fossa less sharply than some of the more cephalad sections of brain. CT scans in the posterior fossa are often degraded owing to the absorption of x-rays by the large amount of

dense surrounding bone; therefore, detail of the cerebellar hemispheres may be obscured. This technique limitation is mitigated to some degree by faster and better scanners, but bone artifact is a limitation of CT scanning.

Proceeding to sections cephalad from the fourth ventricle, one encounters the ambient cistern and cephalad portion of the suprasellar cistern (Fig. 7-3B). The former is an important landmark for the point where the cerebral peduncles (an extension of the brain stem) pass through the tentorium cerebri. Ventral to this landmark and slightly cephalad are located the third ventricle and the anterior horns of the lateral ventricles. At the lateral margins of the anterior horns of the ventricles are the basal ganglia, identifiable as masses of gray matter bordering the lateral and third ventricles (Fig. 7-3C). The caudate nuclei protrude into the anterior horns of the lateral ventricles.

Further cephalad the scans depict the brain cortex and the orderly interfaces between the gray and white matter (Fig. 7-3D). Note that each section of gray matter has an accompanying area of white matter arranged in a predictable pattern. Symmetry is everything in looking at CT scans of the brain. Providing that the patient is properly positioned, structures should match up from side to side.

Despite its immense success, CT has limitations that inhibit its value. For example, CT is inherently limited in its ability to display high degrees of tissue contrast. If two tissues absorb roughly the same number of photons, even though the tissues may be chemically very different, CT cannot discriminate between them. Bone or other high-density items such as aneurysm clips degrade the CT

▶ **TABLE 7-1 Some Common Indications for CAT Scanning and Use of Intravenous Contrast Enhancement**

Indications for CAT Scan	IV Contrast
Trauma	No
Infection	Yes
Congenital anomalies	No
Tumor	Yes
Metabolic disorder	No
Multiple sclerosis	Yes
Hydrocephalus	No

▶ TABLE 7-2 MRI Pulse Sequences

Sequence	Cerebrospinal Fluid Color	Lesion Color
T1-weighted	Black	Variable
T2-weighted	White	White
Inversion recovery	Black	White
Diffusion	Black	White
Gradient (susceptibility)	Black	Black

▶ TABLE 7-3 A Comparison of Indications and Factors Affecting the Choice of CT or MRI

Factor	CT	MRI
Cost	++	+++
Availability	+++	++
Tissue differentiation	+	+++
Multiplanar sequences	+++	+++
Speed of exam	+++	++
Bone reconstruction	+++	+

image. Although the time needed to obtain a section by CT has declined substantially in recent years, there are still physical limitations to CT scanning, and motion artifacts abound in uncooperative or combative patients.

The newest major technique in the imaging of the brain and spinal cord is magnetic resonance imaging (MRI). This technique also had humble beginnings; the first scanners were used to quantify fat in livestock coming to market. MR images are wonderfully detailed, but the studies require more time and are more expensive to carry out than CT scans. MRI has much better tissue contrast than CT, although special resolution is less. The new imaging sequences and enhanced capabilities of MRI to show metabolic, vascular, and functional changes in tissues suggest that it will ultimately be the imaging modality of choice for many conditions.

MRI imaging depends on alterations in the physical behavior of protons (hydrogen is the most abundant natural proton in our water-filled tissues) when first magnetized, then exposed to a pulse of radio-frequency energy. The major variables are therefore the strength of the magnetic field and the way the radio-frequency waves are applied (pulse

sequences). Table 7-2 is a very simplified overview of the current major pulse sequences and the color of lesions and the CSF on the currently used 1.5-tesla MRI scans. There are many exceptions to the data in Table 7-2, and new sequences are rapidly being developed. Therefore, this table should be used only as a rough (90% accurate) guideline to get you in the ballpark when looking at MRI images. Despite the great potential of MRI and its progression from a research device in the early 1980s to a staple of most imaging departments in the United States, at present CT scans still provide the bulk of diagnostic brain images. Table 7-3 compares the strengths and limitations of CT and MRI.

TRAUMA

Perhaps the most common indication for brain imaging is trauma. Human heads are extremely vulnerable to injury; consequently, the trauma CT scanner rarely lacks sufficient business. In assessing a CT performed for trauma, one has a finite number of search parameters for major

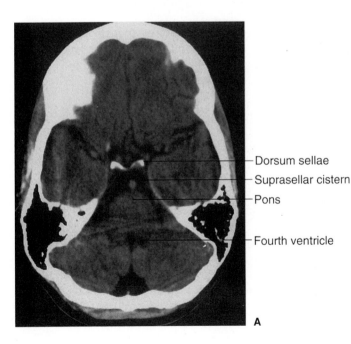

—Dorsum sellae
—Suprasellar cistern
—Pons
—Fourth ventricle

A

FIGURE 7-3. **A:** CT scan of a normal adult at the level of the fourth ventricle. The brain stem structure ventral to the fourth ventricle is the pons. Further anterior lies the five-pointed star representing the suprasellar cistern. Lying within the suprasellar cistern are the vessels of the circle of Willis and the dorsum sella or back of the sella turcica. *(continued)*

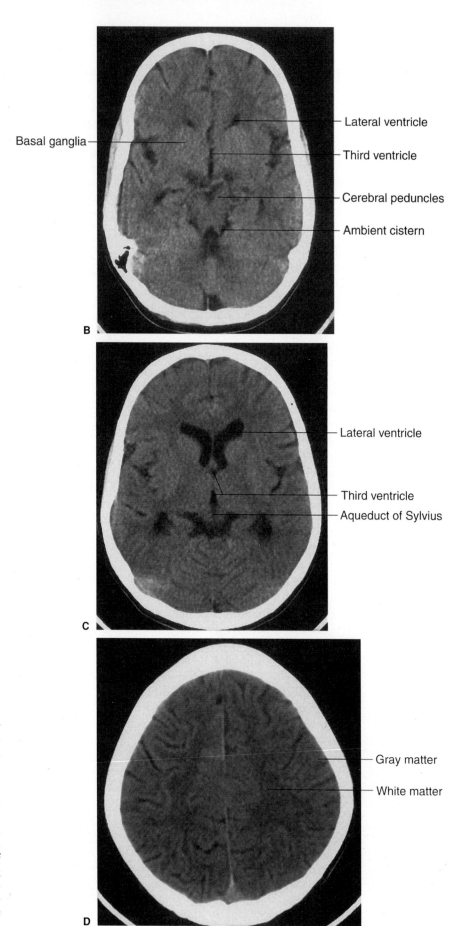

Basal ganglia — Lateral ventricle
Third ventricle
Cerebral peduncles
Ambient cistern

B

Lateral ventricle

Third ventricle
Aqueduct of Sylvius

C

Gray matter
White matter

D

FIGURE 7-3. B: A cut cephalad to A demonstrates the ambient cisterns as curved black cerebrospinal fluid densities just posterior to the cerebral peduncles. If you use your imagination, the cistern is the mouth, the anterior horns of the lateral ventricles the eyes, and the third ventricle the nose of a smiling man! This is an important landmark as it is the point where the cerebral peduncles pass through the tentorium. **C:** Proceeding cephalad we leave the posterior fossa and image the lateral ventricles, third ventricles, aqueduct of Sylvius, and the cerebral hemispheres. **D:** A scan near the vertex of the head depicts the white matter (black on CT) and its relationship to gray matter. Note that each area of gray matter has an associated column of white matter.

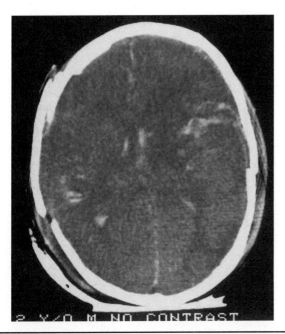

FIGURE 7-4. A child injured in a severe auto accident shows multiple white areas in the brain as well as disruption of the skull. The white areas are intraparenchymal hemorrhage. Note also the disruption of the normal brain architecture (compare to Fig. 7-3D, which shows a section at roughly the same level), reflecting the severe cerebral edema.

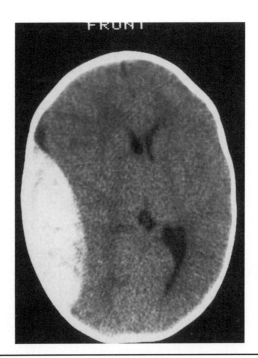

FIGURE 7-5. A large mass of white (blood) density convex toward the brain is characteristic of an epidural hemorrhage. Most of these occur due to traumatic tear of an artery and are surgical emergencies. The brain is shifted by the hematoma as evidenced by the shift of midline.

findings that represent conditions likely to demand immediate intervention.

The presence of blood in the head but outside the vascular system is often a key to the correct diagnosis. Fortunately, when blood is loose in the head, it usually appears as a conspicuous white blob on the CT scan. Therefore, the first rule of looking at trauma CT scans is to look for the white collections inside the skull (Fig. 7-4). Your diagnosis often can be even more specific because the white (or blood) tends to align in certain predictable ways according to its anatomic location. As an overview, the locations of intracranial bleeding are first separated into intraaxial, meaning within the brain tissues themselves, or extraaxial. The extraaxial hemorrhages occur in spaces with characteristic shapes that can assist in localizing the hemorrhage. Fluid in the epidural space, between skull and dura, usually presents as a crescentic mass, convex to the brain (Fig. 7-5). The subdural space between dura and arachnoid membranes, however, is usually concave, paralleling the surface of the skull; therefore subdural hematomas are differentiated from epidural bleeding by their shape (Fig. 7-6). Subarachnoid blood diffuses over the surface of the gyri and fills the cerebrospinal fluid (CSF) cisterns around the brain (Fig. 7-7). Intraaxial bleeding is often confined to the area of the ruptured vessel and is entirely enclosed within the substance of the brain.

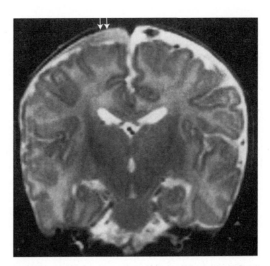

FIGURE 7-6. MRI of the brain, shown to illustrate that MRI is also effective in showing trauma. This is an abused child who has a subdural space hematoma *(arrows)*. Note that the surface is concave, reflecting the contour of the cerebral cortex, but not extending among the gyri. This configuration is typical for a subdural hematoma. Note also that the signal densities are different on MRI. Imaging of bleeding is more complex on MRI than by CAT.

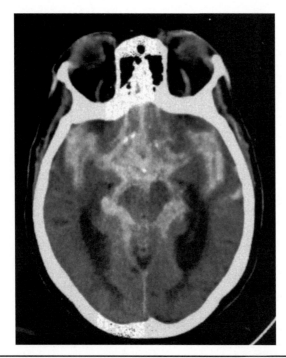

FIGURE 7-7. A CT scan at the level of the ambient cistern showing the cistern as white (blood) instead of black (cerebrospinal fluid; compare to Fig. 7-3B). Note that the white density also surrounds the brain stem. When blood mimics cerebrospinal fluid distribution, it is usually extraaxial and in the subarachnoid space flowing around and over the brain tissues.

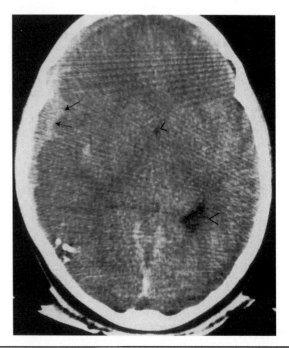

FIGURE 7-8. Intraaxial or intraparenchymal hemorrhage of the brain in a trauma patient. The white densities (blood) do not conform to any definable space and are actually within and between the tissues of the brain. A subdural hematoma *(arrows)* is also present in this patient. Note that the lateral ventricle and its temporal horn *(arrowheads)* are displaced by the mass effect.

Intraventricular hemorrhage lies within the ventricles, often pooling in the dependent portion of the ventricle to form a blood–CSF level. By first finding the "white" blood, then looking at its shape and anatomic location, one can be pretty precise about the diagnosis and the location of the blood. As the hematoma ages, the blood assumes different image characteristics. Table 7-4 provides a description of the differing appearances of blood in the head with age of the bleed.

After looking for bleeding in trauma patients, the next step is to look for mass effect, a clue that there is pressure impinging on an area of the brain. For most injuries, the best way to find significant mass effects is to look for asymmetry with displacement of the midline structures, the most prominent of which are the falx cerebri, lateral ven-

tricles, and interhemispheric fissure (Figs. 7-5 and 7-8). A midline shift away from a lesion, for example, an epidural blood collection, is usually an emergent situation, particularly in the context of trauma. However, a word of caution is advisable: Midline shift does not always signal a need to take out your pocket knife to perform emergent, kitchen-table-type neurosurgery. Diffuse edema of one hemisphere of the brain (Fig. 7-8) or even atrophy of the contralateral hemisphere can cause apparent (or real) shift. The important concept is midline shift. When the brain structures are shifted away from the side of the evident abnormality, such as a hematoma, increase your level of suspicion and urgency in evaluating your patient.

After searching for blood and mass effects on the brain CT scan, the next important step is to assess the densities of the brain tissues themselves. Earlier we described how the gray and white matter components of the brain should be visible on the CT scan (Fig. 7-3D). The lateral ventricles and CSF spaces are black and should be easily distinguished as separate from the tissues of the brain. Variations on this theme are generally bad news. The most prominent and dangerous sign is the obliteration of the distinction between the gray and white matter, which indicates profound edema in the area. If this is a universal pattern, there is a special name for the profound edema that occurs, obliterating all brain landmarks—the "bad black brain" (Fig. 7-9). This finding usually portends a poor outcome,

▶ **TABLE 7-4 Characteristics of Intracranial Blood by Imaging**

| Time of Bleed | CT | MRI | |
		T1-Weighted	T2-Weighted
Immediate	White	Black	Black
Acute	White	White	Black
Subacute	Gray-White	White	White

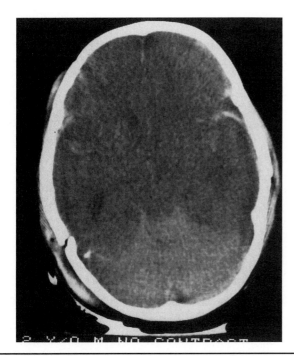

FIGURE 7-9. This severely brain-injured child has neither recognizable ventricles nor gray/white matter differentiation (compare with Fig. 7-3D). In fact, the whole neocortex, except for the areas of hemorrhage, is a uniform shade of black. This severe brain edema portends a poor prognosis.

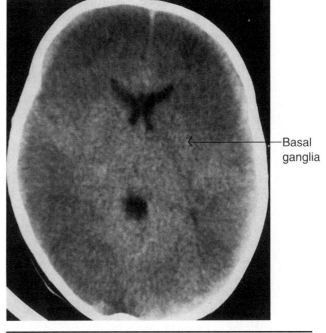

FIGURE 7-10. A child with diffuse hypoxic injury of the brain demonstrates the reversal sign. Note that the basal ganglia are gray and the neocortex black, particularly in the frontal and parietal regions.

representing diffuse breakdown of tissue integrity with ensuing cerebral edema. The cause of this catastrophic chain of events is almost always a limitation of the oxygen supply to the brain tissues, owing to either a compromise of the blood supply or a loss of oxygen to the brain cells. In the latter instance, as the brain swells, cerebral blood supply is compromised by loss of the arterial perfusion gradient, and ultimately there is no circulation to the brain. Owing to different tissue densities and less vulnerable perfusion, the basal ganglia and brain stem are often particularly conspicuous against the uniform density of the bad black brain, and their conspicuity results in the so-called reversal sign (Fig. 7-10).

Please note the intentional lack of a detailed discussion of skull fractures in this section on trauma. That is because, in general, skull fractures aren't very important in the immediate outcome of a patient. It is the effect of the trauma on the brain that does your patient harm, not the crack in the bone (Fig. 7-11). A significant important exception is the depressed skull fracture, a situation where the bone is driven directly back into the meningeal coverings and the brain itself. CT imaging and bone windows are of great importance in documenting the depth and extent of this type of injury, as well as documenting any intracranial air leaks owing to tears of the dura or meninges (Fig. 7-12). In this type of trauma, surgery is usually needed and the identification of the fracture, depth of the fragment(s),

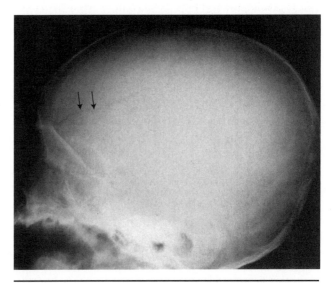

FIGURE 7-11. This child with a linear skull fracture *(arrows)* was completely asymptomatic (except for a palpable bump on his skull) because the brain underlying the skull was not affected. The presence of the skull fracture documents trauma but is of little importance in patient management.

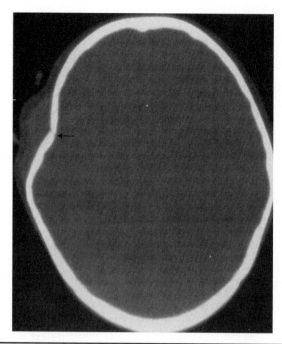

FIGURE 7-12. Bone windows of a CT scan demonstrate the depth of injury in a depressed skull fracture *(arrow)* after this teenager was struck with a hammer.

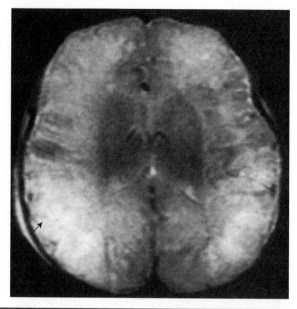

FIGURE 7-13. MRI shows a diffusely increased signal *(white indicated by arrow)* in the posterior parietal lobes of a blunt head trauma victim. This is owing to a cortical contusion that was subtle on the CT scan. Although the finding explained the patient's symptoms and documented the severity of injury, the lesion did not require urgent intervention.

surface brain injury, and pneumocephalus (air inside the skull) are the key observations.

MRI is not to be omitted in any discussion of trauma, but its role, although dramatically increasing, is usually secondary. Owing to the limitations of patient access (ventilator limitations, difficulty in patient observation, etc.) and the longer examination times, MRI is rarely the first imaging modality used for acute trauma. After the acute, life-threatening emergencies have been handled, MRI is extremely sensitive for assessing the extent of parenchymal injury to the brain and for defining more precisely the compartment of localized extraaxial fluid. In each of these instances, the prognosis and etiology of the injury is better defined after MRI. MRI spectroscopy, a study of brain metabolism, holds great promise for predicting the outcome of some injuries. The utility of MRI for finding subarachnoid blood is debatable, but MRI is unparalleled in defining precisely which gyrus was smashed in a previous auto accident (Fig. 7-13). The instances where MRI is critical in deciding the urgent management of a trauma patient are few, but it is an invaluable secondary tool in selected patients.

In summary, a CT scan of an acute trauma patient should be evaluated for the following findings: (a) white densities defining bleeding, including the shape and distribution of the blood collection(s); (b) mass effect, particularly with shift of the midline structures; and (c) loss of normal contrast characteristics (or asymmetry) of the normal tissue and CSF interfaces. These rules won't get

you every answer on every trauma patient, but they will help you in almost 95% of the cases you see. For the other 5%, you may have to do a radiology or neurosurgery residency!

VASCULAR DISEASE

Just after trauma as an indication for brain imaging is vascular disease, and the most prevalent form is stroke. Stroke results from occlusion of the vascular supply (usually arterial but occasionally venous as well) to a focal area of the brain causing tissue ischemia. Many "strokes" are small and not even detected clinically. Most people in their fifth or sixth decade have small areas of abnormal signal called UBOs (unidentified bright objects) on MRI of the brain (Fig. 7-14), and there are some who ascribe the origin of UBOs to silent strokes. We have a lot of brain tissue that we don't fully use, so that loss of these small areas isn't necessarily perceived as a clinical problem.

Only when either a large or a particularly critical area of brain becomes ischemic do emergent symptoms appear and neuroimaging come into play. CT scans are often the first examination; however, their use is problematic as there is a significant incidence of falsely negative CT scans in the first 24 to 48 hours after a stroke. The size, severity, and presence of hemorrhage clearly affect the CT picture of stroke, so that some strokes appear almost

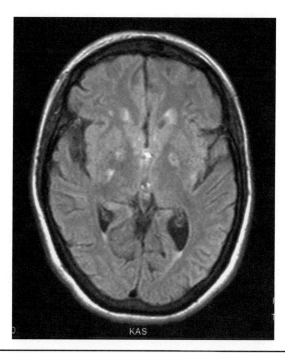

FIGURE 7-14. Widely scattered unidentified bright objects (UBOs) on MRI in the basal ganglia of this octogenarian are not of significance. These UBOs are common near the basal ganglia but can be seen anywhere and are assumed to represent small artery disease with lacunar infarctions.

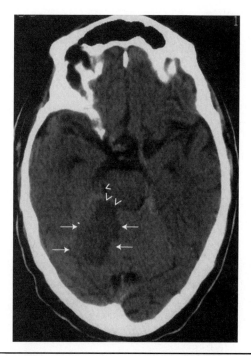

FIGURE 7-15. The low-density lesion in the right cerebellar hemisphere represents an acute stroke owing to arterial occlusion. Note that there is swelling of tissues involved in the stroke as evidenced by effacement of the ambient cistern on the right *(arrowheads)*. The lesion does not contain blood because there is no white signal on CT.

immediately; however, the sensitivity of CT scan for the diagnosis is considerably higher after the first 24 to 48 hours (Fig. 7-15).

The most reliable finding in stroke on CT scan is the loss of the normal architecture of brain substance. The area of the stroke is depicted as a dark (edematous) blotch obliterating the normal tissue density. Occasional strokes will have associated bleeding, particularly in patients with hypertension, and the blood will show up on CT as a white density within the darker area of infarct (Fig. 7-16). A stroke may also change in nature as the tissue is destroyed and revascularization takes place. Bleeding may ensue such that initially nonhemorrhagic strokes can develop high signal characteristic of internal bleeding. This change often portends a poor prognosis.

There is a developing body of knowledge suggesting that early treatment of stroke may restore circulation and limit brain tissue damage. This has led to a change in imaging to emphasize early diagnosis. MRI, particularly with diffusion imaging sequences, is more sensitive to the early changes and has assumed a larger role in the imaging of acute stroke. Diffusion imaging is a series of specific inversion recovery sequences that show Brownian motion of the water molecules released from the damaged brain tissue, which roughly correlates with areas of cell death. This finding is very sensitive and appears within minutes of tissue injury in experimental studies, making it the most useful

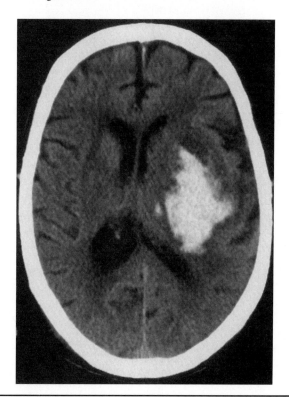

FIGURE 7-16. This huge hematoma in the left side of the brain has an irregular margin and edema surrounding the white area of fresh hemorrhage. This is a 53-year-old hypertensive executive who suffered a fatal acute hemorrhagic stroke.

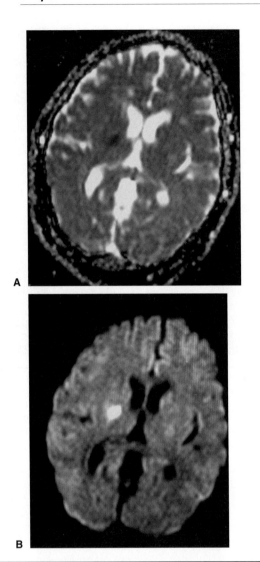

A

B

FIGURE 7-17. A: An acute stroke in the anterior portion of the right thalamus in this 50-year-old hypertensive executive was detected promptly by diffusion-weighted MRI. The acute diffusion coefficient image shows a low-density (black) lesion in the thalamus on the T2 sequence. **B:** The same lesion is white on the conventional inversion recovery sequence.

tool for diagnosing acute stroke (Fig. 7-17). Advances in MRI sequencing are rapid, so it is likely that these sequences will be further refined possibly even to anticipate cell death, but for now diffusion is the most accurate and early sequence for stroke. Eight hours or more after a stroke, the MRI of the damaged tissues shows white (on T2 and FLAIR) owing to the large amount of free water leaked by the ischemic cells. Unfortunately, by this time it is too late to use many of the thrombolytic techniques to limit stroke; therefore, diffusion is critical early in stroke. The use of MRI contrast (gadolinium) has improved detection even further, and MRI may soon be the standard for stroke imaging (Fig. 7-18).

So far we've discussed acute strokes. Chronic strokes result in atrophy of the brain tissue (Fig. 7-19) manifested

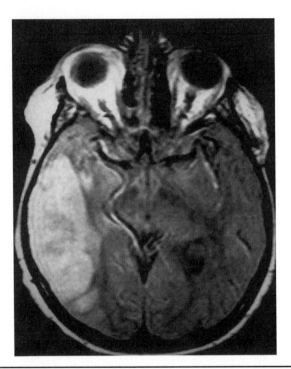

FIGURE 7-18. The white area in the right temporal lobe on this patient is a newly symptomatic stroke as depicted by gadolinium-enhanced MRI.

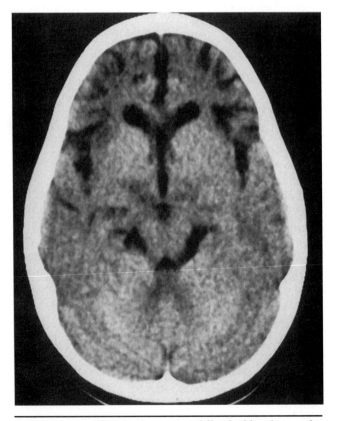

FIGURE 7-19. This elderly man has diffusely dilated ventricles as well as deep sulci over the brain surface because of atrophy presumably associated with multiple prior infarcts.

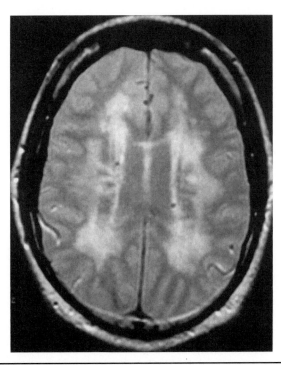

FIGURE 7-20. T2-weighted scan at the level of the lateral ventricles demonstrates multiple high-signal periventricular infarcts owing to lack of perfusion of the deep layers of the brain. These patients present with dementia and movement disorders that may mimic a number of degenerative neurologic conditions.

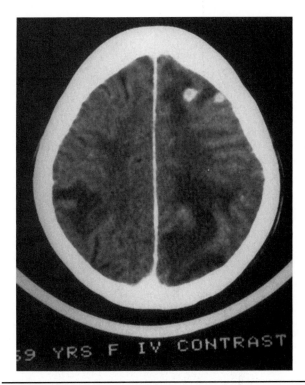

FIGURE 7-21. A contrast-enhanced CT scan of a 59-year-old woman with known lung cancer shows multiple high- and mixed-density lesions. These were metastases from the lung tumor.

by either focal or diffuse shrinkage of the brain owing to cell death. Of special note is diffuse multiinfarct dementia, a condition that is difficult to differentiate from Alzheimer's disease. Here the strokes are small and confined to the areas near the ventricles, so that the ventricles enlarge at the expense of the dead tissue (Fig. 7-20). The patient's CT scan looks like the ventricles are dilated, with the gyri and sulci appearing unusually prominent, a condition sometimes referred to as *hydrocephalus ex vacuo.* These cases are truly a conundrum because Alzheimer's disease, normal pressure hydrocephalus of the elderly, and diffuse brain atrophy from any cause all look the same. Functional brain imaging with spectroscopy, blood perfusion analysis, and/or metabolic measurement is of future consideration for this diagnosis. There is no easy imaging answer, and at present there is no specific treatment with good efficacy for any of these conditions. However, this is a rapidly developing area of medicine and exciting imaging developments are to be anticipated.

TUMOR

The third common application of brain imaging is tumor evaluation. In adults, metastases (Fig. 7-21) constitute the most common tumors, with primary benign or malignant

tumors being somewhat less common. The converse is true in children owing to the lower frequency of primary malignancies that metastasize to brain. The location of the tumors also differs with age. A greater proportion of adult tumors are in the cerebral cortex, whereas in children the proportion of tumors originating below the tentorium is much greater (Fig. 7-22).

CT scanning for tumor follows the same general principles as for trauma, with the major exception that most tumor scans are performed after the administration of intravenous contrast. The theory, which works most of the time, is that the abnormal tumor circulation allows contrast to penetrate the blood–brain barrier and enhance the tumor. Because contrast enhancement is white on a CT scan, the tumor becomes conspicuous. However, tumors can bleed, and the white of the contrast may obscure the white of the bleeding. Because the appearance of blood is an important issue in tumor patients, we often have to study them both with and without intravenous enhancement. In defining tumor and normal anatomy, MRI equals or surpasses CT in efficacy and few neurosurgeons would tackle a brain tumor without the aid of a contrast (gadolinium) MRI.

Just as with trauma, it is important to differentiate intraaxial masses (within the brain tissues) from extraaxial masses, as the differential diagnosis and approach are

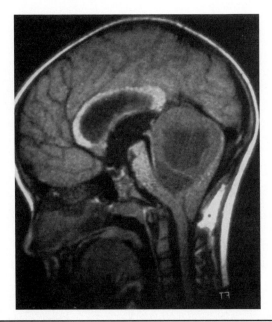

FIGURE 7-22. T1-weighted MRI documents a huge tumor that arises from the cerebellar vermis and pushes the brain stem forward. This is typical behavior of a medulloblastoma.

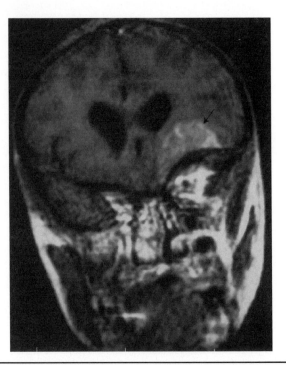

FIGURE 7-23. This large tumor *(arrow)* has a broad base along the roof of the orbit and displaces the frontal lobe of the brain superiorly. This growth is typical of an extraaxial tumor, in this case a meningioma.

different. Determining tumor origin is one of the most difficult diagnostic tasks. In general, an extraaxial tumor will display its widest base at the brain surface and will smoothly indent the brain from without (Fig. 7-23). Extraaxial tumors tend to be related to the meninges or the bones of the skull. Occasionally, a parenchymal brain tumor originates at the brain surface and differentiation is impossible. Conversely, extraaxial tumors sometimes grow from slips of tissues insinuated into the brain, giving the appearance of parenchymal masses.

Tumors that are entirely enveloped within the brain tissues are usually of glial cell origin, with astrocytoma being the most common primary tumor (Fig. 7-24) and metastasis being the most common overall. When the distinction of intraaxial from extraaxial is difficult and critical, using another modality with multiplanar imaging capability, such as MRI, is invaluable. MRI also offers different tissue contrast parameters, and contrast-enhanced MRI adds yet another dimension.

Once the tumor is diagnosed and localized to the proper anatomic location, the next job is to look at the mass effect caused by the tumor and to assess the likelihood of damage to critical centers of the brain requiring emergent action. Here, the principles applied in trauma are useful. Does the tumor cause displacement of the normal structures, such that they are sufficiently compressed to cause compromise of the blood supply or direct pressure damage to the cells of the normal brain tissue? If so, you have to move quickly. Once again, shift away from the tumor and alteration of the normal differentiation of the brain tissues are key to the proper determination.

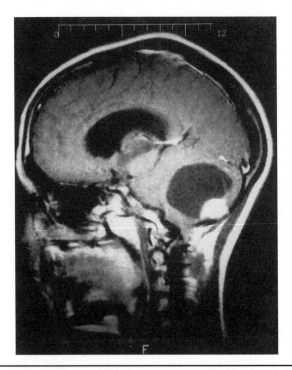

FIGURE 7-24. On gadolinium-enhanced MRI, this cerebellar tumor contains a very bright nidus of tissue within a cystic mass. This is characteristic of a pilocytic astrocytoma.

CONGENITAL ANOMALIES

Although CT is often used for the diagnosis of congenital anomalies of the brain, MRI, with its superior tissue contrast, is invaluable in this area. Congenital anomalies usually present in childhood, either with abnormal physical findings or with seizures. Physical abnormalities most often associated with congenital brain abnormalities include macrocephaly (big head), abnormal appearance of the face (particularly with midline abnormalities such as cleft palate), and meningocele. Each of these findings should tip you off to pursue a specific type of abnormality.

In the case of macrocranium (a big head), the likely diagnosis is hydrocephalus or dilatation of the ventricles because of abnormal CSF circulation. The lateral ventricles stand out so well owing to their CSF content that CT is well adapted to the initial diagnosis and monitoring of treatment for hydrocephalus (Fig. 7-25). The most critical factor is determining the cause of the hydrocephalus so that you can predict whether or not surgical shunting will be of value for the patient. In most instances the method is straightforward: One looks for the most caudal dilated ventricle and assumes that the obstruction is between that site and the most cephalad normal ventricle. For example, if the lateral and third ventricles are dilated but the fourth ventricle is normal, the obstruction is likely at the outflow area of the third ventricle or the aqueduct of Sylvius (Fig. 7-26).

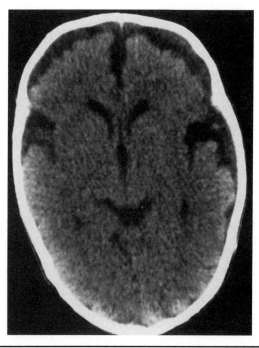

FIGURE 7-25. This child presented with a large head. Family history documented macrocranium in several other family members including the father. The head CT scan shows the ventricles to be slightly enlarged and the subarachnoid spaces to be prominent. This constellation of findings is diagnostic for benign familial macrocranium. In this instance, the child needed no treatment and the CT scan was sufficient to exclude a major problem.

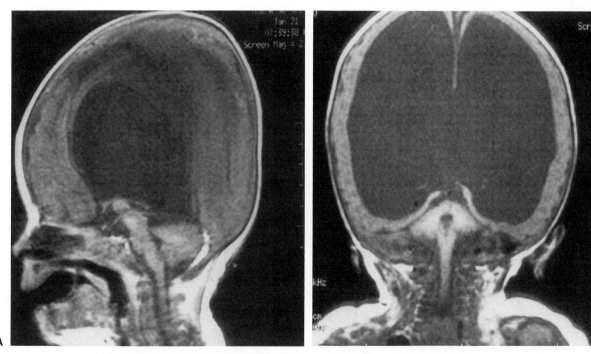

A   B

FIGURE 7-26. A sagittal **(A)** and coronal **(B)** MRI of an infant with a huge head at birth. The child has severe hydrocephalus involving the lateral and third ventricles but a normal fourth ventricle. This is suggestive of an aqueductal obstruction.

Often obstructive hydrocephalus can become static owing to equilibration of the CSF dynamics of production and absorption. In this case, it may not be necessary to place a shunt to drain the CSF. Once the dilated ventricles are detected, the need to shunt can be determined by following the ventricular size over time. This should, of course, be coupled with close observation of the patient's clinical status. Don't ever let the imaging hold you back if your patient is deteriorating. CT scans provide sufficient detail for monitoring progression of hydrocephalus. MRI is often of value in the initial evaluation of hydrocephalus, but follow-up monitoring is the domain of CT. Hydrocephalus can occur on other than a congenital basis, but the rules outlined here for evaluation hold for most instances.

MRI is the best method for initial evaluation of most babies with complex defects of the face and brain because of its multidimensional imaging capability. Holoprosencephaly, or failure of division of the embryonic forebrain, is always associated with facial anomalies and is a good prototype for illustrating the value of MRI. This complex series of anomalies ranges all the way from a totally malformed brain, a condition not compatible with life, to agenesis of the septum pellucidum and optic abnormalities (septooptical dysplasia), conditions compatible with long life (Fig. 7-27). Whereas CT scans are sufficient for the gross defects of holoprosencephaly, MRI can show sufficient detail to define the absence of the septum pellucidum as well as showing the midline defects of the optic tracts. If you have one test to do in these children, MRI is the best.

Meningocele is a common condition caused by failure of closure of the embryonic neural tube. This condition is almost invariably associated with a complex series of abnormalities called the Arnold-Chiari II malformation. The

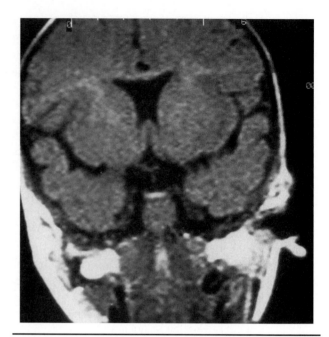

FIGURE 7-27. MRI of an infant with septooptical dysplasia documents the minimal abnormality of incomplete septation of the lateral ventricles by showing a deficiency of the septum pellucidum.

reason all of these brain anomalies are associated with what commonly is a spinal abnormality is complex, but the findings are reproducible and best demonstrated by MRI (Fig. 7-28). The tethering of the spinal cord that occurs with meningocele is associated with protrusion of the cerebellar tonsils below the foramen magnum. As with our other examples, the complex anatomy in developmental brain anomalies is best shown by MRI.

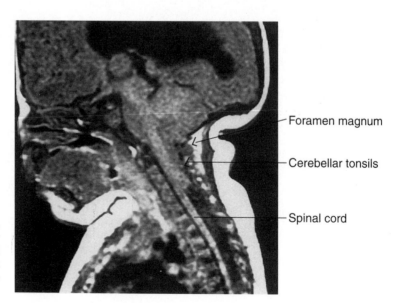

FIGURE 7-28. MRI from a baby with lumbar myelomeningocele. The posterior fossa is small and the cerebellar tonsil protrudes far below the foramen magnum. This is a constant component of the Arnold-Chiari malformation.

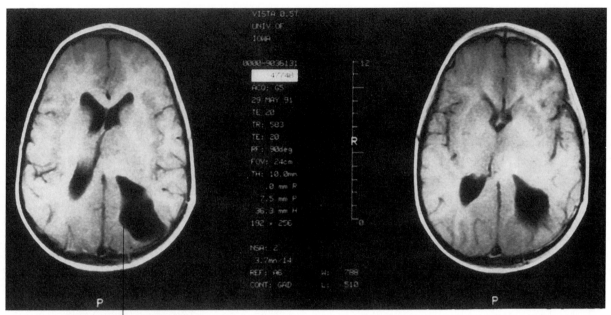

Schizencephalic cleft

FIGURE 7-29. A child with seizures. MRI shows a cleft from the posterior portion of the left lateral ventricle all the way to the brain surface. This condition, caused by a failure of proper migration of neurons as the brain is formed, is called *schizencephaly.*

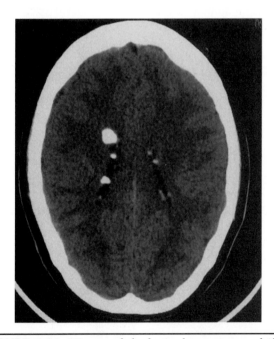

FIGURE 7-30. CT scan of the brain demonstrates calcification in the roof of each lateral ventricle. These calcifications are within the hamartomas or tubers. MRI would also demonstrate the hamartomas as well as showing the lesions that are not calcified.

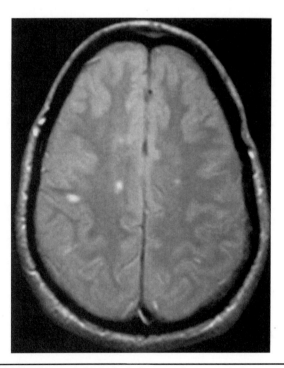

FIGURE 7-31. Multiple high-density white matter lesions are consistent with a myelodegenerative phenomenon, in this case multiple sclerosis. These findings are not specific and must be combined with the clinical and laboratory results to be diagnostic.

The finding of seizures in a child suggests a congenital defect, either structural or owing to a metabolic problem. In either case, MRI is more likely to yield the correct answers. Structural abnormalities include errors of neuronal migration where the brain tissues are arrested in their normal growth, leaving focal islands of tissue in abnormal locations throughout the brain (Fig. 7-29). Other structural abnormalities result from abnormal arrests of tissues proliferating and disrupting the normal brain tissue. A good prototype condition here is tuberous sclerosis (Fig. 7-30), although any other phakomatosis can give similar problems. Metabolic abnormalities causing seizures usually cause demyelination, thereby affecting the white matter either diffusely or as focal lesions (Fig. 7-31). MRI is clearly superior to CT here, although the findings are not specific for one disease process; focal infection or demyelinating disorders such as multiple sclerosis can look the same as metabolic defects.

There are many other potential uses for imaging in neurologic disease. However, if you retain the general principals elucidated here, you can make most of the diagnoses needed for patient care, whether or not you completely master all of the nuances of the differential diagnosis.

KEY POINTS

- Computerized axial tomography (CAT), or computed tomography (CT), is the most commonly performed neuroimaging study in the United States. CT scans can depict the brain in horizontal planes that can be viewed at different levels.
- When assessing a CT scan for potential trauma, begin by looking for blood in the head outside the vascular system. Blood appears on CT initially as a white blob.
- Mass effect is a clue that pressure is impinging on an area of the brain. The best way to find significant mass effect is to look for asymmetry with displacement of the midline structures.
- Obliteration of the distinction between gray and white matter in the brain represents profound edema. If the edema is universal, you are witnessing a "bad black brain," which portends a poor outcome and is almost always caused by a limitation of oxygen in the brain.
- On CT, acute strokes often initially appear as a dark edematous blotch obliterating the normal tissue density. On many MRI sequences with inversion recovery or T2 weighting, the damaged tissues are white because of water leaked by the ischemic cells. Diffusion MRI is the most sensitive imaging test for acute stroke.
- Tumors that are entirely enveloped in the brain tissues are usually of glial cell origin, with astrocytoma being the most common primary tumor.
- Complex anatomy in developmental brain anomalies is best shown with MRI.
- Physical abnormalities most often associated with congenital brain abnormalities include macrocephaly (big head), abnormal appearance of the face (particularly with midline abnormalities such as cleft palate), and meningocele.

SUGGESTED READING

Osborn A. *Diagnostic neuroradiology*. St. Louis, MO: Mosby, 1994.

Head and Neck

Yutaka Sato

In this chapter, a short overview of head and neck imaging is presented. With the recent advancement and widening availability of sectional imagings, such as CT and MRI, the part played by the plain radiographs has decreased significantly.

As an initial screening of sinusitis or facial trauma, radiographs may be used when more sophisticated sectional imagings are not readily available. For facial bone and paranasal sinus evaluation, routine radiographic views include Water's (Fig. 8-1), Caldwell (Fig. 8-2) and lateral (Fig. 8-3) views. Lack of aeration in the sinus antra is suggestive of sinusitis, and a definitive diagnosis can be made when an air–fluid level is present. CT is the primary modality for the evaluation of sinus infection and facial trauma (Figs. 8-4 to 8-6), because bone detail is best evaluated by CT. Because of multiple horizontally-placed buttresses of the facial skeleton, coronal-plane CT images are often used for evaluation (Figs. 8-7 to 8-9).

MR imaging is the modality of choice for the evaluation of neoplastic lesions of the head and neck because of its superior soft tissue characterization and multiplanar capability. MR imaging is essential to evaluate skullbase involvement by head and neck tumors.

SINUSITIS

Clinical presentation of pain, swelling over the paranasal sinuses and leukocytosis are sufficient for the diagnosis of sinusitis; and, in the majority of cases, imaging is not necessary. When intraorbital or intracranial extension of the inflammatory process is suspected and surgical intervention is contemplated, imaging becomes necessary. CT is the modality of choice. Acute fluid collection in the sinus cavity is diagnostic, and associated findings include

mucosal thickening (Fig. 8-10) and erosive or destructive changes of the sinus wall. Extension of the inflammatory process into the orbits (Fig. 8-11) or cranial cavity may be seen and help to determine the therapeutic approach.

For evaluation of children, the developmental sequence of the paranasal sinus should be taken into consideration. Generally, the ethmoid and maxillary sinuses are present at birth but may not be aerated. The sphenoid and frontal sinuses start to be seen at about 3 and 6 years of age, respectively.

TRAUMA

For the evaluation for facial fractures, CT is also the modality of choice. Nasal fractures are the most common, followed by zygomatic fractures. Zygomatic fractures commonly involve the following: (a) the lateral orbital wall at the frontozygomatic suture, (b) the maxillozygomatic suture and (c) the zygomatic arch; they are called trimalar or tripod fractures (Fig. 8-12). If the facial fracture extends posteriorly and violates the pterygoid plate, the fractured facial bones are detached from the cranium. Depending on the level of the fracture line traversing the central midface, these fractures are classified as Le Fort I, II or III fractures (Figs. 8-13 and 8-14). CT is essential to evaluate the entrapped soft tissue and nerves by the fracture fragments, which may require urgent decompression.

Orbital blowout fracture occurs when an object larger than the orbit, such as a fist or a baseball, hits the eye. The impact is transmitted to the orbital contents and raises the intraorbital pressure enough to shatter the weakest wall of the orbit, either the inferior wall into the maxillary sinus (Fig. 8-15) or the medial wall (lamina papyracea) into the ethmoid sinus, without fracturing the orbital rim.

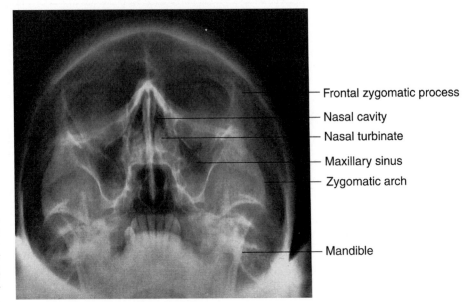

— Frontal zygomatic process
— Nasal cavity
— Nasal turbinate
— Maxillary sinus
— Zygomatic arch

— Mandible

FIGURE 8-1. Normal Water's view of the face, showing the good delineation of the maxilla. The maxillary sinuses are optimally displayed, and the anterior portions of the orbit and the nasal cavity are clearly outlined.

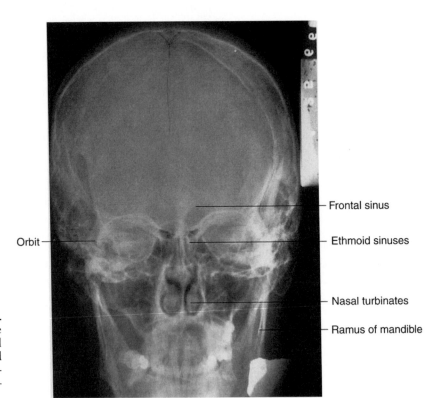

Orbit—

— Frontal sinus

— Ethmoid sinuses

— Nasal turbinates

— Ramus of mandible

FIGURE 8-2. A Caldwell, or PA, view of the face. Note how well the orbits and frontal bone are seen. The maxilla is superimposed on the skull base to some degree. The structures of the internal auditory canals are visible through the orbits.

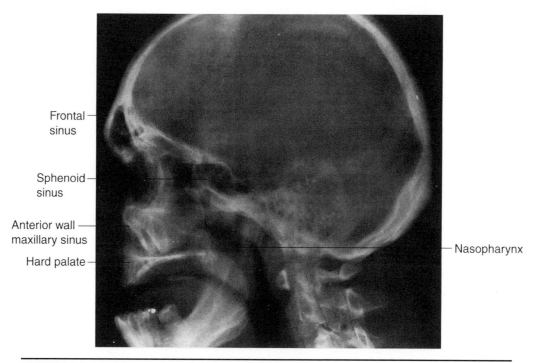

FIGURE 8-3. Lateral view of the skull shows the posteriorly-located sphenoid sinus and the nasopharyngeal airway. This view complements the others, adding the third dimension to the structures of the head and neck.

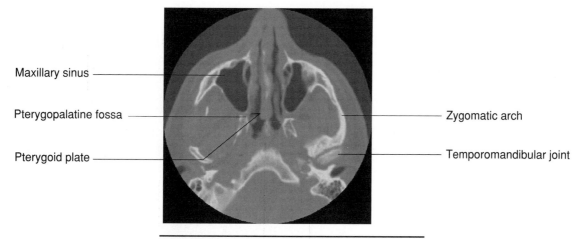

FIGURE 8-4. Normal axial CT image (inferior plane).

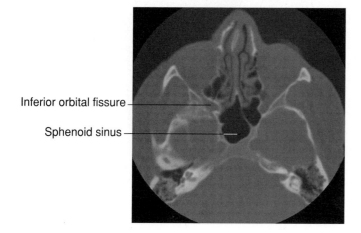

FIGURE 8-5. Normal axial CT image (medial plane).

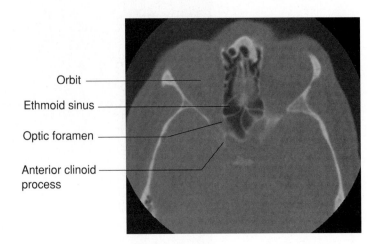

FIGURE 8-6. Normal axial CT image (superior plane).

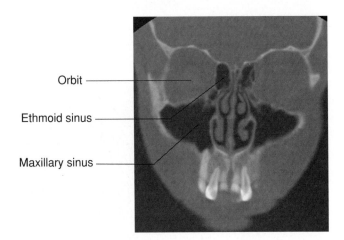

FIGURE 8-7. Normal coronal CT image (anterior plane).

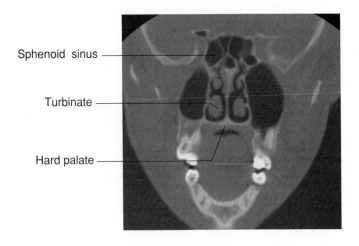

FIGURE 8-8. Normal coronal CT image (medial plane).

Anterior clinoid process

Nasal septum

Mandible

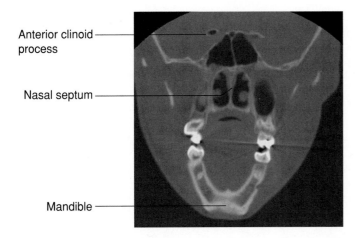

FIGURE 8-9. Normal coronal CT image (posterior plane).

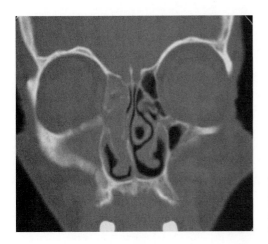

FIGURE 8-10. Chronic maxillary sinusitis. The right maxillary sinus is opacified by thickened mucosa, and mucosal thickening extends into the right nasal cavity. Also, notice sclerotic thickening of the sinus wall, suggestive of the chronic nature of the sinusitis.

Subperiosteal abscess

Lamina papyracea

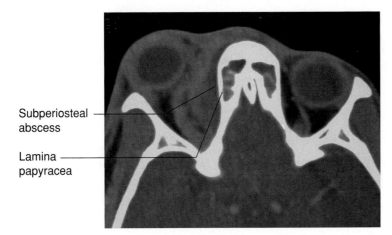

FIGURE 8-11. Orbital cellulitis and subperiosteal abscess. Inflammation of the ethmoid sinus extends into the orbit through the thin wall lamina papyracea, forming a subperiosteal abscess.

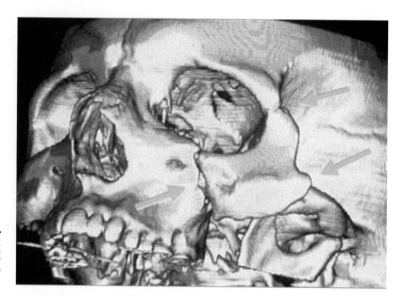

FIGURE 8-12. Tripod fracture. 3D reformatted CT. Note the fractures involved: (a) the lateral orbital wall, (b) the maxillozygomatic suture and (c) the zygomatic arch.

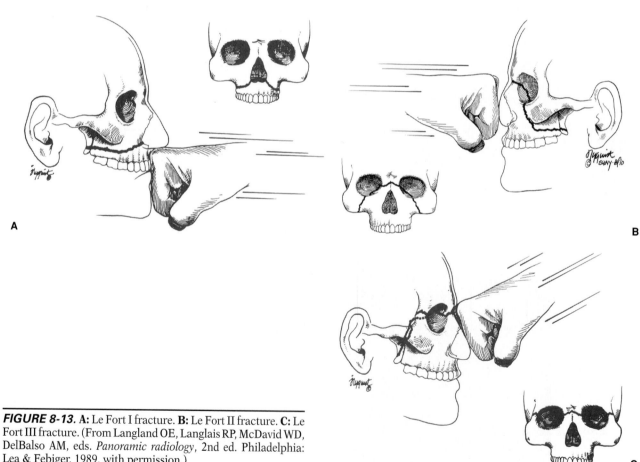

FIGURE 8-13. A: Le Fort I fracture. **B:** Le Fort II fracture. **C:** Le Fort III fracture. (From Langland OE, Langlais RP, McDavid WD, DelBalso AM, eds. *Panoramic radiology*, 2nd ed. Philadelphia: Lea & Febiger, 1989, with permission.)

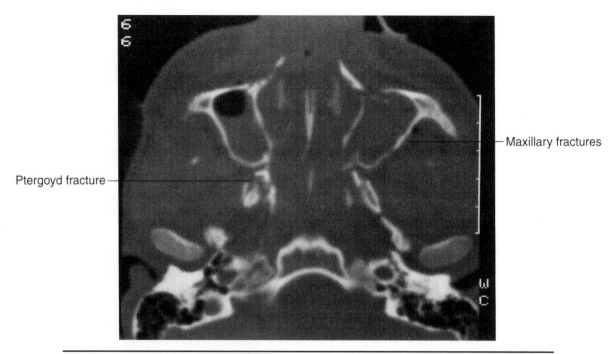

Pterygoyd fracture

Maxillary fractures

FIGURE 8-14. CT scan of an auto accident victim who struck the windshield. There are multiple fractures including disruption of the deeper structures of the face (pterygoid plates illustrated). This is a complex fracture pattern of the Le Forte type and can be defined well only with CT.

The inferior rectus muscle may be trapped and cause paralysis of the inferior gaze of the affected eye.

TUMORS

MRI is the modality of choice for evaluating the neoplastic lesions of the head and neck. The histologic diagnosis of head and neck neoplasms is usually made by fine-needle biopsy, and imagings are primarily used to evaluate the extent of the disease, to delineate the relationship of the tumor to the adjacent anatomic structures and to evaluate metastasis to the regional lymph nodes. All of this information is essential to determine the optimal mode of therapy. MRI is essential, particularly for the evaluation of skull-base involvement by head and neck tumors (Fig. 8-16).

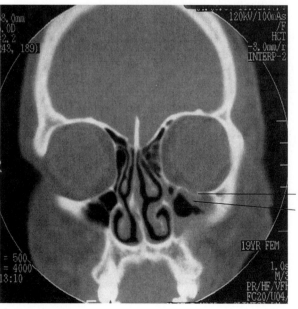

Blowout fracture
Entrapped muscle

FIGURE 8-15. A blowout fracture of the orbit caused by a fist to the eye. Note the soft tissue mass protruding into the maxillary sinus. This woman had no gaze abnormality on presentation for care, but developed one shortly thereafter. The fracture required surgical reconstruction, but the patient now has a normally-functioning eye.

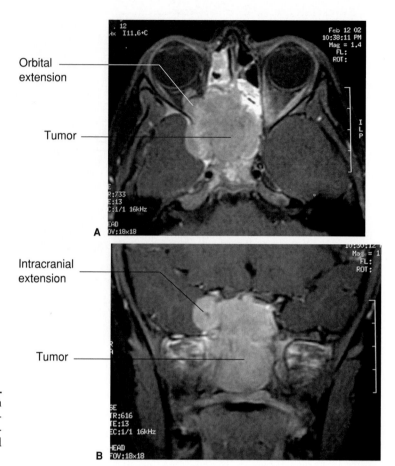

FIGURE 8-16. Rhabdomyosarcoma originating from the nasal cavity. Axial **(A)** and coronal **(B)** contrast-enhanced T1-weighted MR images show an avidly-enhancing tumor extending into the right orbit and into the cranium through the central skullbase.

In adults, squamous cell carcinoma is the most common malignant head and neck mass. Among the pediatric age group, benign masses are more common than malignant ones. Benign masses include congenital cystic lesions, such as thyroglossal cysts and branchial cleft cysts. Benign neoplasms seen in this age group include teratoma and juvenile angiofibroma. Rhabdomyosarcoma is the most common pediatric head and neck malignancy.

KEY POINTS

- CT is the imaging modality of choice in the evaluation of sinusitis and facial bone fractures.
- Imaging features of sinusitis include (a) acute fluid collection of the sinus cavity, (b) mucosal thickening and (c) erosion of the bony wall of the sinus.
- Tripod fractures involve the (a) lateral orbital wall, (b) maxillozygomatic suture and (c) zygomatic arch.

- In Le Fort fractures, the facial bones are detached from the cranium by the fracture of the pterygoid plates.
- In orbital blowout fractures, the inferior rectus muscle may be trapped by the fracture fragments of the orbital floor, requiring surgical release.
- MR is the imaging modality of choice in evaluating head and neck tumors. A skullbase extension of the tumor requires MR imaging.
- In adults, malignant mass lesions are common. In children, benign masses are more common.

SUGGESTED READINGS

Som PM, Curtin HD. *Head and neck imaging,* 2nd ed. St. Louis, MO: Mosby, 2003.
Harnsberger RH. *Handbook of head and neck imaging,* 2nd ed. St. Louis, MO: Mosby, 1995.

Nuclear Imaging

David L. Bushnell, Jr.

Nuclear medicine is an important medical specialty that uses measurements of radioactive tracer behavior in the body to detect and assess various types of diseases. The physiologic images generated by nuclear imaging procedures reveal less anatomic detail than radiologic studies. It is therefore often necessary to correlate the nuclear images with the corresponding radiologic images. Although there are also several therapeutic applications for radioactive agents, the primary emphasis of this chapter will be on diagnostic nuclear imaging.

TECHNICAL ASPECTS OF NUCLEAR IMAGING

When molecules with radionuclide components are prepared for administration to human beings, they are called *radiopharmaceuticals*. The radionuclide portion of the radiopharmaceutical typically emits radiation in the form of gamma rays and/or x-rays that can be detected and used to create the scintigraphic images (often loosely referred to as scans). Radiopharmaceuticals participate in, but do not alter, various physiologic processes. Specific radiopharmaceuticals with particular physiochemical properties are used to study an organ or organ system. Although radiopharmaceuticals can be introduced into the body in several different ways, the most common mode of administration is intravenously through a peripheral vein.

Side effects from the administration of radiopharmaceuticals for diagnostic imaging are extremely rare. The probability of an adverse reaction from the radiation exposure received by a patient or technologist during a diagnostic nuclear medicine procedure is so small that it has not been measurable to date.

Gamma ray imaging systems are used to detect the radiation emitted from the patient and to create images that depict the regional distribution of the radiopharmaceutical within the body. The most common of these imaging systems is the gamma camera. Gamma cameras use a sodium iodide crystal to detect the gamma rays and x-rays. Photons striking the crystal produce light scintillations that are converted to a digital signal. This digital information is stored in a computer and can be transferred to film or interpreted directly from the computer screen (Fig. 9-1). The resultant picture is often referred to as a scan or more appropriately a scintigraphic image. The image is essentially a physiologic map of the radiopharmaceutical distribution within the body. Table 9-1 presents the radiopharmaceuticals and the corresponding imaging procedures that are discussed in this chapter.

VENTILATION AND PERFUSION LUNG IMAGING FOR DIAGNOSIS OF PULMONARY EMBOLISM

Pulmonary thromboembolism (PTE) is a common disorder associated with significant mortality rates, which can be reduced with the appropriate detection and treatment.

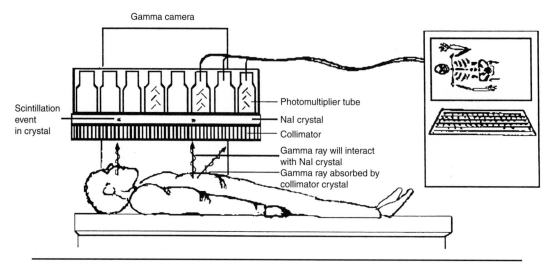

FIGURE 9-1. The basic gamma camera imaging system. The gamma rays that exit the patient perpendicular to the surface of the camera are not absorbed by the collimator and reach the scintillation crystal where they are detected. The pattern of the gamma ray photons striking the crystal is used to create a digital image on the computer. NaI indicates sodium iodide.

Establishing the diagnosis of PTE is often very difficult. Although dyspnea, tachypnea, and sinus tachycardia are present in the large majority of individuals with acute PTE, these symptoms and signs may result from any number of cardiopulmonary disorders. *The diagnosis of pulmonary embolism cannot be made with a high degree of reliability based on clinical findings alone.*

A chest radiograph should be obtained in all patients suspected of having pulmonary embolism. The chest x-ray (CXR) is needed to rule out other causes of the patient's symptoms such as pneumonia, pneumothorax, heart failure, and so on. However, the radiograph may appear entirely normal even when PTE is present. Even if the chest radiograph is abnormal and consistent with PTE, the results are never adequately predictive to form the basis of a therapeutic decision. Consequently, more specific diagnostic procedures are necessary for the workup of individuals who fall into this category.

Perfusion lung imaging is an invaluable tool in the workup of PTE and should be obtained in suspected cases of PTE, particularly when results from the CXR are normal. Scintigraphic perfusion lung imaging has a very high sensitivity for detecting PTE. Images of regional pulmonary perfusion are obtained by intravenously injecting several hundred thousand tiny particles of macroaggregated human albumin that are radiolabeled with technetium-99m (Tc-99m). These particles

▌ **TABLE 9-1 Radiopharmaceuticals Discussed in This Chapter**

Radiopharmaceutical	Imaging Procedure
Tc-99m macroaggregated albumin	Lung perfusion
Xenon-133, Tc-99m diethylenetriamine pentaacetic acid (DTPA) aerosol	Lung ventilation
Tc-99m iminodiacetic acid	Hepatobiliary dynamics
Tc-99m diphosphonate	Skeletal
Tc-99m DTPA	Renal glomerular filtration rate
Thallium-201, Tc-99m sestamibi, Tc-99m tetrofosmin	Myocardial perfusion
F-18 fluorodeoxyglucose (FDG)	PET tumor imaging

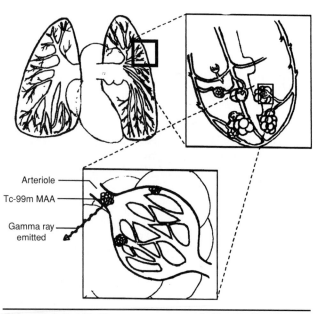

FIGURE 9-2. A Tc-99m macroaggregated albumin (MAA) particle as it becomes trapped in the pulmonary capillaries and emits gamma rays.

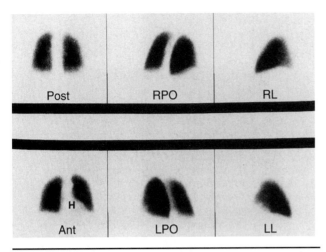

FIGURE 9-3. Normal perfusion lung images in six projections. Ant, anterior; Post, posterior; LPO, left posterior oblique; RPO, right posterior oblique; LL, left lateral; RL, right lateral. "H" designates area of absent activity due to the heart.

have diameters of 10 to 40 μm. Because the diameter of pulmonary capillaries and precapillary arterioles is less than 10 μm, the radioactive particles lodge in these vessels throughout the lung fields in concentrations that are directly proportional to the regional pulmonary perfusion (Fig. 9-2). Because less than 0.1% of the total cross section of the pulmonary vasculature is occluded by the injected radiolabeled particles, complications are extremely rare.

Figure 9-3 shows an example of the normal pulmonary blood flow pattern. Patients with PTE often display diminished or absent blood flow to one or more lung segments (Fig. 9-4A). The emboli are often large enough to occlude the segmental pulmonary arteries, and hence the flow defects on the images will often appear segmental in configuration. However, thromboembolic occlusion of smaller arteries may occur, and the perfusion

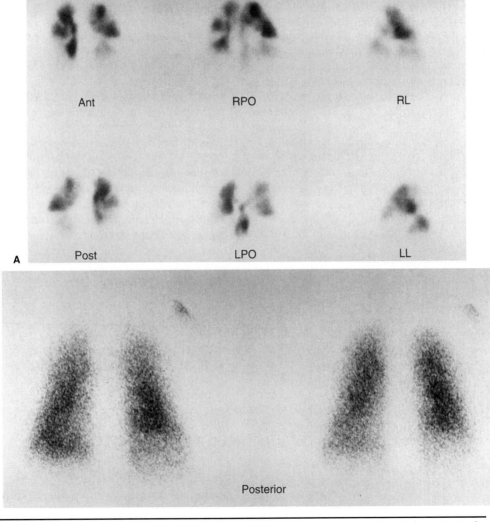

FIGURE 9-4. A: Six-view perfusion scan showing numerous bilateral segmental flow defects. **B:** Single-breath ventilation images showing normal ventilation. This pattern is essentially diagnostic for PTE.

▶ **TABLE 9-2** **Pulmonary Diseases That Cause Decreased Regional Lung Perfusion with Corresponding Abnormal Ventilation**

Pneumonia
Chronic obstructive lung disease
Atelectasis
Asthma

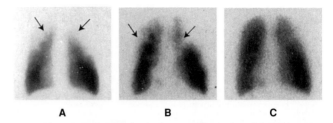

FIGURE 9-6. Patient with chronic obstructive pulmonary disease showing matching ventilation and perfusion defects in upper lobes *(arrows)*. **A:** Posterior perfusion image. **B:** Posterior initial breath hold ventilation image. **C:** Later equilibrium ventilation image showing eventual filling in of defects seen on the initial ventilation image.

pattern may therefore reveal defects that are somewhat smaller.

Lung pathology other than thromboemboli may cause alterations in the regional pulmonary blood flow pattern. Disorders of the lung parenchyma such as pneumonia, chronic obstructive lung disease, and regional atelectasis may lead to abnormalities of lung perfusion due to reflex vasoconstriction in the region of the pathology. As a result, the presence of one or more focal blood flow abnormalities is not necessarily specific for a diagnosis of pulmonary thromboemboli. It is for this reason that scintigraphic ventilation imaging of the lungs is typically combined with the perfusion study in the evaluation of PTE. Determination of the ventilation status of a lung region that shows abnormal perfusion improves the specificity of the test for the diagnosis of PTE. Diseases of the lungs that lead to abnormal regional perfusion and corresponding abnormal regional ventilation are summarized in Table 9-2.

Images of regional pulmonary ventilation are obtained by having the patient breath either radioactive xenon gas or an aerosolized form of Tc-99m diethylenetriamine pentaacetic acid (DTPA). A normal ventilation pattern with xenon is shown in Fig. 9-5.

Areas of the lung with diminished perfusion secondary to nonembolic lung pathology are associated with matching ventilation defects (Fig. 9-6). In contrast, ventilation usually appears normal in regions of the lung that show perfusion defects caused by thromboemboli (Figs. 9-4 and 9-7).

The intrinsic fibrinolytic system will lyse thromboemboli and often restore the pulmonary circulation within weeks and even days in some patients (Fig. 9-8). It is therefore important to obtain the ventilation/perfusion (V/P) examination early in the evaluation of the patient with PTE while the flow defects are still present.

Typically, results from the V/P study are used to estimate the probability that acute PTE has occurred. An entirely normal perfusion pattern indicates virtually no chance that the patient has emboli, and the clinician should then focus on a search for other causes of the patient's symptoms. A finding of multiple (two or more) segmental perfusion defects with a correspondingly normal ventilation pattern indicates a very high probability that the patient has PTE. However, V/P lung imaging does not always lead to a definitive result, particularly when substantial CXR abnormalities are present; then V/P imaging must be followed by ultrafast chest CT with contrast or pulmonary angiography for more conclusive diagnosis of PTE, as shown in Fig. 9-9.

HEPATOBILIARY IMAGING

Patients with acute cholecystitis classically present with right upper quadrant pain/tenderness, fever, and leukocytosis. However, the signs and symptoms of acute cholecystitis often vary, and there are a number of pathologic conditions that occasionally present in a similar fashion. Consequently, the provisional diagnosis of acute cholecystitis typically requires confirmatory testing with ultrasound and/or hepatobiliary scintigraphy.

Hepatobiliary scintigraphic imaging is performed using a Tc-99m-labeled iminodiacetic acid derivative that

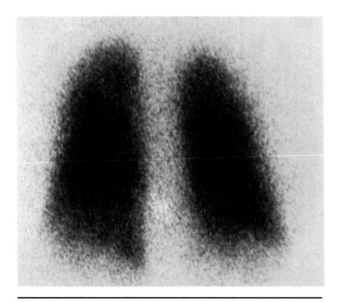

FIGURE 9-5. Normal xenon ventilation study. Posterior view of the initial breath hold image.

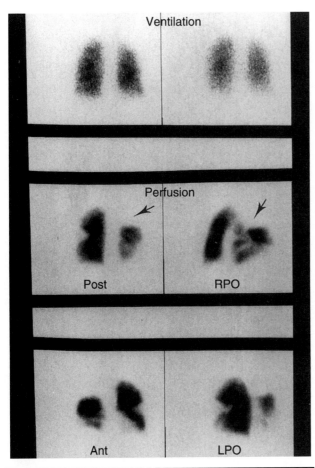

Ventilation

Perfusion

Post   RPO

Ant   LPO

FIGURE 9-7. Top two images are posterior ventilation images with xenon-133 showing uniform ventilation to both lungs. Bottom four images are from the perfusion study showing multiple segmental defects. *Arrow* points to region of absent perfusion in what is probably all three segments of the right upper lobe. Note that the lung regions with flow defects have normal ventilation. This pattern indicates a very high probability for PTE.

is an analog of bilirubin. This radiopharmaceutical is actively transported into hepatocytes by the same system that transports bilirubin and is excreted unchanged into the biliary tract.

In normal individuals, the hepatobiliary radiotracer will flow into the gallbladder within the first hour after intravenous administration (Fig. 9-10). However, in acute cholecystitis the gallbladder fails to fill with the radiotracer because of cystic duct obstruction by a stone. This test is extremely sensitive, and a normal result (i.e., visualization of the gallbladder) virtually excludes the possibility of acute cholecystitis. It is important to note that there are certain conditions that predispose to false-positive results. The most common false-positive result occurs in prolonged fasting of more than 2 or 3 days. Under this condition, the gallbladder rarely contracts and its contents begin to partially solidify into a gelatinous material that

TABLE 9-3 Conditions That May Yield False-Positive Results with Hepatobiliary Imaging in the Evaluation of Acute Cholecystitis

Prolonged fasting (3 days)
Ingestion of food within 2 hours of the study
Chronic cholecystitis
Chronic alcohol abuse
Pancreatitis

can impede or block the entry of the radioactive bile into the gallbladder. The gallbladder also fails to visualize in many patients who have ingested food within 2 hours of the hepatobiliary study as a result of the high level of circulating cholecystokinin causing gallbladder contraction, which limits entry of the radioactive bile. For this reason, scintigraphic hepatobiliary imaging should not be performed within 2 hours of a meal. Conditions that lead to false-positive (gallbladder nonvisualization) results are summarized in Table 9-3.

The use of morphine with hepatobiliary imaging has been found to be helpful in reducing the number of false-positive results, thereby improving the specificity of the test. Morphine causes constriction of the sphincter of Odi and leads to a rise in biliary system pressure. This augments bile movement through the cystic duct, improving gallbladder visualization. For this reason, the use of morphine has become standard practice with this procedure. Figure 9-11 shows a case in which a normal gallbladder became visible only after administration of morphine. Figure 9-12 shows a patient with acute cholecystitis and gallbladder nonvisualization both before and after administration of morphine.

Hepatobiliary imaging can be used in infants to help distinguish biliary atresia from neonatal hepatitis, and it is a very sensitive test for detecting acute common bile duct obstruction in adults. The study has also been used successfully to identify biliary leaks due to trauma, surgery, or acute cholecystitis.

SKELETAL IMAGING

Skeletal scintigraphic imaging, more commonly referred to as the bone scan, is a valuable tool for investigation of a number of disorders of the skeletal system. A Tc-99m-labeled diphosphonate derivative is used to perform skeletal scintigraphy because this radiolabeled agent is adsorbed onto the surface of newly forming hydroxyapatite crystal in the bone. New bone formation occurs in response to the presence of almost all skeletal pathology. Consequently, scintigraphic images will demonstrate increased gamma ray emissions localized to the site of bone abnormality.

(text continues on page 350)

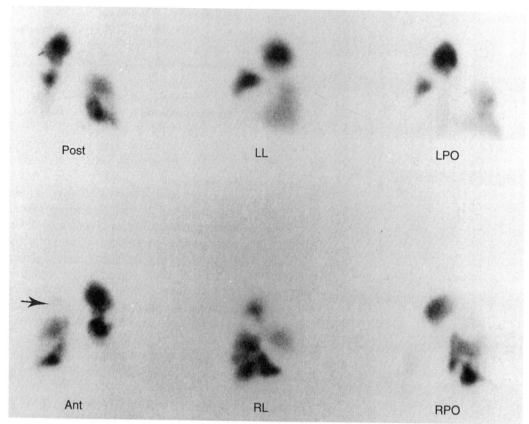

A

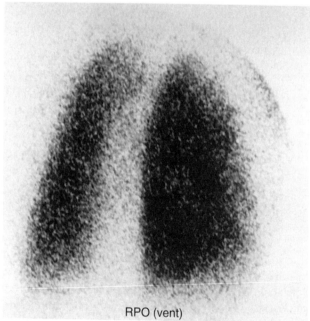

B

FIGURE 9-8. Patient with PTE showing resolution of flow defects over time. **A:** Lung perfusion study shortly after onset of patient's respiratory symptoms. Chest x-ray and ventilation study **(B)** were essentially normal. The diagnosis of PTE was established from these images and the patient was placed on heparin. Ten days later the patient had additional respiratory symptoms and the lung scan was repeated. **C:** The repeat study again showed multiple segmental defects of perfusion in the same locations as seen on the first exam. However, blood flow was almost completely restored to at least one large area (right upper lobe indicated by *arrow*).

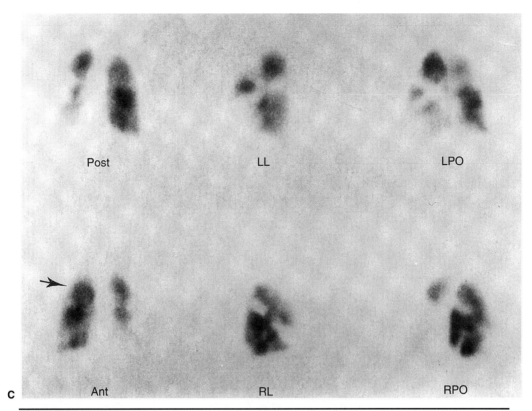

Post   LL   LPO

c   Ant   RL   RPO

FIGURE 9-8. (*Continued*)

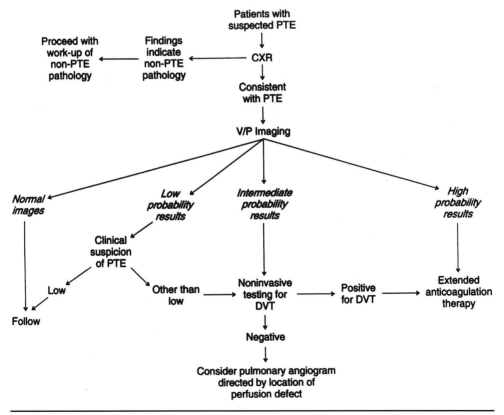

FIGURE 9-9. Flow diagram for use of test results in diagnosis and treatment of PTE.

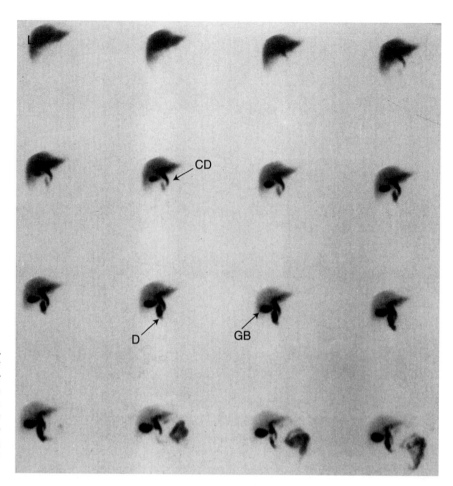

FIGURE 9-10. Normal hepatobiliary study. Images obtained in the anterior view every 2 minutes (moving from left to right and top to bottom) following injection of the hepatobiliary radiotracer show good extraction of the agent by the liver (L). The common bile duct *(arrow CD)* is seen along with the duodenum *(arrow D)* and gallbladder *(arrow GB)*.

It is important for clinicians to know whether skeletal metastases are present in patients with malignant tumors. Evaluation of patients for possible metastases is carried out predominantly in those individuals who have tumors that tend to metastasize to the bone, such as breast, lung, prostate, and renal carcinomas. Well-differentiated thyroid cancer is also prone to disseminate to sites in bone, but these lesions are probably better detected with iodine-131 imaging.

The normal bone scan appearance is shown in Fig. 9-13. The bone scan in a patient with skeletal metastases typically reveals numerous foci of excessive tracer accumulation, most commonly in the axial skeleton, but also to a lesser extent present in the appendicular skeleton (Fig. 9-14). Skeletal metastases usually arise as a result of hematogenous seeding of tumor cells in the bone marrow. Because most of the adult marrow resides in the axial skeleton, it makes sense that *the large majority of metastatic lesions are detected in the axial skeleton.*

The bone scan is very sensitive for detecting metastatic lesions and in general will identify a metastasis before a conventional radiograph can detect it. However, it is often not possible to ascertain whether lesions seen on a bone scan are malignant or benign, and this is particularly true for a single lesion, which often is caused by a benign process. *Numerous focal lesions are much more often due to metastatic disease.* In a patient with a single vertebral lesion on bone scan and a normal radiograph, it is often prudent to obtain an MRI study to better determine if a marrow metastasis is present.

Other skeletal abnormalities are also readily detected with a bone scan. Like metastases, osteomyelitis can be detected earlier with a bone scan than with a radiograph (Fig. 9-15). The bone scan is particularly useful in childhood osteomyelitis where early treatment is very important. The bone scan may also be useful to detect a nondisplaced fracture or traumatic lesion of a type not easily seen on radiographs. For example, lesions that originate from intense physical activity, such as stress fractures (Fig. 9-16) and shin splints (Fig. 9-17), are readily detected on a bone scan and may not be seen on a radiograph. In most cases, fractures through the full thickness of the bone cortex are readily detected by a plain radiograph. Some full-thickness fractures, such as those in the sacrum, scapula, femoral neck, and small bones of the wrist and ankle, are occasionally difficult to visualize on a radiograph, but are detectable by a bone scan.

(text continues on page 354)

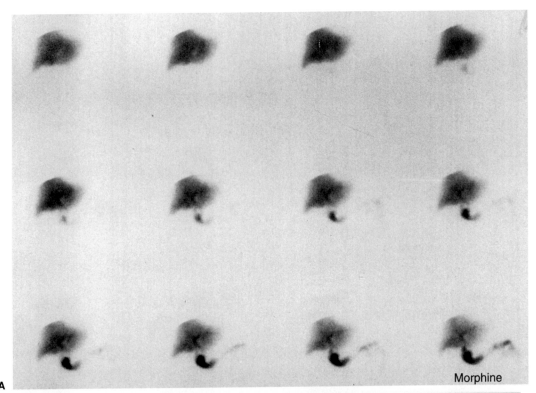

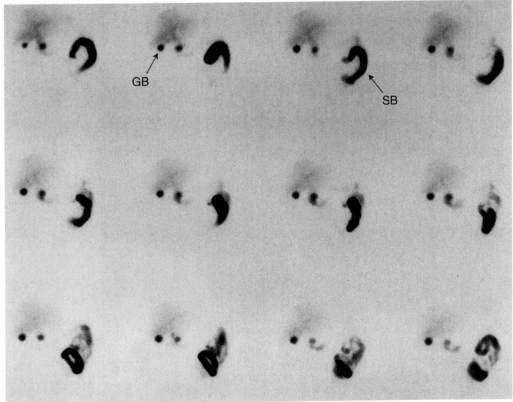

FIGURE 9-11. Hepatobiliary examination in a patient with right upper quadrant pain. **A:** Initial set of images show normal uptake and excretion by the liver, but over time the gallbladder is not visualized and consequently morphine is given at approximately 40 minutes into the study. **B:** Images obtained immediately following administration of morphine show the gallbladder visualization *(arrow GB)*, which effectively rules out acute cholecystitis. Note activity in the small bowel *(arrow SB)*.

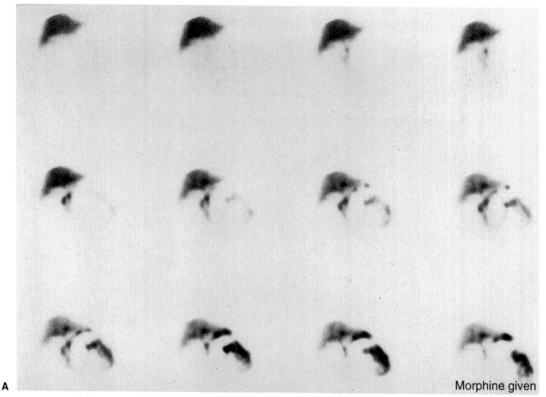

A

Morphine given

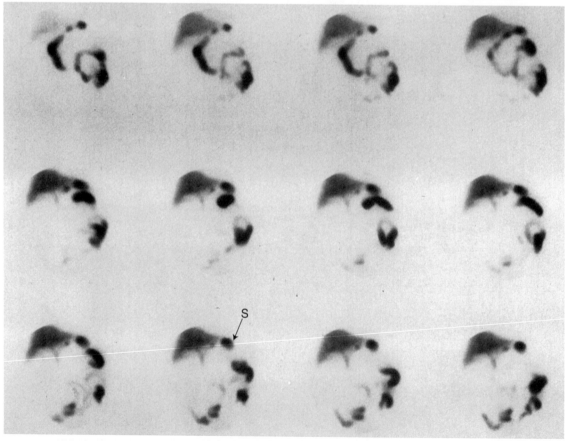

B

FIGURE 9-12. Hepatobiliary study in a patient with fever and right upper quadrant pain. **A:** Initial set of images show normal uptake and excretion by the liver, but the gallbladder is not visualized and consequently morphine is given at approximately the time of the image at bottom right. **B:** Images obtained immediately following injection of morphine continue to show absence of gallbladder activity, indicating cystic duct obstruction and very probably acute cholecystitis. Note the reflux of radioactive bile into the stomach *(arrow S).* The patient was taken to surgery and found to have acute cholecystitis.

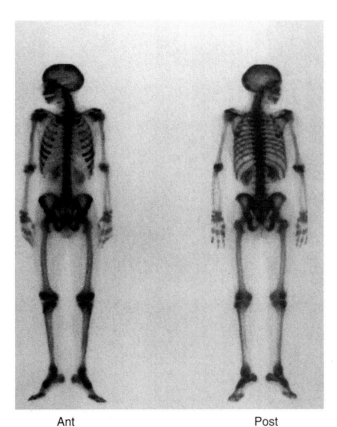

Ant   Post

FIGURE 9-13. Anterior and posterior whole-body images of a normal bone scan.

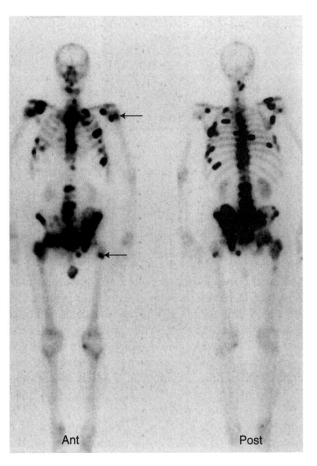

Ant   Post

FIGURE 9-14. Whole-body bone scan in anterior and posterior projections of a 65-year-old man with diffuse skeletal metastases from prostate carcinoma. Images reveal numerous metastatic lesions (black foci), primarily in the axial skeleton on both anterior and posterior views. However, lesions are also seen in the proximal femurs and humeri *(arrows)*.

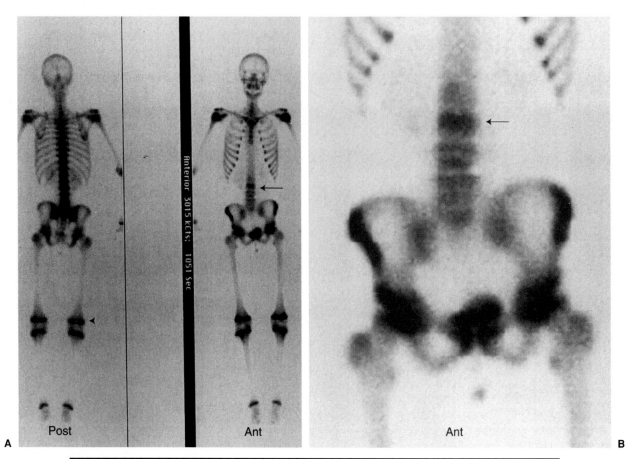

FIGURE 9-15. Skeletal scintigraphic images (whole body, **A**; regional view, **B**) from an 18-year-old girl with diabetes who presented with 3 to 4 weeks of low back pain. Radiographs of the vertebra were unremarkable. The images show abnormally increased technetium-99m (MDP) activity in the L-3 vertebral body *(arrow)*. Biopsy of the site confirmed osteomyelitis. Notice the normal intense uptake of Tc-99m MDP at the growth plates in the lower extremities *(arrowhead)* on the whole-body images.

ANGIOTENSIN-CONVERTING ENZYME INHIBITOR RENAL SCINTIGRAPHIC IMAGING

Scintigraphic imaging procedures can be used to evaluate renal perfusion and various aspects of renal function. Technetium-99m-labeled molecules that are filtered by the renal glomerulus can be used to assess glomerular filtration rate (GFR). Scintigraphic imaging of GFR combined with administration of an angiotensin-converting enzyme (ACE) inhibitor, such as captopril, is used to identify patients with hypertension caused by renal artery stenosis.

In patients with renal vascular hypertension (RVH), renin secretion is enhanced secondary to the hemodynamic effects of a functionally significant stenosis in the renal artery (Fig. 9-18). Decreased perfusion pressure as a result of the stenosis causes the juxtaglomerular cells to increase secretion of renin. Renin acts on angiotensino-

gen to form angiotensin I. Angiotensin I is converted to angiotensin II by ACE. Angiotensin II stimulates release of aldosterone and also acts as a potent vasoconstrictor of the peripheral vasculature, also including vasoconstriction of the efferent renal arterioles distal to the glomerulus in the under-perfused kidney with the stenosis. The efferent vasoconstriction acts to preserve the transglomerular pressure gradient and therefore helps to preserve the GFR in the affected kidney. If an ACE inhibitor such as captopril is administered in this setting, angiotensin II levels will drop and the efferent arterioles will dilate, leading to a fall in GFR in the stenotic kidney.

In patients with RVH, scintigraphic images of the kidneys obtained during ACE inhibition demonstrate this deterioration in GFR in the stenotic kidney (Fig. 9-19). In contrast, patients with essential hypertension will have no effect from captopril on the renal scintigraphic images (Fig. 9-20).

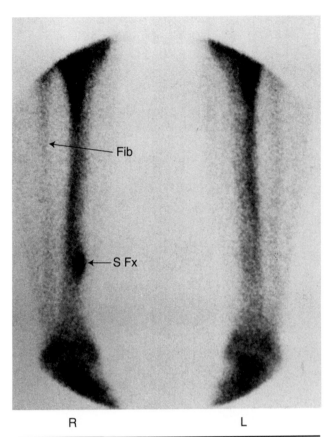

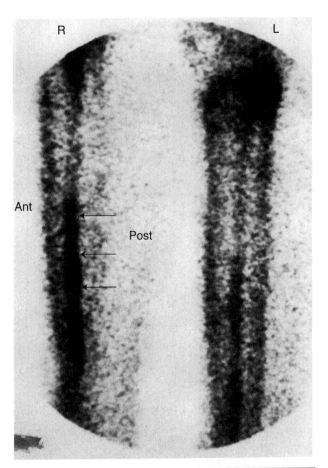

FIGURE 9-16. A 20-year-old woman with pain in the right distal lower extremity. Patient was an athlete in training with an extensive running regimen. Radiographs shortly after the onset of pain were normal. Scintigraphic images of the distal lower extremities show focal lesion in the posterior medial aspect of the right distal tibia consistent with a stress fracture *(arrow)*. Notice that the lesion does not involve the full thickness of the tibia. Fibula indicated by *long arrow*.

FIGURE 9-17. Bone scan in a patient with shin splints showing linear pattern of increased radiopharmaceutical concentration *(arrows)* along the posterior aspect of the tibia.

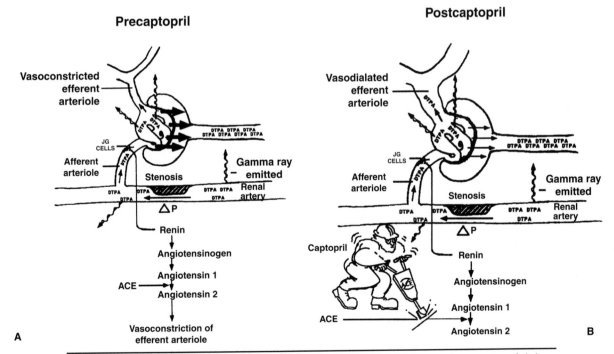

FIGURE 9-18. Effect of angiotensin-converting enzyme (ACE) inhibitor, such as captopril **(B)** on glomerular filtration rate in the setting of renal artery stenosis and renal vascular hypertension. **A:** Without ACE inhibitor.

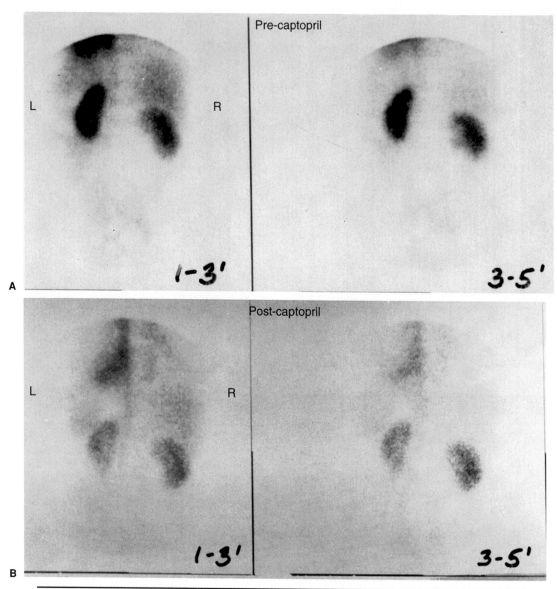

FIGURE 9-19. **A:** Scintigraphic images of the kidneys in the posterior projection, 1 to 3 minutes and 3 to 5 minutes following IV injection of a Tc-99m-labeled agent that is filtered by the glomerulus. **B:** Repeat images following administration of captopril show a significant decrease in the concentration of this agent (and therefore decrease in GFR) in the left kidney compared to the precaptopril study. This finding indicates renal artery stenosis causing renal vascular hypertension.

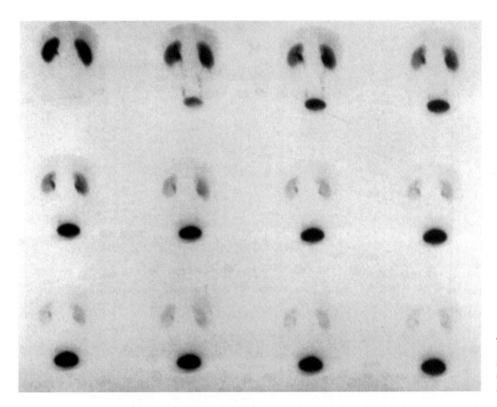

FIGURE 9-20. Patient with essential hypertension showing no effect of captopril on renal images.

Patients with a strongly positive scintigraphic ACE inhibitor study are very likely to experience improvement or cure in their hypertension if the stenosis is repaired. Conversely, patients with a completely normal result are very unlikely to respond to repair of the renal artery stenosis.

MYOCARDIAL PERFUSION IMAGING

Perfusion imaging of the myocardium can be performed using intravenous injected thallium-201 chloride or Tc-99m-labeled agents known as sestamibi or tetrofosmin. These substances accumulate in the myocardium in direct proportion to the regional myocardial blood flow and the number of viable myocytes. SPECT (single photon emission computed tomography) imaging is used to obtain perfusion images of the heart in three dimensions using one of these agents (Fig. 9-21). SPECT is a technique that yields a three-dimensional pattern of radiopharmaceutical distribution in the body with images displayed in cross section much like CT or MRI. A normal cardiac SPECT thallium-201 study shows uniform perfusion throughout the myocardium (Fig. 9-22).

Myocardial perfusion stress imaging can be performed with either exercise or a pharmacologic agent such as adenosine. Application of the cardiac stress improves the sensitivity of myocardial perfusion imaging for

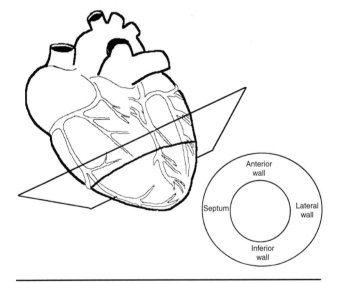

FIGURE 9-21. Single photon emission computed tomography (SPECT) short-axis cross section from the left ventricle. The short-axis cross-sectional view is obtained by slicing the three-dimensional image of the heart muscle in planes perpendicular to the long dimension of the heart.

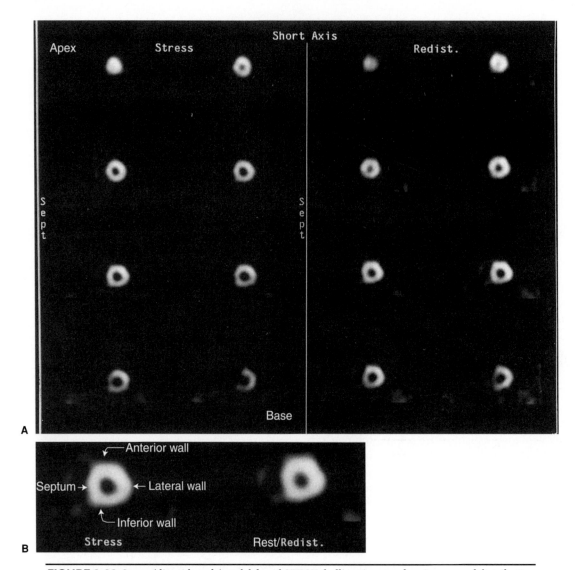

A

B

FIGURE 9-22. Stress (dipyridamole) and delayed SPECT thallium images showing normal distribution of thallium-201 in the left ventricular myocardium. **A:** All short-axis images from the apex of the heart to the base of the heart. **B:** Selected short-axis images from the midregion of the heart.

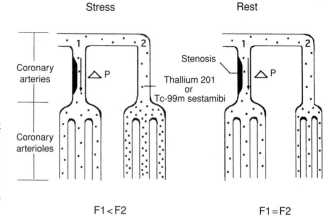

FIGURE 9-23. Diagram showing the effects on the caliber of coronary arterioles from a pressure gradient. Blood flow through the stenosed artery, F1, is essentially the same as flow through the normal artery, F2, at rest due to arteriolar vasodilatation. However, in the presence of a stress (exercise or pharmacologic), F2 increases to a greater extent than does F1, creating a discrepancy in regional myocardial perfusion.

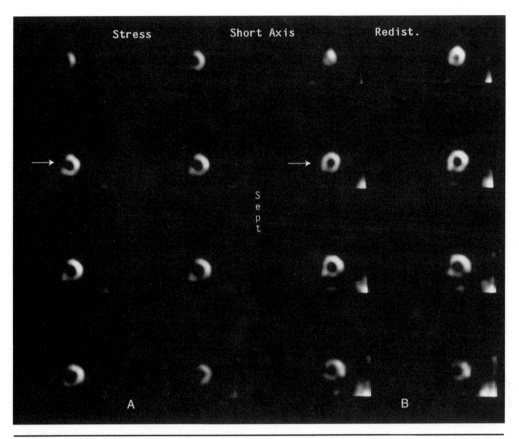

FIGURE 9-24. Thallium images from a patient with tight stenosis of the left anterior descending coronary artery; short-axis stress images **(A)** showing a severe perfusion defect in the septum, which is reversible on rest/redistribution images **(B)**.

detecting coronary artery disease. Arterioles distal to a normal coronary artery will dilate substantially in response to either exercise or pharmacologic stimulation. As a result, perfusion (and therefore radiotracer concentration) will increase considerably in the myocardium distal to a normal vessel, whereas myocardial perfusion will change little if at all distal to a significant stenosis (Fig. 9-23). Therefore, significant coronary artery disease will result in a perfusion defect on the cardiac images immediately following the stress (Fig. 9-24).

Perfusion defects seen on the stress images that become less severe or normalize on delayed images are referred to as reversible and almost always contain viable myocardium (Fig. 9-24). Defects that do not change from stress to the delayed images (termed "fixed") usually contain scar tissue. However, in some instances fixed defects might still contain viable tissue. This information is very important for making decisions about possible coronary bypass surgery. Figure 9-25 shows an example of a fixed thallium defect representing scar tissue from previous infarction.

Myocardial stress imaging can be used to select appropriate candidates with suspected coronary artery disease for coronary arteriography. In addition, this technique can provide information on the hemodynamic severity of coronary lesions already seen on the angiogram and thus assist in selecting patients for coronary revascularization procedures.

POSITRON EMISSION TOMOGRAPHY (PET)

PET differs somewhat from the more conventional nuclear medicine procedures because the radioisotopes that are used emit positrons and the imaging machine is consequently designed differently. After a positron is emitted, it travels a very short distance in body tissue (a few mm), combines with an electron, and the mass of the positron and electron are converted into energy in the form of two gamma rays that travel in opposite directions along a line. These gamma rays are detected by the PET machine, which then creates a three-dimensional

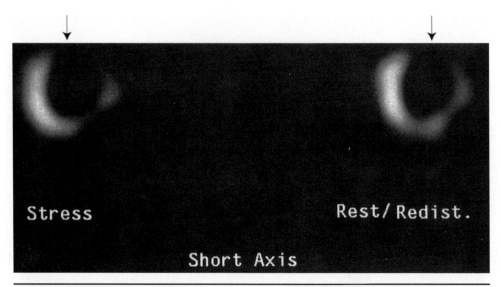

FIGURE 9-25. Thallium images from a patient with past infarction of the anterior wall, of the heart. Short-axis images show severe defects in the anterior wall *(arrows)* and lateral wall, both of which are fixed (unchanged from stress to rest/redistribution images). These findings are consistent with scarring in the anterior and lateral walls.

image set of the distribution of the radioisotope in the body.

Positron emitting radioisotopes include C-11, N-13, O-15, and F-18. These radioisotopes can in theory be labeled to virtually any organic molecule. Currently the primary PET radiopharmaceutical used in clinical practice is F-18-labeled fluorodeoxyglucose (FDG). PET imaging with FDG depicts the distribution of glucose metabolism in the body.

The large majority of malignant tumors demonstrate enhanced metabolism of glucose relative to normal organs, and consequently FDG PET imaging can be used to detect sites of malignancy throughout the body. A PET image of a patient with primary lung cancer is shown in Figure 9-26, and an image of a patient with lymphoma is presented in Figure 9-27.

RADIONUCLIDE THERAPY

Although a detailed discussion of the therapeutic applications of internally administered radionuclides is beyond the scope of this chapter, it is important to recognize this aspect of nuclear medicine. Generally, the radioactive isotopes being used now for therapy emit beta particles, and in the future alpha particle emitters may also be used. Currently the most common radioisotope used in therapy is I-131. In its elemental form this agent is used to treat thyroid disorders such as Graves disease and thyroid cancer. Because the iodine is trapped by the abnor-

mal thyroid cells, the radiation effect is concentrated at the desired site. A relatively new way of delivering a radioisotope to a selected target in the body is through the use of radiolabeled monoclonal antibodies (MoAb). The MoAb carrying the radioemitter will bind to a particular tumor cell surface antigen and thus deliver the radioisotope and its radioactive emissions directly to the tumor site. Two radiolabeled MoAbs are now available for clinical use in treating patients with non-Hodgkin's lymphoma (NHL). One is labeled with I-131 and the other is labeled with Y-90. Treatment with these agents, after standard chemotherapy has failed, leads to disease remission in 70% to 80% of patients with NHL. Table 9-4 lists some of the therapeutic uses of internally administered radioisotopes.

▶ **TABLE 9-4 Some Radioisotopes Used in Therapeutic Applications**

Radioisotope	Disease
Iodine-131, yttrium-90-labeled monoclonal antibodies	Lymphoma
Samarium-153, strontium-89	Skeletal metastases
Phosphorus-32	Polycythemia vera
Iodine-131	Thyroid cancer, Graves disease

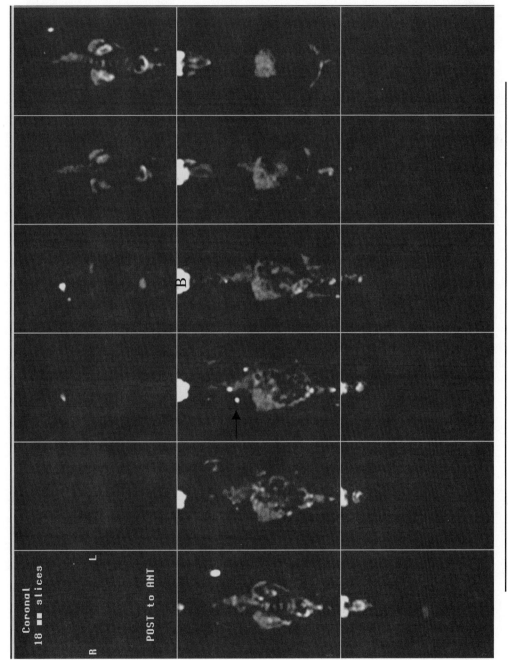

FIGURE 9-26. Tomographic coronal plane FDG PET images of a patient with primary lung cancer. The tumor has metastasized to numerous locations (white/bright foci). The primary lung tumor is noted by the *white arrow* in the right lung. Metastatic lesions are located in the proximal left humerus, posterior right third rib, left adrenal, mediastinum, and left lung base. Note the intense FDG metabolism in the brain (marked with a "B")

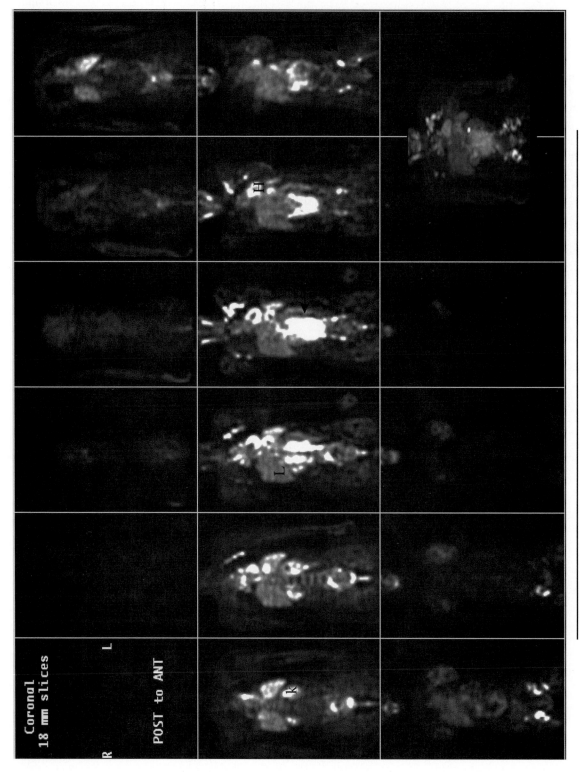

FIGURE 9-27. Tomographic coronal FDG PET images of a patient with non-Hodgkin's lymphoma prior to therapy. Widespread disease is seen in the chest and abdomen and other lymph node sites. *Horizontal arrow* indicates very large mass of tumor in retroperitoneal lymph nodes. Tumor in left inguinal node is also noted by *white arrow*. Note the high FDG metabolism in the heart (marked with an "H"). Liver (L) and left kidney (K) are also marked.

KEY POINTS

- Nuclear imaging is performed using radiolabeled molecules injected into the body to create images of organ physiology.
- Ventilation-perfusion lung imaging plays an important role in the workup of patients with suspected PTE.
- Normal pulmonary perfusion essentially rules out the diagnosis of PTE.
- Visualization of the gallbladder with hepatobiliary scintigraphy almost always rules out the diagnosis of acute cholecystis.
- Bone pathology (e.g., metastases) causes increased bone hydroxyapatite formation, leading to increased uptake of the bone scan radiopharmaceutical.
- Bone scintigraphy is a sensitive test for detecting skeletal metastases, osteomyelitis, and fractures.
- Captopril renal imaging accurately detects hemodynamically significant renal artery stenosis in patients with renovascular hypertension.

- Myocardial stress perfusion imaging is an accurate technique for detecting coronary artery disease.
- PET imaging with FDG can detect many types of malignant tumors.

ACKNOWLEDGMENTS

The author thanks Brian Clarke, CNMT, for his original drawings of Figs. 9-1, 9-2, 9-18, 9-21, and 9-23; Dr. Parvez Shirazi for supplying the images for Fig. 9-17; and Ms. Maryann O'Brien, MA, CNMT, for her assistance in preparing this manuscript.

SUGGESTED READINGS

Henkin RE, Boles MA, Dillehay GL, Halama JR, Karesh SM, Wagner RH, Zimmer AM, eds. *Nuclear medicine*. St. Louis, MO: Mosby, 1996.

Wagner HN, Szabo Z, Buchanan JW, eds. *Principles of nuclear medicine*. Philadelphia: WB Saunders, 1995.

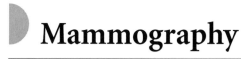

Chapter 10

Mammography

William E. Erkonen, Laurie L. Fajardo, and John W. Boardman

This chapter is short, but its importance is unrelated to its length. There are a number of good textbooks on this subject that are more encyclopedic, and you can and should refer to these (e.g., 1). The purpose of this chapter is to stress the importance of mammography in the management of breast disease and the screening for early cancer detection.

Approximately one in eight females in the United States will develop cancer of the breast during her lifetime, and this incidence appears to be increasing. Breast cancer currently involves over 180,000 women per year in the United States, and it causes approximately 44,000 deaths per year. An effective strategy to decrease the mortality associated with this disease is to find the lesions at an early and curable stage. Mammography can detect early invasive lesions or carcinomas *in situ* that measure only a few millimeters before they become symptomatic and or palpable. It is generally believed that the earlier breast cancer is diagnosed, the smaller the chance of metastases. Consequently, mammography is widely used as a routine screening tool to detect occult breast cancer in the general asymptomatic female population. *However, screening mammography must always be used in conjunction with monthly breast self-examination and an annual breast examination performed by a physician.* A National Cancer Institute review showed that this approach significantly reduces breast cancer deaths for women of all ages.

Mammography is also a key tool in the evaluation of known or suspected breast disease in both males and females. A variety of special diagnostic mammographic studies such as spot compression or magnification mammography are used to supplement a routine screening exam when symptomatic patients are evaluated.

There is little doubt that mammograms must be interpreted by qualified radiologists, and the radiologist's role in breast disease continues to increase. Radiologists are more frequently being called on to perform breast procedures such as percutaneous breast biopsies and cyst drainage. Given the prevalence of breast problems, all doctors should be aware of the basics of breast imaging, including the limitations of mammography.

GUIDELINES FOR MAMMOGRAPHY

Some generally accepted guidelines for mammography are listed in Table 10-1. These guidelines provide you with something on which you can hang your hat, but there isn't unanimous agreement about them. Unfortunately, only about 50% to 60% of women over the age of 50 have annual mammograms, and only 50% to 60% of physicians use these guidelines for screening asymptomatic women. As indicated in the guidelines in Table 10-1, risk factors are important and influence the timing for mammography. Some of the common risk factors are listed in Table 10-2. Depending on the risk factors, the time tables may be advanced to younger ages by approximately 5 to 10 years.

▶ **TABLE 10-1 General Mammography Guidelines**

1. Baseline between 35 and 40 years for future comparison; baseline before age 35 if mother or sister had premenopausal breast cancer
2. Every 1–2 years between ages 40 and 49 depending on risk factors (see Table 10-2)
3. Annual mammograms for all women over 50
4. At any age when there are symptoms or clinical findings suspicious for malignancy

▶ **TABLE 10-2 Risk Factors That Can Influence the Timing for Mammography**

1. Prior personal history of breast cancer
2. Family history of premenopausal breast cancer in mother or sister
3. Presence of BRCA-1 and BRCA-2 genes
4. Previous biopsy findings: ductal carcinoma *in situ,* atypia, juvenile papillomatosis, lobular neoplasia (1)
5. Age (incidence increases with age)
6. Years of menstruation: early age menarche, late age menopause
7. Nulliparous, late age first birth
8. Never breast-fed
9. Postmenopausal obesity
10. Others (1)

TECHNIQUE

The importance of a well-performed mammogram cannot be overemphasized. A standard mammogram consists of a *mediolateral oblique* (MLO) view with the central x-ray beam traversing the breast obliquely in a medial to lateral direction (Fig. 10-1A) and a *craniocaudal* (CC) view (Fig. 10-1B) with the central x-ray beam traversing the breast in a head-to-foot direction. It is necessary to compress the breast during the examination to optimally image all the breast tissue, and this may cause mild to moderate discomfort. The technical aspects of mammography are very complicated, and it is extremely important that the mammographer be properly trained and qualified. Mammography quality controls are mandatory and regulated by the federal government under the Mammography Quality Standards Act (MQSA) of 1993.

Normal MLO and CC views of the breast are shown in Fig. 10-2. Notice that breast images are a combination of fat (black) and water density soft tissues (gray to white). This background of black and gray, especially the black, enhances visualization of the white calcifications. The major portion of the breast tissue is connective tissue and fat. Breast tissue is composed predominately of connective tissue in young women and gradually replaced with adipose tissue in older women. Only a very small amount of the breast volume is made up of epithelial tissues (lobules and ducts).

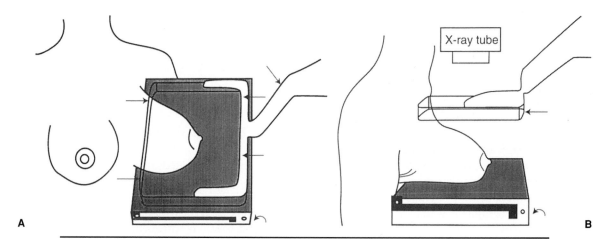

A   **B**

FIGURE 10-1. **A:** Illustration of how the patient is positioned for a mediolateral oblique (MLO) mammogram. The x-ray beam passes obliquely through the breast in a medial to lateral direction. The breast is routinely compressed between the compression device *(straight arrows)* and the radiographic cassette *(curved arrow).* The cassette contains a radiographic film on which the image will be recorded. Compression improves the diagnostic quality of the images by thinning the breast to a more homogeneous thickness. **B:** Illustration of how the patient is positioned for a craniocaudal (CC) mammogram. The x-ray beam passes through the breast in a head-to-foot or cephalad to caudad direction. The compression device *(straight arrow)* is more easily visualized in this illustration. Again, the image will be recorded on the film in the radiographic cassette *(curved arrow).*

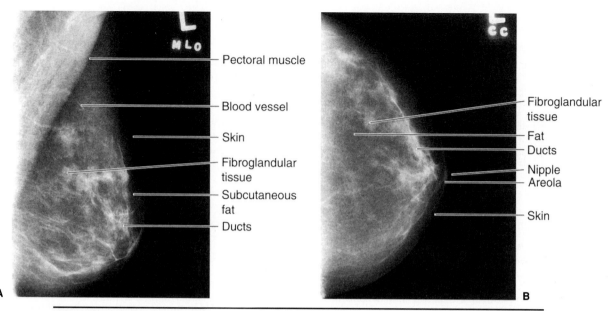

FIGURE 10-2. **A:** Left breast mediolateral oblique (MLO) mammogram. Normal. **B:** Left breast cranio-caudal (CC) mammogram. Normal.

MASSES

Benign

Benign disease (Table 10-3) may or may not be symptomatic or have associated masses. A fibroadenoma (Fig. 10-3) is a benign lesion that must be differentiated from a malignant mass. It generally occurs in young women and may be multiple or single. On physical exam, fibroadenomas are hard and often movable. The mammographic appearance is a mass sometimes associated with coarse "popcorn" calcifications. On sonography, these fibroadenomas will usually appear hypoechoic.

Another common clinical problem is benign cystic disease, and this problem occurs at all ages. Cysts may present as a palpable mass that may or may not be tender, or an incidental mammographic finding. The mammographic appearance of a cyst is usually a mass of water density with well-defined sharp borders (Fig. 10-4A). Rarely, cysts have mural calcifications. Ultrasonography (Fig. 10-4B) usually shows a well-defined anechoic mass with posterior acoustic enhancement. Cysts may require aspiration depending on the clinical situation, and aspiration under ultrasound-guided aspiration is quite effective.

Breast augmentation implants (Fig. 10-5) are relatively common; over 2 million women now have them (1). The augmentations may be for cosmetic reasons or for post-surgical reconstruction. Special views are required to visualize the breast tissue surrounding the implant and to evaluate for implant rupture. Breast implants vary in appearance from water density saline to dense silicone.

Malignant

Common mammographic findings of malignancy are listed in Table 10-4. Calcifications are important as they may represent the first sign of malignancy, especially if they are new, punctate (small spots), pleomorphic, or branching (Fig. 10-6). It should be emphasized that most

▶ **TABLE 10-3 Partial List of Benign Breast Disease Etiologies**

1. Cystic disease
2. Sclerosing adenosis
3. Fibroadenoma
4. Lipoma
5. Foreign body reaction to augmentation

▶ **TABLE 10-4 Mammographic Findings Suspect for Malignancy**

1. Mass on mammogram with:
   a. Ill-defined or spiculated borders
   b. Malignant calcifications
   c. Skin retraction or thickening
2. Microcalcifications with or without a mass
   a. Linear or branching
   b. Clusters
   c. Punctate
3. Mammographic architectural distortion (asymmetry)
4. Hypoechoic solid mass on ultrasound

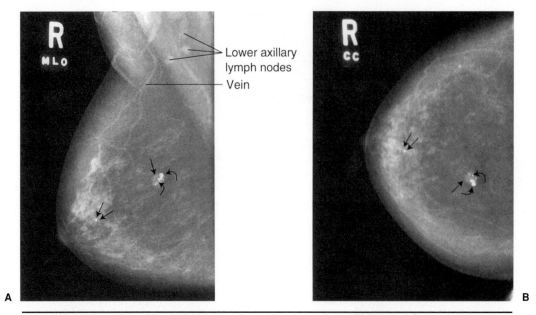

Lower axillary
lymph nodes

Vein

FIGURE 10-3. Right breast mediolateral oblique **(A)** and craniocaudal **(B)** mammograms. Calcified benign fibroadenoma. The fibroadenoma mass is only faintly visible *(single straight arrows)*. The benign calcifications within the fibroadenoma are typically globular, coarse, and variable in size *(curved arrows)*. Note the single benign globular calcification incidentally found without a mass associated *(double straight arrows)*.

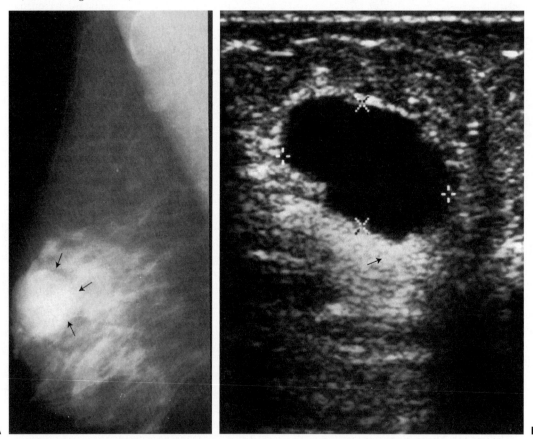

FIGURE 10-4. A: Right breast mediolateral oblique mammogram. Benign cyst. The water density cyst *(straight arrows)* has sharp borders and no calcifications. Note the difference between the smooth sharp borders of this benign cyst compared to the irregular and poorly defined borders of the carcinoma in Fig. 10-6. **B:** Right breast sonogram of the lesion in A. This is the classic appearance of a benign breast cyst. The cystic fluid is the anechoic or black area, and the thin cyst walls are the hyperechoic or white areas. The Xs and *crosses* are electronic caliper marks on the cyst's wall that are used in measuring the dimensions of the cyst. Posterior acoustic enhancement *(straight arrow)* is commonly found immediately posterior to a cyst.

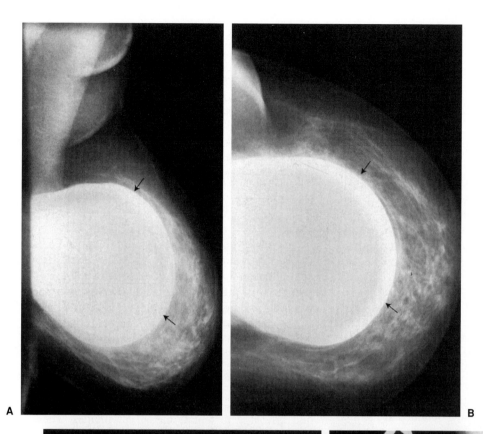

FIGURE 10-5. Left breast mediolateral oblique **(A)** and craniocaudal **(B)** mammograms. Bilateral breast augmentations. The bright white areas represent the surgically implanted silicone augmentations *(straight arrows)*.

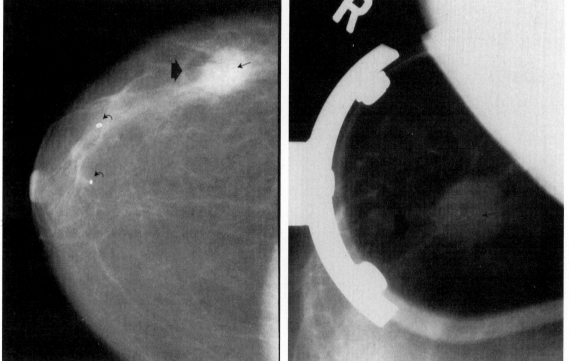

FIGURE 10-6. **A:** Right breast craniocaudal mammogram. Carcinoma of the breast with malignant calcifications. The water density malignant mass lesion *(arrowhead)* has spiculated and poorly defined borders. The outline or border of this mass is in contrast to the sharp and well-defined border of the benign cyst in Fig. 10-4A. The malignant calcifications *(straight arrow)* are punctate and centrally located. In the same breast there are coarse benign calcifications *(curved arrows)* that are larger and more globular in appearance. **B:** Right breast spot magnification view of the lesion in Fig. 10-6A. This clearly demonstrates the classical appearance of malignant calcifications *(straight arrow)* in the mass *(arrowhead)*. Note the difference between the coarse benign calcifications in the fibroadenoma in Fig. 10-3 and the more delicate punctate malignant calcifications in this patient. Also, the spiculated and poorly defined borders are more obvious in this magnification view.

calcifications are benign. Therefore, it is essential that the radiologist distinguish between benign and malignant calcifications. Some calcifications are so small that a magnifying glass is needed when viewing mammograms. After being detected on a screening mammogram, calcifications are frequently evaluated in more detail using special magnification mammography images. Once suspicious calcifications have been biopsied, the biopsy specimen can be radiographed to make sure that the calcifications have been adequately sampled and/or removed.

Asymmetric masses and architectural changes are also suspicious for malignancy, especially if they have appeared recently.

MALE BREAST

All of the diseases that occur in the female breast can potentially occur in the male breast. The incidence of male breast carcinoma is approximately 900 cases per year in the United States, and this, of course, is dramatically lower than that in the female population. The indications for male mammography and the image obtained are similar to those for females.

▶ **TABLE 10-5 Some Causes of Male Gynecomastia**

1. Common in the neonatal male
2. Common in pubertal males
3. Adult men
   a. Any underlying disease causing hormone imbalance (e.g., liver cirrhosis)
   b. Drugs (digitalis, steroids)
   c. Androgen deficiency as in aging

One male breast clinical situation that can be confusing is gynecomastia (Fig. 10-7). The etiologies for male gynecomastia are listed in Table 10-5. Usually, adult men present with a tender subareolar breast mass, and it is generally unilateral. On mammography, there is breast tissue in the subareolar zone that may rarely contain calcifications. The need for biopsy will be determined by a combination of symptoms, physical findings, and mammographic findings. There is probably no correlation between gynecomastia and carcinoma.

Male breast carcinomas are similar in appearance and histology to female breast carcinomas. They most commonly present as irregular or ill-defined solid masses.

SUGGESTED WORKUP OF COMMON CLINICAL PROBLEMS

Suggested algorithms for the workup of two common clinical scenarios are shown in Fig. 10-8.

OTHER TECHNOLOGIES

Magnetic resonance is used to image implants and evaluate for rupture and to evaluate the extent of disease in some women diagnosed with breast cancer, especially in women with dense breast tissue that is not well imaged by mammography.

Small-field digital imaging is used for stereotactic core biopsies. Full-field digital mammography is being used in some field trials and in the future may replace film-screen mammography in a filmless radiology department.

There are now several digital mammography systems approved for both screening and diagnostic mammography. Advantages of digital mammography include the ability to (a) use image-processing techniques to aid in evaluating the images, (b) apply computer-assisted techniques to aid in detecting abnormalities, (c) transmit images rapidly to another location for a second opinion, and (d) store images electronically (i.e., digital images cannot be lost or misplaced as may occur with film images).

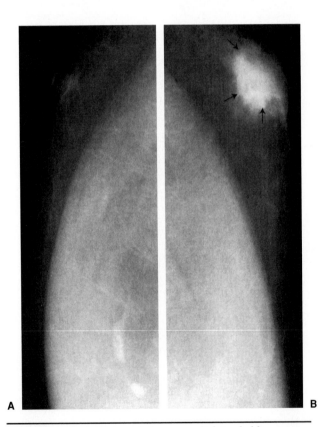

FIGURE 10-7. A: Right male breast mediolateral oblique mammogram. Normal. **B:** Left male breast mediolateral oblique mammogram. Benign gynecomastia. The *straight arrows* indicate the typical increased but normal appearing subareolar soft tissue without calcification.

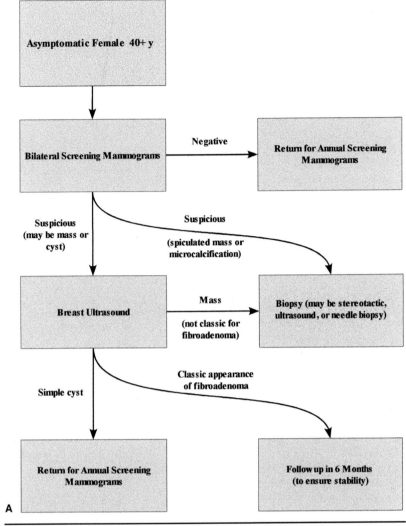

FIGURE 10-8. Examples of possible work up algorithms. **A:** Screening for breast carcinoma. *(continued)*

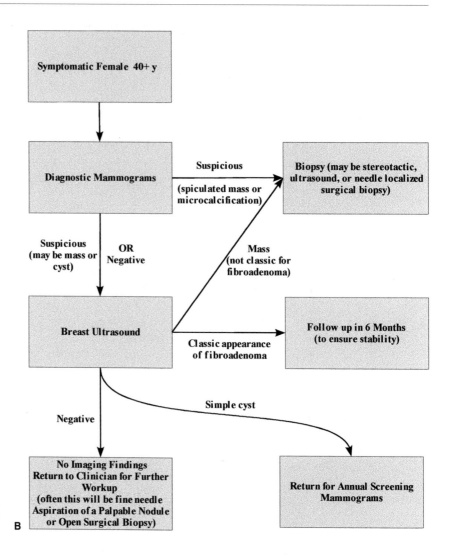

FIGURE 10-8. B: Work up of a palpable breast mass.

Positron emission tomography (PET) is a functional or molecular imaging technique that is performed after the intravenous injection of fluorodeoxyglucose (FDG). FDG is taken up by cancer cells because of increased metabolic activity and detected on the PET scan. In some centers PET imaging is being evaluated as a technique for staging breast cancer and/or detecting distant metastases.

KEY POINTS

- Approximately one in eight females in the United States will develop carcinoma of the breast at some time.
- Mammograms must be interpreted by qualified radiologists. Mammograms of high quality are imperative.
- A routine mammogram consists of mediolateral oblique and craniocaudal views.
- Screening mammography, monthly breast self-examination, and annual breast examinations by a physician can improve the survival rate of breast cancer.

- Mammographic findings suspect for malignancy include an irregularly outlined mass, skin retraction or thickening, architectural distortion (asymmetric compared to opposite breast), and/or a hypoechoic mass on ultrasonography.
- Calcifications that are suspicious for malignancy include new calcifications, irregular punctate calcifications, pleomorphic calcifications, and small branching calcifications.
- Ultrasonography is often useful in differentiating solid from cystic breast masses.

REFERENCE

1. Cardenosa G. *Breast imaging companion*. Philadelphia: Lippincott-Raven Publishers, 1997.

SUGGESTED READING

Cardenosa G. *Breast imaging companion*. Philadelphia: Lippincott-Raven Publishers, 1997.

Chapter 11

Interventional Radiology

Thomas A. Farrell and Monte L. Harvill

OVERVIEW

Interventional Radiology (IR) is a diverse practice of patient care using minimally invasive, imaging-guided procedures to diagnose and treat disease nonoperatively. Percutaneous diagnostic and therapeutic procedures are performed using fluoroscopy, ultrasound, computed tomography (CT), or magnetic resonance imaging (MRI) for guidance. These procedures, which may be categorized as vascular (i.e., arteriography, venography) and nonvascular (e.g., decompression and drainage of obstructed kidneys and bile ducts), are performed in an interventional radiology suite, and are often done on an outpatient basis. Many procedures that were previously performed surgically are now accomplished by an interventional radiologist with less morbidity and a shorter hospital stay.

Since 1958, when Dr. Seldinger described a method of percutaneous vascular access using a hollow-core needle, guidewire, and catheter, interventional radiology has continued to evolve, as new techniques and devices are developed to enhance patient care. Technical advances have led to significant improvements in patient safety and procedural diversity. As these rapid changes in endovascular technologies continue to expand, so will the possibilities of image-guided, minimally invasive procedures.

Because IR is procedural, interventional radiologists tend to be more involved in patient care. Referred patients are routinely worked up by the IR service and are subsequently followed up postprocedure. The preprocedure workup consists of patient assessment, as well as evaluation of previous imaging studies (Table 11-1). Postprocedure follow-up is essential to determine if the procedure has been successful and free of complications. This all-inclusive clinical service underlines that there is more to IR than simply doing procedures. Because procedures performed by interventional radiologists are invasive, there are associated risks for developing complications. It is important that the patient be aware of these risks so that an informed decision can be made by weighing the possible risks of a procedure against its benefits. A physician should never place a patient in a position of risk unless the risks, benefits, and alternatives of the planned procedure have

▶ **TABLE 11-1** **Interventional Radiology Preprocedure Checklist**

Discuss indication for procedure/question(s) to be answered from procedure
Discuss contraindications for procedure
Review prior imaging and noninvasive studies
Check for contrast allergy
Discuss and obtain written informed consent
Check coagulation parameters and serum creatinine
Need for prophylactic antibiotics
Ensure that patient is fasting and well hydrated
Discontinue heparin infusion

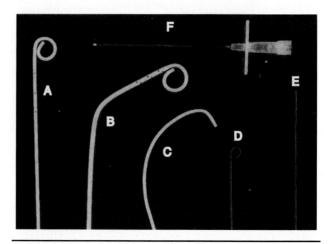

FIGURE 11-1. Tools of the trade. **A:** Pigtail catheter. **B:** Angled pigtail catheter. **C:** Cobra catheter. **D:** J-tipped guidewire. **E:** Straight (Bentson) guidewire. **F:** An 18-gauge needle for vessel puncture.

been discussed, understood, and consented to before the procedure. It is in the physician's best interest to be honest and forthright when dealing with patients and their expectations about the outcomes of a procedure.

The aim of this chapter is to explain the background, indications, and basic techniques of the procedures commonly performed in interventional radiology so that the reader will gain an understanding of how IR contributes to patient care.

INSTRUMENTS AND TOOLS OF THE TRADE

Interventional radiologic procedures are performed in imaging suites with fluoroscopy and digital subtraction angiography. Ultrasound, CT, and MRI are also used by the interventional radiologist.

Each angiography/interventional suite is staffed by the operating radiologist and at least one assistant. A radiology technologist provides imaging expertise and a nurse provides patient sedation, monitors vital signs, and attends to patient needs during the procedure.

Endoluminal procedures require administration of a contrast agent. Nonionic radiographic contrast is most frequently used to delineate, radiographically, the lumen of an artery, vein, biliary duct, gastrointestinal tract, or urinary tract. Carbon dioxide or gadolinium can be used in patients with renal insufficiency or allergy to radiographic contrast agents.

There are a wide variety of commercially available catheters, sheaths, guidewires, balloon catheters, vascular stents, and caval filters. Familiarity with these instruments requires significant training and experience. There are numerous preformed shapes and types of angiographic catheters, most of which are made from flexible plastic material such as polyethylene or polyurethane. Wire braiding may be incorporated into the catheter shaft to increase stiffness and improve its torque. Catheter diameters are measured in French (F) size, where 3F equals 1.0 mm (outside diameter). Most angiographic catheters are in the

4F to 7F range. Aortic angiography is performed with pigtail catheters that have several side holes proximal to the tip, allowing rapid flow of a contrast bolus while the pigtail loop stabilizes the catheter, preventing recoil (Fig. 11-1A, B). Selective angiography (renal, celiac, and superior mesenteric arteries) is performed with a curved end-hole catheter such as a Cobra C2 (Fig. 11-1C). A variety of catheters and guidewires may be necessary during a procedure, and placement of a vascular sheath with a hemostatic valve at the site of access reduces vessel trauma and facilitates rapid catheter and guidewire exchange.

Catheters used in the drainage of abscesses, obstructed kidneys (percutaneous nephrostomy), and bile ducts are made of polyurethane and are of greater diameter than angiographic catheters (8 to 12 French). These drainage catheters are usually placed using the Seldinger technique after which they are secured in position by deploying a locking pigtail mechanism formed by pulling on a suture that runs in most of the catheter shaft and is attached to its tip. The pigtail loop itself contains large side holes for drainage. The smaller diameter catheters occlude more easily with debris and should be routinely changed over a guidewire every 6 to 8 weeks when continued drainage is required.

Guidewires increase the ease and safety of catheter placement. The outer shell of a guidewire consists of a very tightly wound but flexible metal spring coil. A stiff central core provides rigidity over a variable length of the guidewire. The balance between these two components dictates the handling characteristics of the guide wire. For example, the distal 15 cm of a Bentson guidewire is floppy, allowing easy coiling (Fig. 11-1E). A J-tipped guidewire reduces the risk of damaging the vessel wall because of its blunt tip (Fig. 11-1D). Guidewires usually range in diameter from 18 thousandths of an inch (0.018 in.) to

38 thousandths of an inch (0.038 in.). The standard length for most wires is 145 cm, although longer guidewires (260 cm) are available to facilitate catheter exchange. Needles used in arteriography range in size from a 21-gauge needle through which an 0.018-in. guidewire will pass to an 18-gauge needle that accepts a 0.035-in. guidewire (Fig. 11-10F).

ANGIOGRAPHY

Angiography is a technique of imaging blood vessels, usually by injecting contrast material via an intraluminally placed catheter. Blood vessels may also be visualized noninvasively using computed tomography angiography (CTA) or magnetic resonance angiography (MRA), which takes advantage of the inherent contrast between flowing blood and stationary tissue.

Diagnostic Percutaneous Arteriography

Diagnostic arteriography begins by catheterizing an artery using *Seldinger technique* (Fig 11-2). This technique of vascular catheterization was initially described by a radiologist, Sven Seldinger. After a hollow-core needle is placed into an artery (femoral or brachial), a guidewire is inserted through the needle and into the artery. Sonographic and fluoroscopic guidance is often necessary. The needle is exchanged for a vascular catheter or vascular introducing sheath. Subsequent catheter movement and exchange is performed over a guidewire. Large vessel arteriography is performed using flush catheters (pigtail, tennis racquet). Smaller arteries are selectively imaged using catheters of various shapes and sizes. Microcatheters are used for sub- or superselective arteriography.

After the catheter is safely positioned in the artery of choice, the guidewire is removed and a contrast agent injected through the catheter during image acquisition. Mask images obtained before injection of contrast allows for subtraction of nonvascular structures, producing the arteriogram. Many images are acquired as the contrast agent flows through the lumen of the vessel. The catheter can be exchanged or repositioned for additional imaging. After completion of the procedure, the catheter is removed and hemostasis obtained at the arterotomy site using manual compression or a percutaneous closure device. Recovery time for the patient is 2 to 6 hours.

Noninvasive angiography (MRA/CTA) will eventually replace most percutaneous diagnostic arteriography, except where intervention is expected or other exams are indefinite. Pulmonary arteriography, performed by venous catheterization and crossing the right side of the heart, has largely been replaced by computed tomography angiography (CTA).

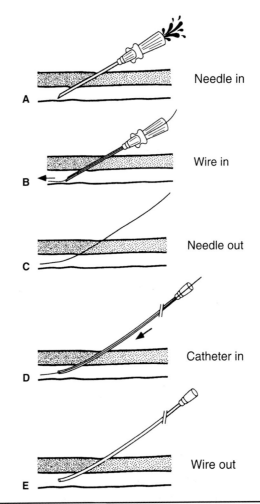

Needle in

Wire in

Needle out

Catheter in

Wire out

FIGURE 11-2. Seldinger technique. **A:** The vessel is punctured with the needle. **B:** A guidewire is advanced through the needle into the vessel. **C:** The needle is removed, leaving the guidewire in place. **D:** A catheter is advanced over the guidewire into the vessel. **E:** The guidewire is removed and the catheter flushed.

Peripheral Arterial Disease

Generally, the diagnosis of peripheral arterial disease (PAD), or peripheral vascular disease (PVD), has already been made by the time an arteriogram is requested. The patient evaluation includes an assessment of the patient's symptoms, a physical examination, and a review of the noninvasive imaging tests, such as CT, MR, duplex ultrasonography, and segmental limb pressures before proceeding to angiography. Rather than being an endpoint, the angiogram helps formulate a comprehensive plan in the patient's subsequent treatment as it evaluates the extent and severity of disease and provides a road map for intervention (balloon angioplasty, stenting, surgery, etc.). Diabetic patients may present with a more advanced stage of ischemia as they are prone to developing peripheral neuropathy that may mask the PAD symptoms. Diabetics also tend to have a greater prevalence of small vessel disease, which is more difficult to treat surgically and contributes to a less favorable long-term prognosis compared to other causes of PAD.

Arteriographic evaluation of patients with PAD may be divided into three anatomic regions: aortoiliac, infrainguinal, and infrageniculate. Aortic aneurysms occur most commonly below the level of the renal arteries. The number of renal arteries should also be noted, as should the presence of stenoses in these vessels. Bilateral oblique views of the pelvis should be obtained during the arteriogram, as hemodynamically significant stenoses can be missed if only a frontal view is performed.

In general, arterial stenoses are not regarded as significant unless they reduce the lumen diameter by 50% angiographically. Measuring a pressure gradient across it can more accurately assess the significance of a stenosis. The presence of a 10-mm Hg gradient or greater across a stenosis is regarded as significant and worthy of further treatment such as angioplasty or stenting. If the gradient is less than 10 mm Hg, a vasodilator such as nitroglycerin may be given intraarterially to simulate exercise and possibly unmask a significant stenosis. Most endovascular interventions are performed in the carotid, renal, aortoiliac, and femoropopliteal arteries. In the absence of satisfactory femoral pulses bilaterally, either the brachial or axillary arteries can be punctured.

Venography

Diagnostic venography is performed in all extremities, as well as centrally, for surgical planning or evaluation of deep venous thrombosis when vascular ultrasound is indeterminate. Most venography is performed in conjunction with interventional procedures (placement of caval filters and central venous catheters, renal vein sampling).

Complications

Complications of diagnostic angiography (Table 11-2) are infrequent, with access vascular injury and hematoma comprising the overwhelming majority. Risk factors for this complication include hypertension and obesity. Prevention involves meticulous technique including vessel puncture over the femoral head and constant manual pressure directly over the puncture site after removal of the catheter until hemostasis is achieved. The hematoma may extend into the retroperitoneum when the puncture site is above the inguinal ligament. Incomplete or intermittent compression over the puncture site may also result in the formation of a pseudoaneurysm. Complications following brachial or axillary arterial puncture are more common than with femoral artery puncture because of the smaller vessel size and the close proximity of the vessels to nerves within a common sheath in the arm. Dissection, thrombo-

▶ **TABLE 11-2 Complications of Angiography**

Systemic
Allergic contrast reaction
Renal failure

Local
Puncture site:
  Hematoma
  Pseudoaneurysm
  Arteriovenous fistula
Intraluminal:
  Subintimal dissection
  Thrombosis
  Distal embolization

sis, or pseudoaneurysm of the access artery may require endovascular intervention or surgical repair.

Contrast-related nephropathy refers to transient renal insufficiency and occasionally, acute renal failure that is a result of contrast use. Contrast-induced renal failure is usually mild and self-limiting, with serum creatinine levels peaking by 3 to 5 days and returning to normal within 2 weeks. The pathophysiology of this complication is thought to be due to a combination of vasoconstriction and direct toxicity of contrast on the renal tubules. Diabetics and patients with preexisting renal impairment (serum creatinine greater than 2 mg%) are at increased risk for developing contrast-induced renal failure. Clinical judgment, adequate hydration, renal protective drugs, or alternative contrast agents (CO_2, gadolinium) should be used in high-risk patients (elderly, Cr greater than 1.5, diabetes mellitus). Alternative imaging modalities (ultrasound, MRA) should also be explored to avoid this potential complication. Transient renal insufficiency usually returns to baseline in 10 to 14 days.

Systemic allergic or idiosyncratic reactions to radiographic contrast media are rare, with severity depending on the type, dose, route, and rate of contrast delivery. Reactions may be categorized as mild, moderate, or severe (Table 11-3). The prevalence of most reactions is greater with the intravenous route. Many studies suggest a lower incidence of severe reactions when nonionic iodinated contrast is used. The mortality rate, which is equivalent for high and lower osmolar contrast agents, is approximately 1 per 45,000 examinations. Moderate contrast reactions characterized by hypertension, hypotension, wheezing, and laryngospasm occur in 1% to 2% of examinations. Idiosyncratic reactions are usually mild (nausea, cough, hives, and flushing), are even more common, and can be treated symptomatically. Premedication with steroids for 24 hours prior to angiography has reduced the incidence of idiosyncratic contrast reactions.

▶ **TABLE 11-3 Allergic Contrast Reactions**

Type	Mild	Moderate	Severe
Incidence (%)	5–15	1–2	0.1
Clinical features	Nausea	Bronchospasm	Laryngospasm
	Vomiting	Dyspnea	Facial edema
	Urticaria	Vasovagal reaction	Cardiorespiratory arrest
		Hypertension	Seizures
Treatment	Monitor vital signs	Oxygen	Oxygen/IV fluids
	Observe for clinical deterioration	β_2 agonist	Epinephrine SC or IV
			β_2 agonist
			Diazepam
			Cardiopulmonary resuscitation

VASCULAR INTERVENTIONS

Thrombolysis

Thrombolysis is the process of removing a blood clot to establish patency of an occluded (thrombosed) vessel. Thrombolysis can be achieved using mechanical devices or pharmacologic agents—urokinase, tissue plasminogen activator (t-PA), retaplase (r-PA), tenectaplase (TNK). Several mechanical devices are available and can be used in conjunction with the pharmacologic agents. Thrombolytic drugs are infused directly into the thrombosed grafts and vessels to ensure a very high local concentration of the drug. Active internal bleeding, recent intracranial hemorrhage, or surgery are absolute contraindications for thrombolysis (Table 11-4).

Complications include bleeding and distal embolization of thrombus. The cumulative probability of major complications increases with duration of infusion, rising from less than 10% after 16 hours to more than 30% at 40 hours. Once thrombolysis is complete, balloon angioplasty or surgery can be used to treat any underlying vessel stenoses that contributed to the occlusion.

▶ **TABLE 11-4 Contraindications for Arterial Thrombolysis**

Absolute
Active gastrointestinal (GI) or genitourinary (GU) bleeding
Recent (<2 months) cerebral hemorrhage/infarct/surgery
Irreversible limb ischemia

Relative
History of GI or GU bleeding
Recent thoracic/abdominal surgery
Recent trauma
Severe uncontrolled hypertension

Percutaneous Transluminal Angioplasty (PTA)

Balloon Angioplasty

Percutaneous transluminal balloon angioplasty (PTA) has become an established technique in the treatment of vascular stenoses due to atherosclerotic plaque and fibromuscular dysplasia. The precise pathophysiologic mechanism of PTA in atherosclerotic plaque is controversial. However, most agree that PTA results in a controlled plaque and intimal fracture with localized dissection into the underlying media, thereby increasing the intraluminal diameter. The plaque, intima, and media are subsequently remodeled to give a smoother endoluminal surface. The appropriate angioplasty balloon catheter should be chosen so that its inflated diameter is the same size or slightly larger than the adjacent nondiseased vessel. Initially, the stenosis is crossed with a guidewire that is left across the lesion until the procedure is finished. Heparin and nitroglycerin may be given intraarterially to prevent thrombosis and vessel spasm, respectively. The angioplasty balloon is advanced across the stenosis and inflated and deflated slowly under fluoroscopic guidance. Repeat angiography and pressure measurements should be obtained to evaluate the results of angioplasty. Suboptimal angioplasty results may require placement of an endovascular stent.

Iliac artery angioplasty improves inflow to the lower limb and requires balloons that are 7 to 10 mm in diameter. Again, a guidewire is left across the stenosis during the procedure, the success of which is judged on angiographic and hemodynamic criteria. Stent placement should be considered if the postangioplasty pressure gradient is greater than 10 mm Hg, there is residual stenosis of greater than 30%, or if a flow-limiting dissection is present (Fig. 11-3). Simultaneous PTA of both common iliac arteries, known as the kissing-balloons technique, is effective in treating bilateral proximal common iliac artery stenoses.

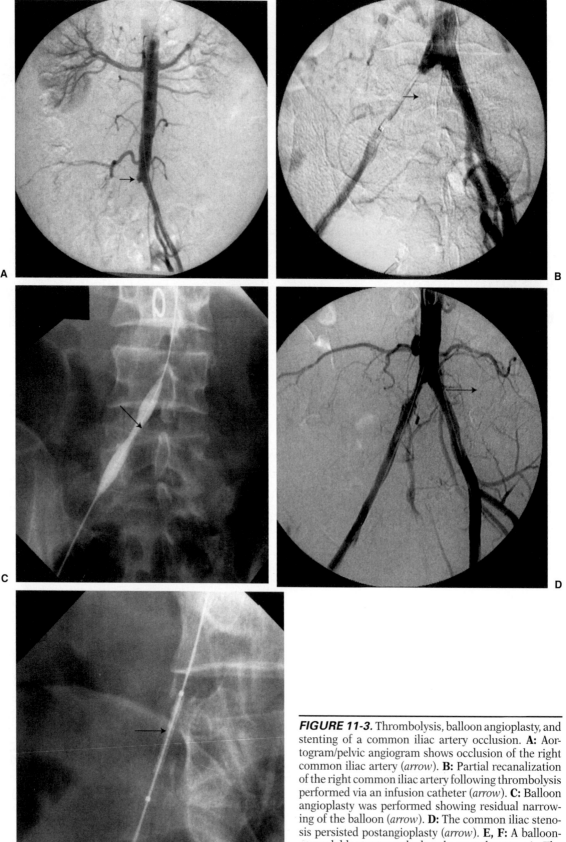

FIGURE 11-3. Thrombolysis, balloon angioplasty, and stenting of a common iliac artery occlusion. **A:** Aortogram/pelvic angiogram shows occlusion of the right common iliac artery (*arrow*). **B:** Partial recanalization of the right common iliac artery following thrombolysis performed via an infusion catheter (*arrow*). **C:** Balloon angioplasty was performed showing residual narrowing of the balloon (*arrow*). **D:** The common iliac stenosis persisted postangioplasty (*arrow*). **E, F:** A balloon-expandable stent was deployed across the stenosis. The undeployed stent (*arrow*) can be seen on the distal portion of the angioplasty balloon. **G:** Poststenting, no residual stenosis is present.

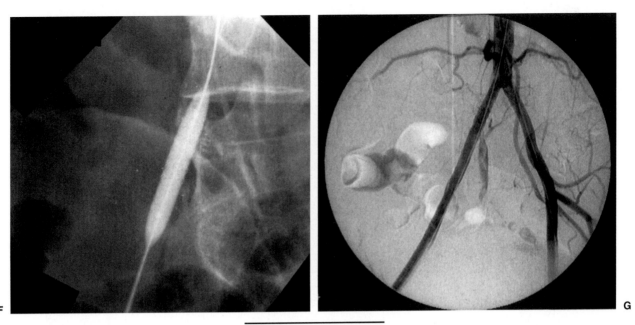

F   G

FIGURE 11-3. (*Continued*)

Infrainguinal angioplasty (superficial femoral and popliteal arteries) is gaining clinical acceptance as patency outcomes for PTA and stenting rivals outcomes of surgical bypass procedures. Infrageniculate angioplasty (anterior/posterior tibial and peroneal arteries) is usually performed for limb salvage or to reduce the extent of an impending below-the-knee or forefoot amputation for ischemia. This technique requires a fine guidewire (0.010 in. to 0.018 in.) and angioplasty balloon (2 to 3 mm in diameter) because of the smaller vessel size. An antegrade common femoral arterial approach, where the artery is punctured in a downstream direction, is helpful, as are higher doses of heparin and nitroglycerin to prevent vessel thrombosis and spasm.

Renal artery angioplasty is usually performed with a 5- to 7-mm-diameter balloon. Atheromatous disease usually involves the proximal or ostial portion of the vessel in contrast to fibromuscular dysplasia, which usually affects the midportion of the vessel. The improvement in renal function and hypertension following renal artery angioplasty is equivalent to that obtained after surgical revascularization (Fig. 11-4). Renal artery stenting is performed if

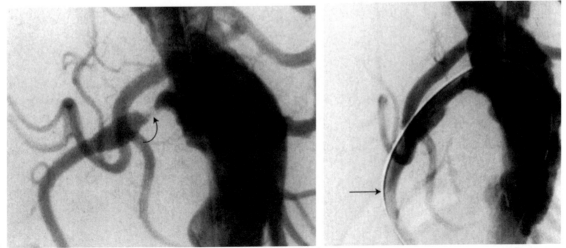

A   B

FIGURE 11-4. Renal artery angioplasty. **A:** Flush aortogram with a pigtail catheter (*arrow*) showing right renal artery stenosis (*curved arrow*). **B:** Residual stenosis persists post–balloon angioplasty. Note that the guidewire (*arrow*) is left across the stenosis.

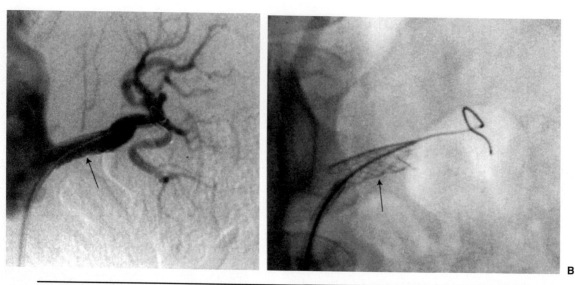

FIGURE 11-5. Renal artery stenting. A Palmaz stent (*arrow*) has been placed across a left renal artery stenosis.

there is a residual stenosis or significant dissection postangioplasty (Fig. 11-5). Ostial lesions are often stented primarily, without predilatation.

Endovascular Stents

Peripheral Endovascular Stents

There are two main indications for endovascular stent placement: (a) a residual pressure gradient of more than 10 mm Hg postangioplasty, which is regarded as an indication for either repeat angioplasty or stent placement; and

(b) postangioplasty flow-limiting dissection, where the goal of stent placement is to appose the dissected flap against the wall and improve flow. The balloon–stent combination is placed across the stenosis and the balloon is inflated, thus opening and deploying the stent. The balloon is then deflated and removed (Fig. 11-6).

There are two general types of metallic endovascular stents, balloon-expandable and self-expanding. Deployment of the balloon-expandable stent was just described. Deployment of the self-expanding stent, which does not require delivery on an angioplasty balloon, involves withdrawal of a covering sheath, after which the stent

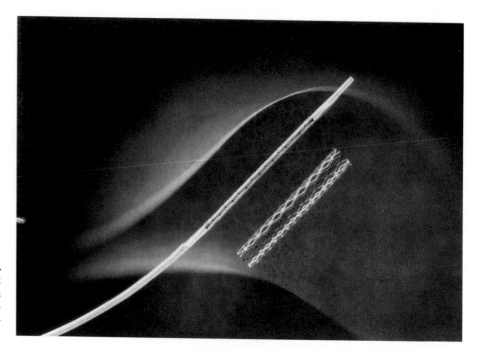

FIGURE 11-6. Palmaz stent mounted on an angioplasty balloon and in its expanded form. (Photograph courtesy of Cordis Corporation.)

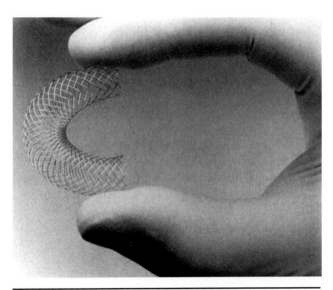

FIGURE 11-7. The Wallstent is self-expanding and flexible. (Photograph courtesy of Schneider, Inc.)

expands. Postdilatation with an angioplasty balloon may be necessary. Self-expanding stents are usually more flexible than balloon-mounted stents, which is an advantage when stenting tortuous vessels (Fig. 11-7). Covered Polyte-trafluoro ethylene (PTFE, Dacron) stents are available for treatment of vascular injury resulting in pseudoaneurysm, hemorrhage, or arteriovenous fistula. Drug- or radiation-emitting stents are currently being investigated to determine efficacy in treatment of arterial stenosis. These stents are designed to reduce neointimal hyperplasia, which develops and covers the inside the stent.

Aortic Stent Grafts

Stent grafts have revolutionized the treatment of abdominal aortic aneurysms (AAA), reducing the severity and duration of the procedure and postprocedure morbidity and hospital stay. Ninety percent of patients are discharged home within 48 hours of the procedure, which is usually done in the operating room or combined operative/fluoroscopy suite under general or epidural anesthesia. Through bilateral femoral artery surgical, cutdowns, the various components of the aortic stent graft are introduced and deployed in the abdominal aorta and iliac arteries under fluoroscopic guidance. A preprocedure CT scan of the aorta is essential for precise vessel measurement and localization of arterial branches. The device(s), which is composed of woven polyester on a Nitinol wire exoskeleton frame, is placed in the infrarenal aorta and extends down to the common or external iliac arteries (Fig 11-8). Postprocedure follow-up with CT scans every 6 months is important for the detection of an endoleak, which is a leak into the aneurysm sac. In the absence

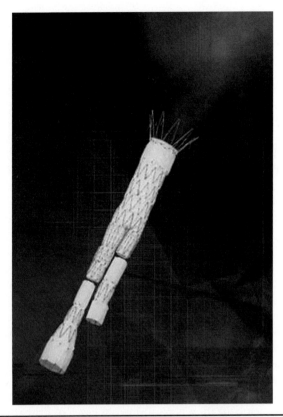

FIGURE 11-8. Aortic stent graft device is composed of three components—a main body and two iliac extensions, which can be custom made to suit each patient. The components are placed through femoral artery cutdowns. (Photograph courtesy of Cook, Inc.)

of such an endoleak, the aneurysm sac should reduce in size.

Embolization

Gastrointestinal Hemorrhage

Selective angiography and therapeutic embolization have become important techniques in the management of patients with gastrointestinal (GI) bleeding. Initially, a nuclear medicine study using radiolabeled red cells should be done to confirm the presence and anatomic location of the bleeding vessel. Selective angiography of either the celiac, superior mesenteric, or inferior mesenteric arteries is then performed. Once a bleeding site has been demonstrated, the catheter can be used to control bleeding either by selectively infusing vasopressin to constrict the vessel or by injecting embolic materials such as gelatin sponge pledgets or coils to mechanically occlude flow. The specific treatment depends on the nature and location of the hemorrhage. Both upper and lower GI bleeding are now most commonly treated by embolization via a coaxial microcatheter.

Uterine Fibroid Embolization

Fibroids commonly present as pain, menorrhagia, or pressure symptoms related to mass effect. Traditionally, patients were treated with hysterectomy or myomectomy. Uterine fibroid embolization offers an effective and less invasive treatment option. After selective catheterization of the uterine arteries, inert particles up to 900 microns (0.9 mm) in size are injected, infarcting the fibroids, eventually reducing their size and improving symptoms. The fibroid size reduces by 60% at 6 months and up to 90% of patients notice an improvement in their pain, menorrhagia, or pressure symptoms.

Oncology Therapy

Arterial embolization is expanding as an option for regional cancer therapy. Bland embolization of primary or metastatic tumors is performed to decrease blood flow to a tumor, depriving the tumor of nutrient sources. Bland embolization is usually performed for vascular tumors, bleeding from tumor or adjacent invaded organs, and for palliation. In the case of renal cell carcinoma, the kidney or metastatic lesion is often embolized prior to surgery to decrease bleeding during nephrectomy or resection. Chemoembolization is performed in cases of primary or metastatic cancer, subselectively embolizing the hepatic tumor with chemotherapeutic drugs and inert particles. Portal vein embolization using a percutaneous, transhepatic approach is sometimes performed prior to partial hepatectomy. Embolization of the portal vein branches supplying the hepatic lobe that contains tumor provides the nondiseased portion of the liver time to hypertrophy prior to tumor resection, as well as decreased bleeding during surgery. Other forms of regional oncology therapy are discussed in the nonvascular intervention section later in this chapter.

Trauma

The interventional radiologist has an important role in the management of trauma patients. Most emergent trauma procedures referred to IR involve bleeding or injury to the vascular system. Vessel injury with bleeding, intimal injury, pseudoaneurysm, or fistula can be diagnosed and immediately treated in the angiography suite, often using covered stents or embolization techniques.

Hemorrhage Associated with Pelvic Fracture

Prior to the introduction of external fixation devices, much of the early mortality associated with pelvic fractures was due to internal hemorrhage. Presently, up to 20% of patients with pelvic fractures require the services of interventional radiology for the diagnosis and treatment of hemorrhage. In general, surgery is not a satisfactory treatment option for this problem as exploration will decompress the pelvic hematoma, reduce the tamponade effect, and lead to further blood loss. A diagnostic pelvic angiogram is performed with a pigtail catheter placed above the aortic bifurcation. Active hemorrhage is diagnosed by extravasation of contrast. The bleeding vessel may then be embolized with either a stainless steel Gianturco coil or pledgets of gelatin sponge, both of which can be placed through a selective 5F angiographic catheter. Gelatin sponge results in temporary vascular occlusion that recanalizes within 2 to 3 weeks, whereas a Gianturco coil usually results in a permanent occlusion. Pelvic ischemia following selective arterial embolization is unusual because of the extensive collateral blood supply.

Traumatic Aortic Injury

Eighty percent of those who sustain a laceration to the thoracic aorta following blunt trauma die at the scene of the accident, en route to the hospital, or shortly after arriving in the hospital. The cause of death in most cases is exsanguination from aortic transection. The precise mechanism of aortic transection is uncertain. It may be due to sudden deceleration where the mobile descending aorta shears from the relatively fixed aortic arch, as the most common site for aortic transection is just distal to the origin of the left subclavian artery. As in all trauma patients, clinical evaluation is important, but up to 50% of patients surviving accidents with blunt aortic injuries have no external physical signs of injury. Multidetector CT of the chest is rapidly replacing catheter aortography as the gold standard for diagnosing aortic arch injury. An arch aortogram is performed by advancing a 6F or 7F pigtail catheter carefully through the common femoral artery and across the aortic arch so that the catheter tip lies just above the aortic valve. The left anterior oblique (LAO) projection provides an optimal view of the aortic arch. A second view in an orthogonal plane, right anterior oblique (RAO), should detect an injury in the posteromedial wall that was not seen on the initial LAO projection. One should be aware of a normal anatomic variant in the aortic arch that may be misdiagnosed as traumatic aortic injury—the so-called ductus bump, which lies proximally on the inferior surface of the aortic arch and represents the site of attachment of the ductus arteriosus (Fig. 11-9).

Venous Access

Central Venous Access

Central venous catheters are placed for a variety of indications including administration of antibiotics, chemotherapy, and hemodialysis. There are essentially two types of catheters: tunneled and nontunneled. Tunneling refers to

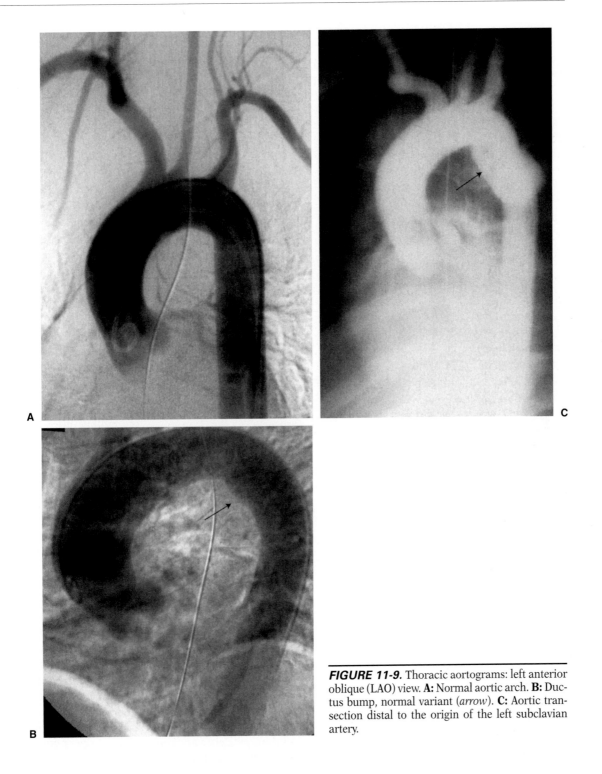

FIGURE 11-9. Thoracic aortograms: left anterior oblique (LAO) view. **A:** Normal aortic arch. **B:** Ductus bump, normal variant (*arrow*). **C:** Aortic transection distal to the origin of the left subclavian artery.

the creation of a subcutaneous tract in which the catheter lies before it enters the vein. The tunnel acts as a physical barrier reducing the incidence of catheter-related infection and also enhances catheter security. A Dacron cuff is present on some catheters, causing a localized fibrotic reaction and stabilizing it within the subcutaneous tissues. Most long-term catheters are made of polyurethane, a biocompatible material. The optimal position for placement

of the catheter tip is at the junction of the superior vena cava (SVC) and the right atrium. The right internal jugular vein is the preferred site for these catheters. Another type of tunneled venous access is a port device consisting of a subcutaneously implanted reservoir in the chest wall or upper arm to which the catheter is connected. Ports can be accessed percutaneously with a noncoring needle.

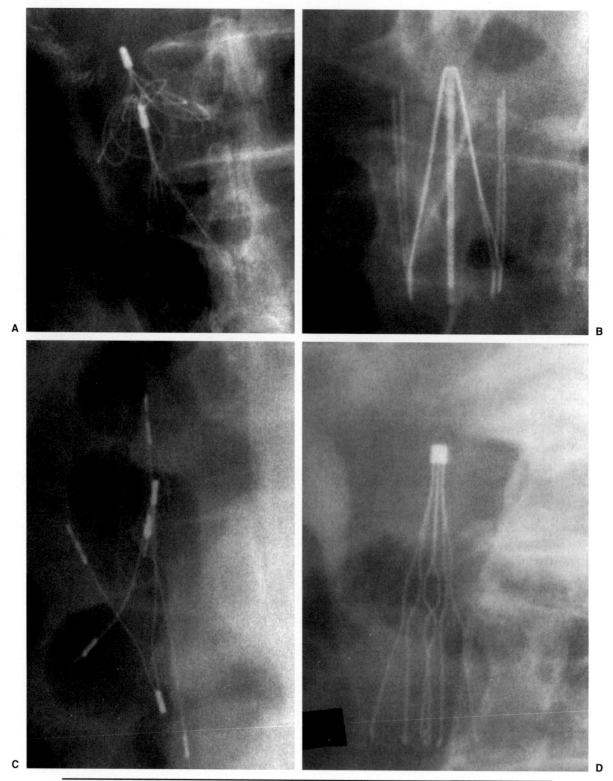

FIGURE 11-10. Intravenous catheter filters. **A:** Simon Nitinol filter. **B:** Braun Venatech filter. **C:** Bird's nest filter (*arrow* represents wire mesh). **D:** Greenfield filter.

For short-term venous access (less than 90 days), a non-tunneled catheter such as a peripherally inserted central catheter (PICC) is appropriate. A PICC is inserted by direct percutaneous puncture of either arm or forearm veins and advanced under fluoroscopic guidance until the tip lies in the SVC.

Venous Interventions

Vena Cava Filters

The purpose of an inferior vena cava (IVC) filter is to prevent pulmonary embolism by trapping a clot before it gets to the lungs. The filter is usually placed in patients in whom anticoagulation is contraindicated or ineffective; it is usually placed percutaneously via a common femoral or internal jugular vein approach. Currently, there are several types of permanent filters available (Fig. 11-10), all of which are made from either stainless steel or Nitinol, an alloy of nickel and titanium. The filter designs depend primarily on their legs to trap clots in the infrarenal IVC to reduce risk of renal vein thrombosis. Retrievable IVC filters may be placed in trauma patients or others at short-term risk of pulmonary embolism (PE). These devices may be retrieved up to 6 months after placement. Their design is similar to existing filters apart from a hook at the top to facilitate retrieval with a loop snare. If the indication for

filter placement remains at the end of this time, then the filter may be left in place as a permanent filter.

Venous Thrombolysis

Deep venous thrombosis can be treated using catheter-directed thrombolysis in a manner similar to arterial thrombolysis. Complete thrombolysis may take two to three days of continuous infusion. An underlying venous stenosis can be subsequently treated with angioplasty and stent placement.

Venous Ablation

Lower extremity venous insufficiency with reflux can be treated by sclerosing or ablating the greater saphenous vein via popliteal venous access. Ablation is achieved using lasers or radiofrequency energy and is performed as an outpatient procedure.

Foreign Body Retrieval

Occasionally it may be necessary to retrieve an object regarded as a foreign body (Fig. 11-11) from within the vascular system. These procedures sometimes necessitate the full use of the interventionalist's armamentarium of skills as well as equipment!

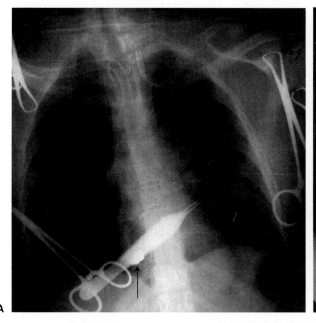 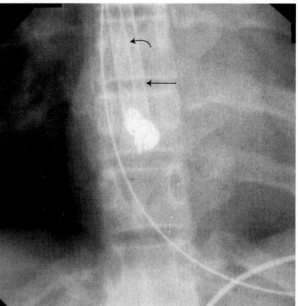

A   B

FIGURE 11-11. A bullet is lodged deep in the subcutaneous tissue below the right clavicle after deflecting off the patient's chin. Attempted removal of the bullet in the emergency room pushed it deeper into the subcutaneous tissue. A chest radiograph **(A)** showed that the bullet (*arrow*) had migrated to the right atrium. A 24F (8-mm diameter) vascular sheath (*arrow*) was advanced into the right atrium via the right internal jugular vein and a loop snare (*curved arrow*) was placed through this to retrieve the slug **(B)**. This case demonstrates the usefulness of interventional radiology in a situation that would otherwise have required cardiac surgery.

Hemodialysis Access Interventions

Using the percutaneous skills described previously, including thrombolysis, angioplasty, and stent placement, hemodialysis access (arteriovenous) fistulae and grafts are declotted and maintained, preserving graft function and longevity. Proper graft or fistula maintenance can add many years to the life of a dialysis-dependent patient. When a dialysis fistula fails to mature, venous collaterals can be embolized to help mature the surgically created dialysis fistula.

NONVASCULAR INTERVENTION

Urological

Percutaneous nephrostomy is a valuable tool in the treatment of urinary obstruction, which is most commonly caused by calculi, neoplasms, and benign strictures. With the patient in the prone position, the obstructed renal pelvis is accessed using the Seldinger technique during which an 8F or 10F pigtail drainage catheter is passed over a guidewire and the loop formed and secured in the renal pelvis. Further intervention such as ureteral stenting or stone removal (nephrolithotomy) may be performed through this renal access. Mild hematuria is not uncommon after percutaneous nephrostomy and usually resolves within 72 hours.

Biliary

Obstructive jaundice may be further evaluated by a percutaneous transhepatic cholangiogram (PTC) whereby a long 22-gauge needle is advanced through the liver parenchyma from a site in the eleventh intercostal space in the right midaxillary line or through the left lobe, using a subxiphoid approach and ultrasound guidance. The needle is then slowly withdrawn while injecting it with contrast to opacify any bile ducts that may have been traversed. Successful PTC is more likely if the ductal system is dilated. Once a duct is opacified, a larger (21- or 18-gauge) needle is then used to percutaneously access one of the opacified ducts peripherally. The tract is dilated over a guidewire and an attempt to traverse the biliary obstruction is made, followed by placement of an internal-external biliary drainage catheter (PTBD) to decompress the ductal system. Permanent self-expanding metallic stents may be placed percutaneously or endoscopically when internalized biliary drainage is desired, as in the case of a malignant obstruction. Alternatively, temporary short plastic stents may be placed in the common duct when surgery is planned or in patients with benign strictures.

Percutaneous Feeding Tubes

Radiologically guided placement of percutaneous gastrostomy and gastrojejunostomy tubes for enteral nutri-

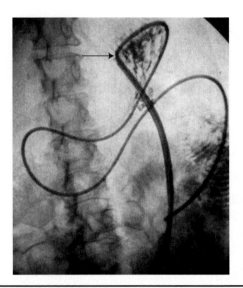

FIGURE 11-12. Double-lumen gastrojejunostomy tube allows delivery of enteral nutrition through the distal tip of the catheter into the small bowel while the gastric contents are drained through the proximal portion (*arrow*), preventing aspiration of gastric contents into the lungs.

tion has gained widespread acceptance in the management of patients who cannot eat or swallow because of stroke, or head injury, or head and neck tumors. The stomach is accessed percutaneously under fluoroscopic guidance using the Seldinger technique and the tract dilated over a guidewire. A 12F or 14F self-retaining pigtail feeding tube is placed over a guidewire and secured within the stomach. If delivery of liquid feeds directly into the small bowel rather than the stomach is preferred, then a gastrojejunostomy tube can be placed in a transgastric fashion as just described and the tip directed through the pylorus to the distal duodenum (Fig. 11-12). The jejunum may also be punctured percutaneously directly and a feeding tube placed within its lumen for feeding.

Abscess Drainage

The Seldinger technique is used to percutaneously drain abscesses and other fluid collections. Ultrasound and CT are often used for guidance of the needle placement. CT and ultrasound guidance are also often used for needle (fine or core) biopsies of deep structures in the chest, abdomen, and pelvis.

Regional Oncology Therapy

Radiofrequency Ablation (RFA) of Tumors

This minimally invasive technique is often used in the treatment of liver, lung, and bone tumors and results in a reduced hospital stay and complication rate. RFA involves the deposition of energy at 480 KHz, causing

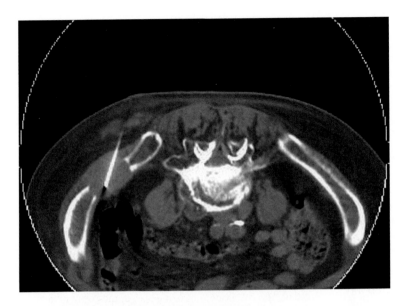

FIGURE 11-13. Radiofrequency ablation. CT pelvis shows an RFA needle in a bony metastasis in the right iliac bone, with the patient in the prone position. The heat generated locally will kill the pain fibers, improving the patient's symptoms.

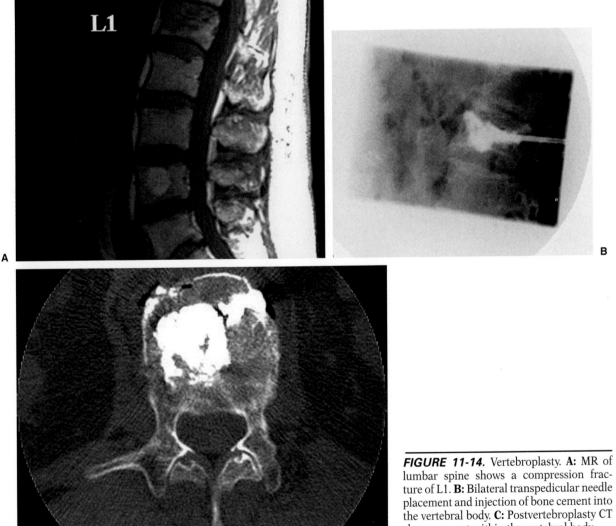

FIGURE 11-14. Vertebroplasty. **A:** MR of lumbar spine shows a compression fracture of L1. **B:** Bilateral transpedicular needle placement and injection of bone cement into the vertebral body. **C:** Postvertebroplasty CT shows cement within the vertebral body.

coagulation necrosis by heating the tissue. Under CT or ultrasound guidance, a probe is percutaneously inserted into the tumor that is then heated to 60°C at which temperature cell death occurs. Tumors such as hepatoma, certain hepatic metastases, lung carcinoma (primary and secondary), and painful bony metastases whose diameter is less than 3.5 cm are suitable for this treatment (Fig. 11-13).

Vertebroplasty

In the United States, osteoporosis causes more than 1.5 million fractures a year of which 700,000 are spinal or vertebral compression fractures. Vertebroplasty is the percutaneous injection of bone cement into a vertebral body fracture, thereby stabilizing it and rendering it less painful. With the patient in the prone position and under fluoroscopic guidance, an 11- or 13-gauge needle is advanced percutaneously through the pedicle into the vertebral body where 3 to 5 cc of liquid bone cement is then injected. The cement hardens and stabilizes the fracture (Fig. 11-14).

KEY POINTS

- Interventional radiology is a specialty of medicine that provides patients diagnostic and therapeutic minimally invasive procedures using imaging guidance.
- Written informed consent is necessary for most angiographic and interventional procedures. The benefits, risks, and possible complications must be discussed with the patient.

- The Seldinger technique is a method for gaining vascular or visceral access using a needle, a guidewire, and a catheter.
- Most arteriograms are performed via the common femoral artery, which should be punctured over the femoral head.
- Iodinated contrast is nephrotoxic, particularly in diabetics and patients with preexisting renal impairment.
- Computed tomography angiography (CTA) has superseded pulmonary angiography and ventilation/perfusion scintigraphy in the diagnosis of pulmonary embolism.
- Most currently available IVC filters are permanent and are placed below the renal veins.
- A positive nuclear medicine scan is helpful in patients with GI bleeding because it not only confirms the diagnosis but also directs the angiographer to the site of bleeding.
- Arterial embolization is an important therapy for traumatic vascular injury, gastrointestinal bleeding, uterine fibroids, and certain oncology tumors.

BIBLIOGRAPHY

Ansell G, Bettman M, Kaufmann J, Wilkins RA. *Complications in diagnostic imaging and interventional radiology*, 3rd ed. Boston: Blackwell Science, 1996.

Baum S, Pentecost MHJ, eds. *Abrams angiography*, 3rd ed. Boston: Little, Brown and Company, 1997.

Cope C, Burke D, Meranze S. *Atlas of interventional radiology*. Philadelphia: JB Lippincott Co, 1990.

Kadir S. *Atlas of normal and variant angiographic anatomy*. Philadelphia: WB Saunders, 1991.

Kandarpa K, Aruny JE. *Handbook of interventional radiologic procedures*, 2nd ed. Boston: Little, Brown and Company, 1996.

NOTE: An *f* after a page number denotes a figure; a *t* after a page number denotes a table.